Make YOU Happen!

10 Weeks to a New You

To David Platt!
I'm so glad you have passion for health & fitness. I look forward to our continued success!
Your trainer for life,
7-9-08

Published by Aura Publications
PO Box 820505
Vancouver, WA 98682
www.aurapublications.com

Go to MakeYouHappen.com to check out the magazine!

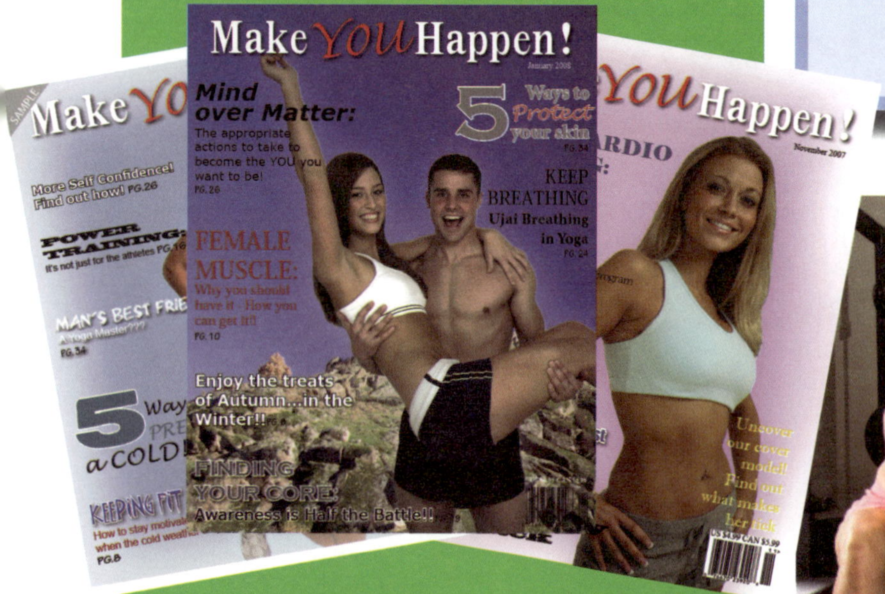

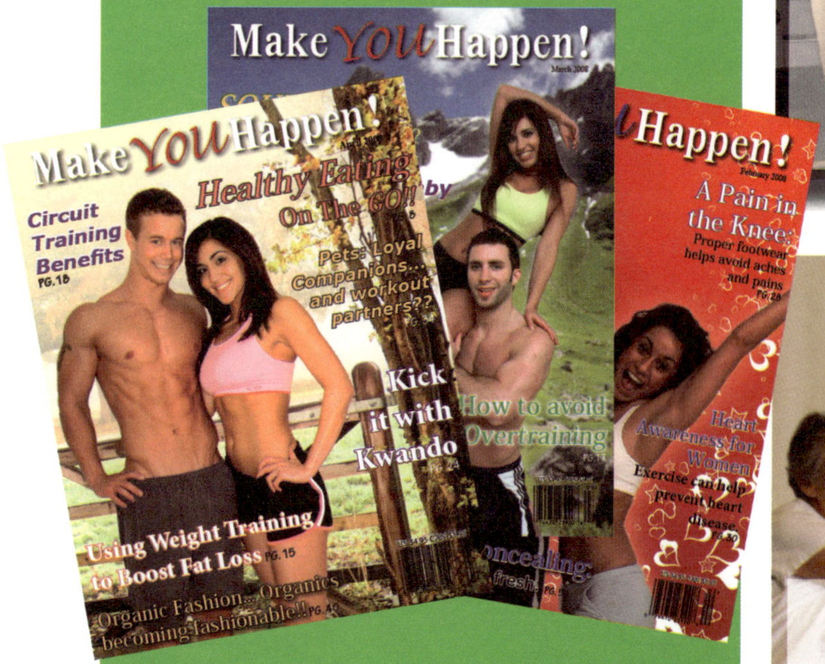

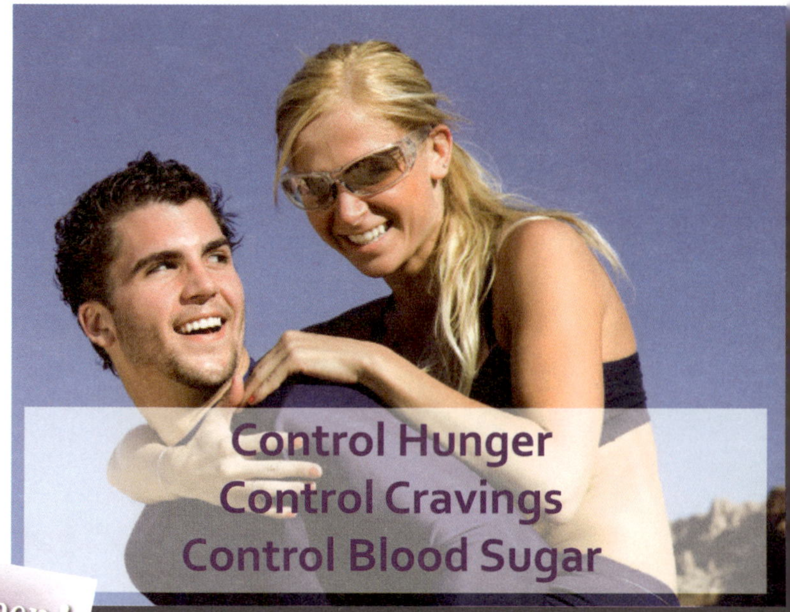

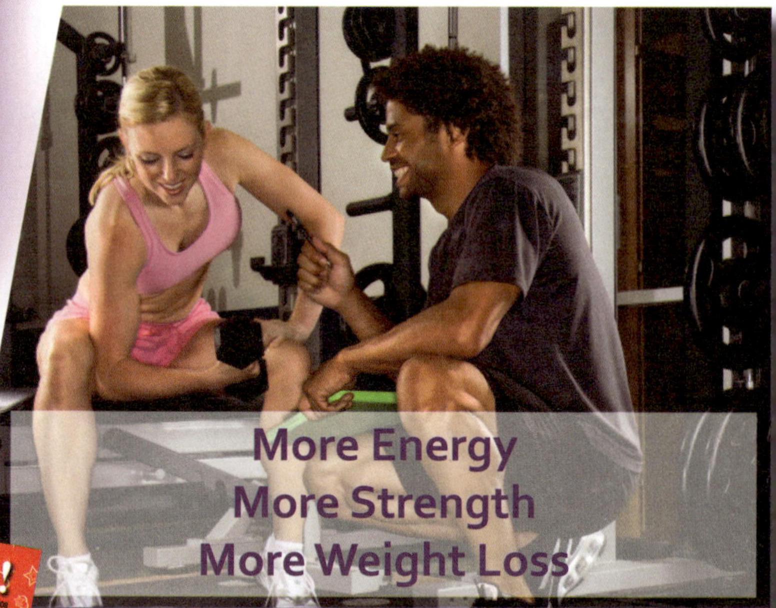

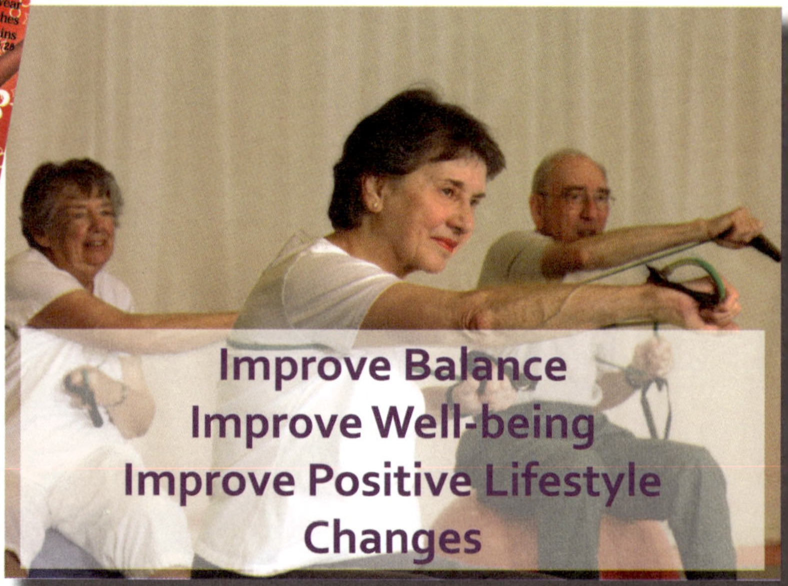

"Kevin is a professional certified personal trainer of the highest caliber. He encompasses the technical knowledge and surpasses most in his field in health and fitness as well as an approachable demeanor that makes him well liked by clients as well as members and fellow peers."

-Mina Clouten, District Manager at 24HR Fitness

Other books that will be available soon are:

- Make You Happen: Everyday Healthy Cooking
- Make You Happen: Slimming and Toning
- Make You Happen: Strength Performance
- Make You Happen: Endurance Performance
- Make You Happen: Rehabilitation
- Make You Happen: Self-Empowerment

Also available is the Make You Happen magazine. For more information visit www.makeyouhappen.com.

Published by Aura Publications
PO Box 820505
Vancouver, WA 98682
www.aurapublications.com

To publish your success story, please mail to the above address or E-mail submissions@makeyouhappen.com.

Printed in the United States of America

Editor: Melinda Walsh
Assistant Editors: Amanda LaPore, Linda Detmers
Cover Models: Sunny Anderson, Nick Swanegan, Brodi Ayers
Models: Amanda LaPore, Christine McAniff, Bob McCabe
Interior Photography: Aura Publications and Becky Cole
Photo Editor: Erich Wehrmann, Jordan Niswender
Layout Editor: Erich Wehrmann
Cartoons and Illustrations: Joshua Cleland

Library of Congress Cataloging-in-Publications Data

Make You Happen / Kevin M Orr
Includes Index
ISBN 978-0-9816731-03 Paperback

Make You Happen: 10 Weeks to a New You is available for bulk purchase, special promotions and premiums. For more information on reselling and special purchase opportunities, please E-mail us at customerservice@makeyouhappen.com.

Distributed by Aura Publications
Printed in the United States of America

Acknowledgements

"Success is one percent inspiration and ninety-nine percent perspiration."
~Thomas A. Edison

I would like to thank God, my family, friends, clients, and associates. You have convinced me that I have something important to share with others. You have persuaded me to jump into the world of writing and to publish this book. This project has taken several years from conceptualization to completion. Without your continued support and encouragement, I could not have finished the process. I would also like to give the following people special thanks for contributing their success stories, reading and critiquing each page, and working with me to ensure that this book became a reality.

Thank you

Adam Stratton
Al Epperson
Alina Pitchenko
Amanda LaPore
Amy Gurske
Ann Stillman
Beth Johnson
Becky Cole
Bob McCabe
Brodi Ayers
Cailyn McIntosh
Carol Davis
Charlotte Williams
Cheryl Tangocci
Christine McAniff
Dan Mitchell
Dave Cole
Dave Tremain
Dave Williams
David Lathrop
Deborah Goedecke
Denise Manes
Diana Edgerton
Dolly Bales
Dwight Karlsen
Erich Wehrmann
Forrest Belmont
Gal Westbrook
Hallie Kofstad
Heather Cowell
Igor Lupekha
Jaime Hongel
Jim Hicks
Jordan Niswender
Joshua Cleland
Joyce Scalice
Julie Merryman
Justin Miller
Karen Tallman
Kathaleen Crawford
Ken Taylor
Kim Smith
Lacey Richards
Lily Samarsky
Lily Sourichone
Linda Detmers
Marcie Mueller
Mark Bergmann
Mary Unruh
Melinda Walsh
Meriza Rodrigues
Mike Halladay
Mike Orr
Millie Rable
Mina Clouten
Mort Kelsey
Michelle Ackerman
Nina Kolafa
Nick Swanegan
Otoniel Rosales
Patricia Hale
Rita Paulson
Sally Sheffield
Seth Kelsey
Sherene Jennings
Stephanie Rotondo
Sunny Anderson
Susie Falter
Terra Crooker
Teri Erickson
Terri Maxwell
Tim Adamsen
Tim Fetters
Tim Kofstad
Tom Knox
Tyrone Whalen

Table of Contents

Foreword

In the fall of 2001, I was overweight, unhealthy, and depressed. My blood pressure and cholesterol were through the roof. I was borderline diabetic, my joints hurt, and the big 5-0 was looming on my horizon. I was a mess both physically and emotionally. My doctor insisted that I start eating more sensibly and get some exercise. I was told, in no uncertain terms, to lose weight. I didn't have a clue how to do that successfully. So I joined the gym and started working with a personal trainer (not Kevin!). I HATED it and the worst part was I wasn't seeing any results. One afternoon, I forced myself, yet again, to meet with my trainer and she wasn't there! I was livid. The fitness manager was apologetic and suggested I work with another trainer. Furious, I was ready to walk out the door knowing full well that if I did, I would NEVER step foot in that place again. But to my great fortune, Kevin Orr overheard our conversation and said, "I'll do it." I started to say, "Forget it," but there was something very reassuring in his eyes. I took a leap of faith and said, "OK."

And then he changed my life.

Kevin became my personal trainer. Inch by inch, pound by pound, he supported, encouraged, affirmed, and challenged me. When we first met, I told him that the gym felt like a foreign country to me. I didn't understand the language or the culture. He took the mystery out of "sets" and "reps" and the names of muscles. He made me believe that I could reach my goals and be a healthy person. He taught me how to take control of my diet and to maximize my time in the gym, so that every drop of sweat and every meal could propel me toward my goals.

I began meeting my goals. My depression lifted and my self-confidence slowly returned. Most importantly, I got my health back. All those bad numbers: blood pressure, cholesterol, and blood sugar went back where they belonged. By the time I turned 50, I was feeling great and I still feel great! I am in better shape now than I have been for many years. I have been able to maintain my results and thanks to Kevin, I will continue to maintain them throughout my lifetime.

I am proud to be a part of the creation of this book. We have developed a resource for you that is like having Kevin as your own personal trainer. It will take you step-by-step through the same nutrition and exercise techniques that Kevin taught me and his other clients that will make you healthy and strong. This book will give you the confidence to make real and lasting lifestyle changes.

So, get started! Make you happen!

Melinda Walsh
Editor
June 2007

From the Author

I have been a professional personal trainer for many years. In that time, I have come to deeply understand that the way we live our lives determines our health and well-being. I have met so many people who felt trapped in their bodies and thought that successfully making positive changes was impossible. They lived chaotic lives and couldn't imagine adding one more commitment. They felt they didn't have the time or the energy to change. What they found, however, was that adopting positive lifestyle habits provided them with more time and energy. Once they became healthy and fit, they had consistent energy and were able to accomplish far more than they imagined.

Many of my clients lived in a state of unbalance due to negative lifestyle habits. Negative habits gave them low energy and dramatically decreased their mental and physical productivity. They found it difficult to focus which led to unhappiness, dissatisfaction, frustration, and even frequent illness.

My clients inspired me to write this book. Over the years, they collected pages of nutrition and fitness information that I had given them. They continued to refer to that advice for support and guidance between sessions and when they were planning their own workouts to complete independently. One of my clients brought me a stack of those notes and jokingly said she had enough pages to fill a book. Well, I took that seemingly off-hand comment to heart.

Without guidance and support, it is not easy to make positive lifestyle changes and it's even harder to make them stick. Knowing that my clients were relying on my notes to continue to successfully meet their fitness goals on their own, convinced me that there was a need for this book. That is why I have written *Make You Happen*.

Make You Happen is a compilation of the proven step-by-step routines, guidelines, and techniques that I have used with hundreds of clients to help them reach their fitness and nutrition goals. I want to guide you to that same kind of success by helping *you* establish a healthy lifestyle in the same way that I helped my clients during our training sessions.

This book will take you through ten step-by-step personal training sessions. It will provide you with clear and concise instructions for building a healthy lifestyle. Each session will set you up to succeed and will create a solid foundation to launch you to the next steps toward meeting your fitness goals. It is easy to follow with exercise do's and don'ts, visualization techniques, and most importantly, a nutrition plan.

If you want to look and feel your best, add years and quality to your life, boost your energy and mental clarity every day, then this book is for you. Whatever your motivation, I am positive this book will help you to accomplish your goals. Let's Make You Happen!

Kevin Orr

Getting Started

Each week in *Make You Happen* is designed to resemble a personal training session and will provide essential information on the five major components necessary to help you reach your fitness goals:

1. ☐ **Nutrition** to optimize your metabolism

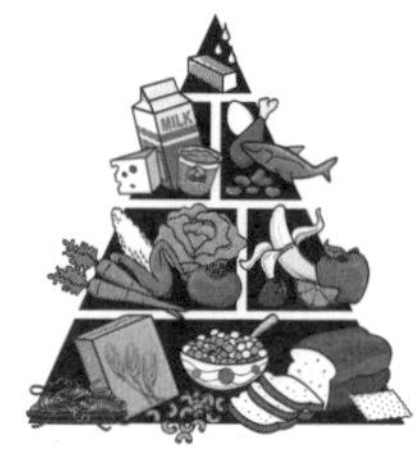

2. ☐ **Weight training** to build muscle to burn calories 24/7

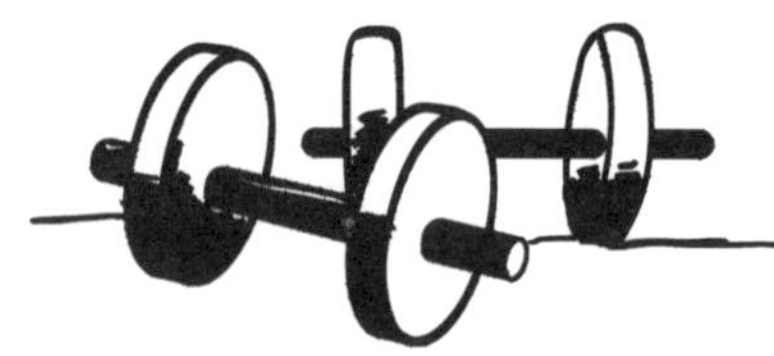

3. ☐ **Cardio training** to boost your metabolism

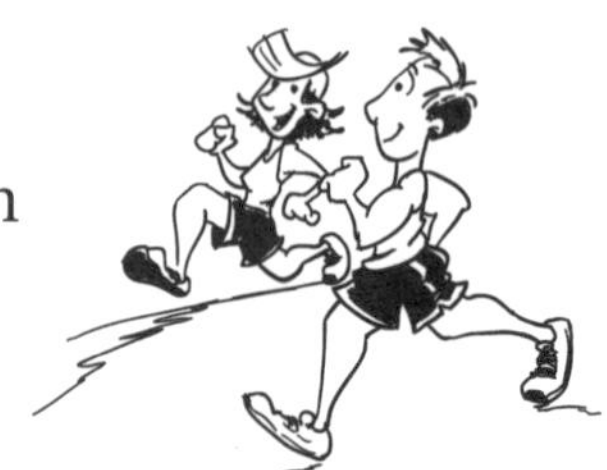

4. ☐ **Planning ahead** to organize your schedule

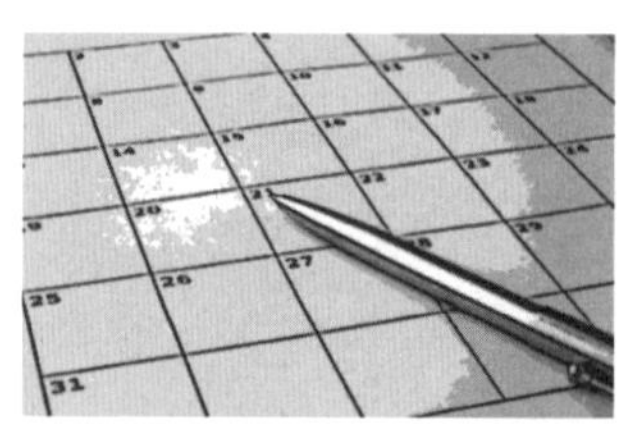

5. ☐ **Executing** your plan for results!

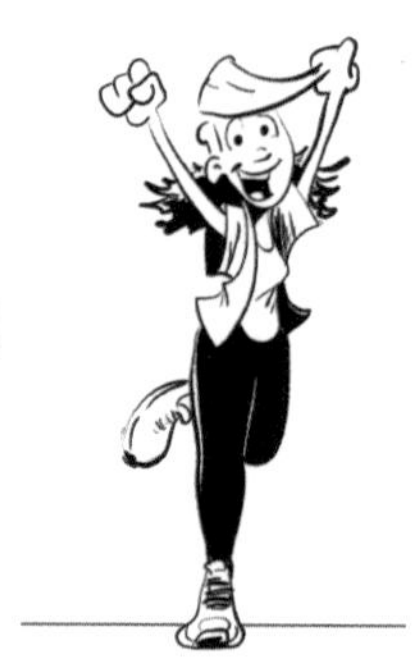

Week by week, you will follow the formula for success to learn and master the skills needed to build a foundation for fitness.

Nutrition is 80% of your success. As you progress, you will master the key concept of maintaining a blood sugar balance, which will allow you to optimize your mental and physical performance, and improve your health and well-being.

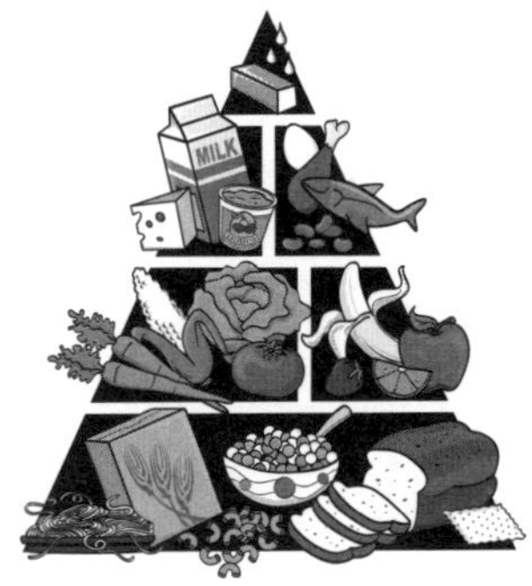

=80%

Weight training is 15% of your success. In each session, you will learn a series of visualization techniques and exercise do's and don'ts to help reshape your body, increase performance, and burn more calories 24 hours a day.

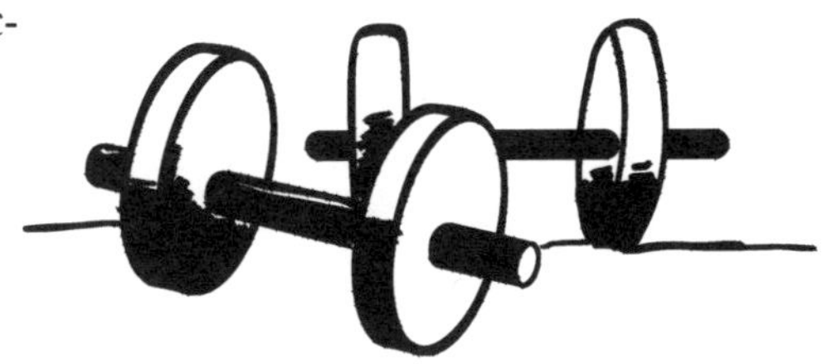

=15%

Cardio training is the remaining 5%. Improving your cardio capacity and burning extra calories are imperative to your success. Similar to your weight training exercises, you will learn the visualization techniques and cardio do's and don'ts to intensify your cardio workouts without overtraining.

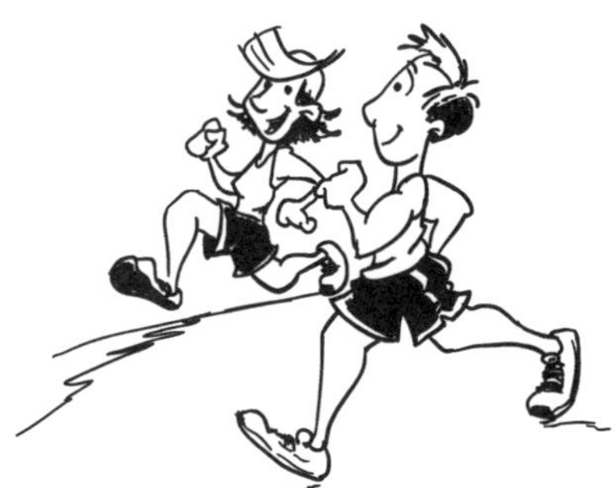

=5%

Start with a Goal. The first step to changing your life starts with a goal. Do you want to lose body fat? Gain strength? Increase your endurance? Increase your energy? Fit into those tight jeans? You can do it! However, crossing the finish line is so much easier if you know where it is. Goals give us a reason to wake up in the morning and help us focus when temptation is in front of us. Once you know what you want, you can go after it.

Write it Down. Write your goal on the top of your exercise schedule (page 249) and in other places where you can keep it in sight throughout the day. Seeing your goal several times a day will serve as a constant reminder to keep you on track. Goals are the key to transforming your dream to reality.

Workout with a Partner. Accountability and motivation keep you on track. Sometimes having a partner helps you reach your goals. Some individuals are more likely to follow through if somebody else is counting on them. Try working out with a friend, family member, co-worker, or your spouse. Go for a run together or meet them at the gym. Finding someone with similar goals can make the difference.

Track Your Progress. It helps to have statistical goals to track. Weigh yourself once a week on the same scale and at the same time of day. Take your measurements once a month. You can also go to your local gym and find out if they can assist in measuring your body fat with body fat calipers. Record your "stats" in your exercise journal (page 249). Seeing is believing.

Visualize Your Goals. Visualize being leaner or more muscular, or performing one more rep or running just a little further. How about visualizing being more energetic and healthier? In order to cross the finish line, you must first visualize it. This will help you achieve both short- and long-term goals.

Be Realistic. Getting to your finish line will not be a straight path. "Life", such as work, family, friends, or school will sometimes get in the way. Be flexible. If you are unable to work out one day, reschedule for the next day. There is no reason to feel guilty if you miss a day. Be sure to set realistic goals for your healthy lifestyle. Incorporating healthy lifestyle changes into your life should be a gradual and steady process. It takes motivation and self-discipline to stay consistent with your healthy habits. One by one, the habits will build upon each other, creating a solid foundation of fitness for the healthy new you. Don't expect to be perfect. Just stay the course as best you can. If something comes up and you slip or give in, regroup and get back on track with your next meal or workout. Later, reflect on your slip. Try to figure out what triggered it and how you can avoid it next time. At the end of each day, try to realize which steps you have taken toward your goal and which steps you have taken that move you further away from your goal. Use this as a way of giving credit to yourself when it is due and planning for obstacles so that you don't make the same mistakes over and over again.

Read Every Weekly Chapter and Follow Through with Each Goal. Follow the step-by-step, week-by-week progression. Begin by following instructions from each chapter once a week. Depending on your level of conditioning and training, you may need to complete two chapters weekly. Each week will help you develop positive lifestyle habits and a new life routine, and will create a solid foundation to launch you to the next steps toward meeting your fitness goals. Ease your way into the nutritional changes and exercise routines. Use the nutrition log (page 248) and exercise schedule (page 249). Write down everything:. The day and time of when, what, and how much you eat and when you work out. Be complete and honest with yourself. Stick with your goals week by week and you will see the results. This is the most important task in setting yourself up to succeed.

Congratulations! You are ready, so let's get started!

The first ten weeks focus on balance and positive lifestyle changes. As noted below in the example weekly progression, begin by following each chapter once a week. You may, however, need to complete two chapters weekly, depending on your level of conditioning and training.

Weekly Chapter Progression

	Sunday	Monday	Tuesday	Wednesday	Thursday	Friday	Saturday
Week 1		Chapter 1					
Week 2		Chapter 2					
Week 3		Chapter 3					
Week 4		Chapter 4					
Week 5		Chapter 5					
Week 6		Chapter 6					
Week 7		Chapter 7					
Week 8		Chapter 8					
Week 9		Chapter 9					
Week 10		Chapter 10					

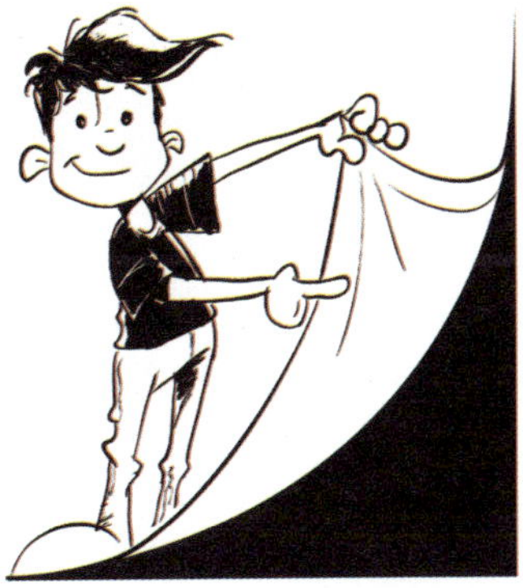

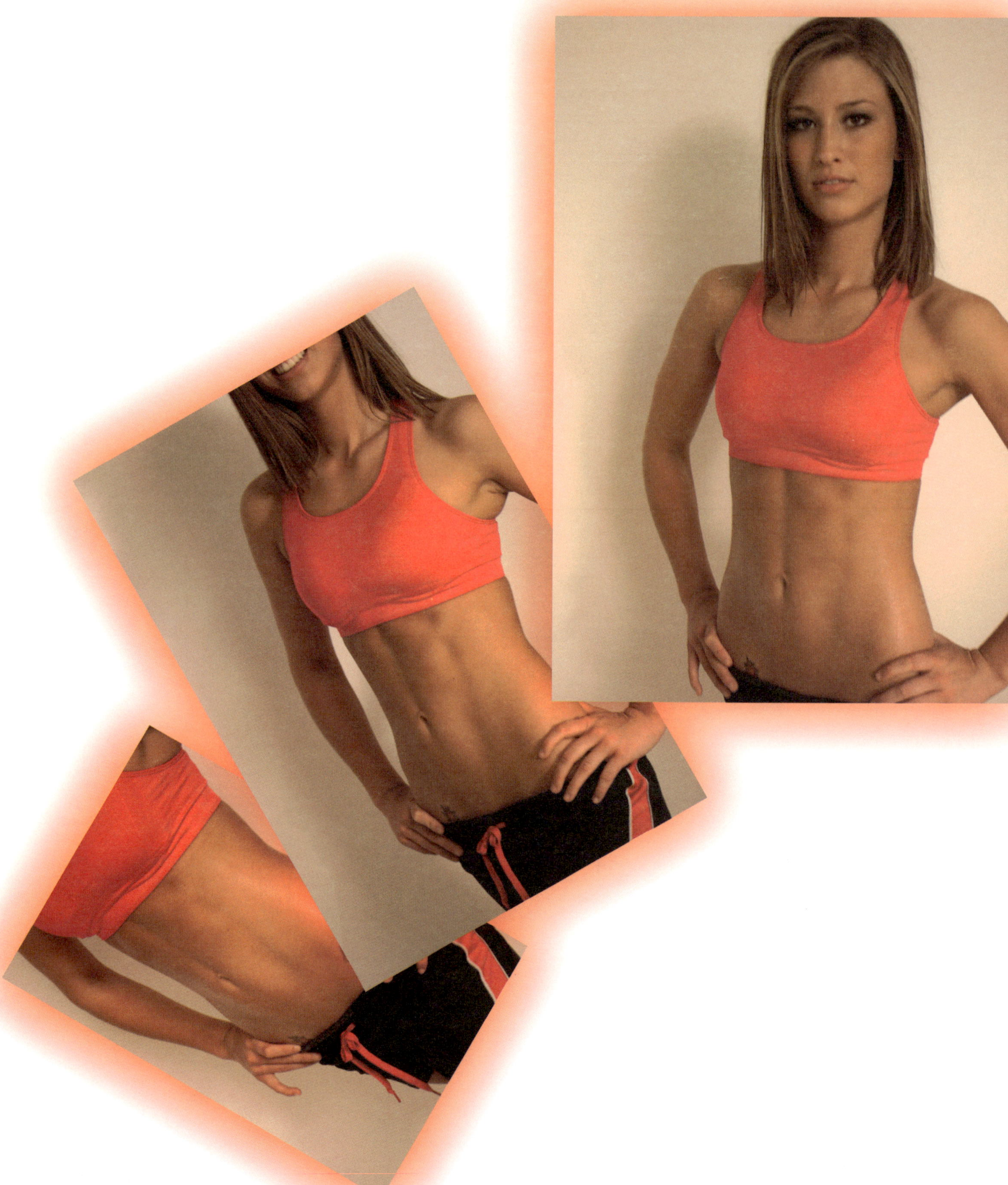

Week 1

You're on your way!

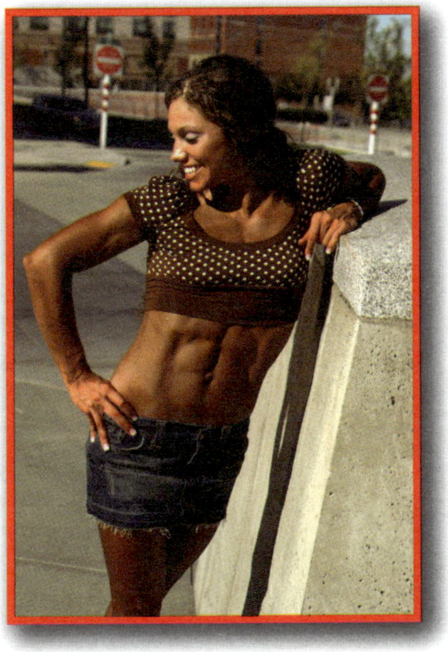

There is no better feeling than achieving a healthy and fit body. I am not going to lie to you–it takes work. But, as I am sure many of you already know, nothing worth doing is easy. Kevin Orr changed my life forever. He gave me the keys to success and now he wants to share them with you! Kevin's book offers the knowledge of nutrition and training that I used to transform my body. He is handing you the tools, and now it is up to you. Set your mind to it and find the courage and conviction to follow through. I have no doubt that Kevin's program will give you the results you are waiting for.

-Amanda LaPore, figure competitor

Goal:

Eat a small meal or snack about every three hours. This may be the most important change that you make!

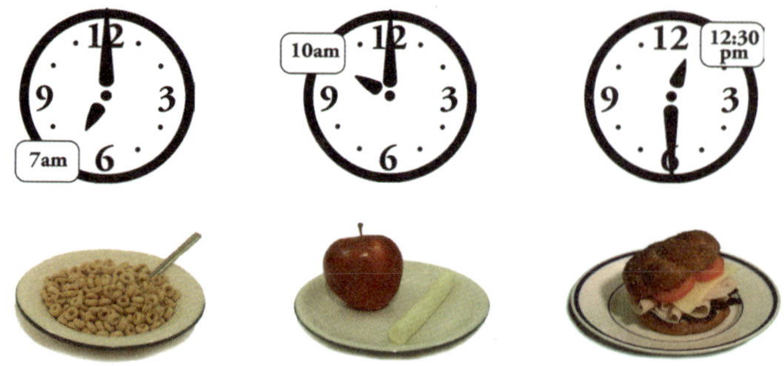

Why?

Eating *something* is better than eating *nothing*. Really! Consuming food once every three hours balances your blood sugar which helps you increase energy and maintain a higher metabolism. When you don't eat anything for four hours (or longer), your body believes that it is experiencing a period of famine and reacts as if you are starving! This leads to a blood sugar low which, in turn, results in lower energy. Your energy level is your best indicator of how eating something every three hours makes a difference for your body. If your energy level drops, ask yourself, "When did I last eat something?"

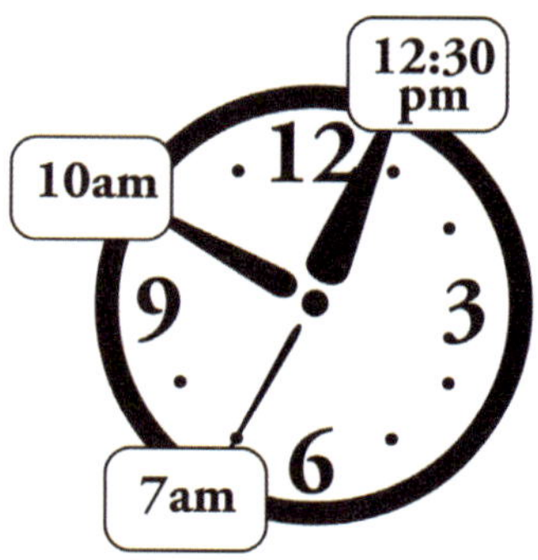

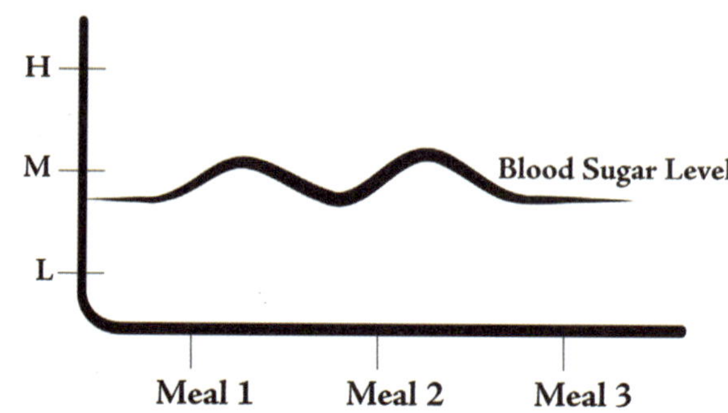

Meal Consistency = Optimal Metabolism and Energy

How?

Plan to eat breakfast, your first meal of the day, within an hour of waking.

Look at the chart on your right. If breakfast is at 7:00 a.m., then plan to eat a meal or snack at 10:00 a.m. and about every three hours the rest of the day. You should feel a little bit hungry when it's time for your next meal. If you're not hungry three hours later then your "small meal" probably contained too many calories. If you're extremely hungry three hours later, then you're probably not eating enough. It's a little bit of trial and error at first, but you'll learn how much you need to eat to satisfy your hunger for three hours. Always try to eat within a half hour of your scheduled meal. A week of practicing this schedule will help you with portion control to avoid over or under eating. This is a critical first step before moving on to other nutrition goals. And remember, eating any form of calories (within reason) once every three hours is better than eating nothing.

For Example:

Time	Food and Amount
7:00 AM	2 Cups of Cheerios, 1 cup milk
10:00 AM	1 String Cheese, Apple
12:30 PM	1 Sandwich
3:00 PM	1 cup Cottage Cheese, Banana
6:00 PM	Work Out
8:00 PM	4 oz. Chicken, Salad, Vegetables

Questions and Answers

What if I'm not hungry in the morning?

If you're not hungry for breakfast in the morning, you may have eaten too much for dinner the night before. You will need to decrease your portion sizes at dinner enough to be hungry when you wake up in the morning. Skipping breakfast tends to make people very hungry towards the late afternoon and evening. When this happens, they naturally feel the need to overeat in the evening. Overeating in the evening suppresses your appetite and you will be much less hungry in the morning. This cycle leads to low energy and body fat storage. In order to break the cycle and start your day off right, begin each morning with a light breakfast. To find out exactly how much you need to eat for dinner, decrease your intake slowly and progressively until you begin to feel hungry in the morning. For example:

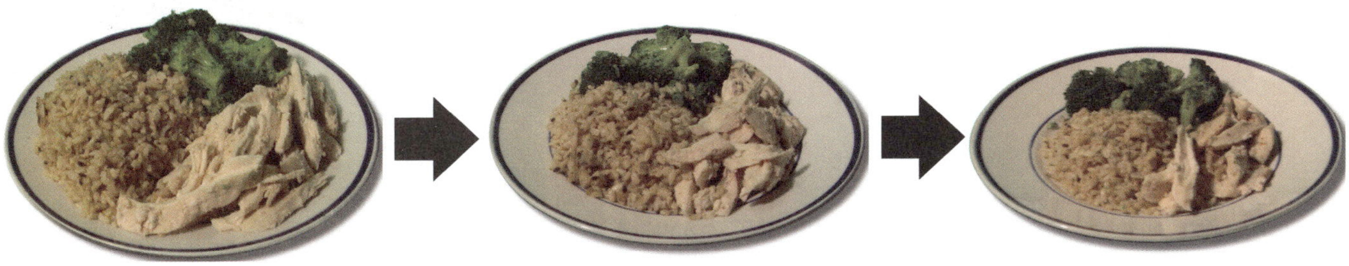

Decrease the portion size of your dinner. If you find that you are still satisfied in the morning, continue to adjust your portion sizes until you find just the right amount for your body. You will know you have found the right amount when you are ready to eat first thing in the morning.

Why do I have to eat breakfast?

It is important to establish new eating habits beginning with your first meal of the day. Breakfast fuels your mind and body. It helps your cells to function correctly and maintain the proper hormonal balance. This balance increases your metabolism as well as your mental alertness and physical performance. Eating breakfast sets you up to succeed.

Eating every three hours leaves me feeling stuffed all day! Am I eating too much?

If you are feeling full, you have eaten too much. You need to eat just enough food to satisfy your hunger for three hours. In order to avoid feeling full, you will need to decrease your portion size enough to be hungry three hours later.

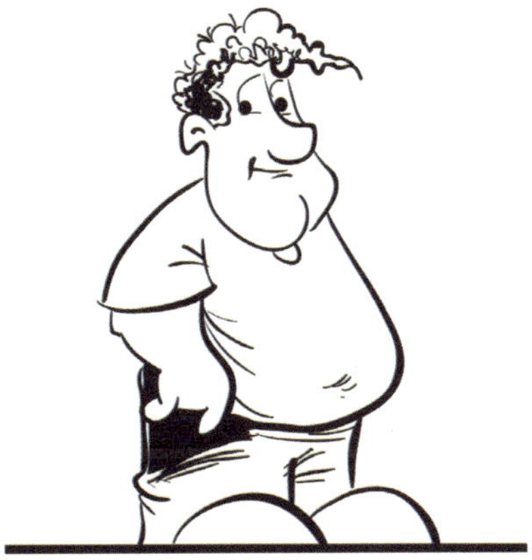

If you eat too many calories at one meal and feel full, your blood sugar rises. The higher the calorie consumption, the faster your blood sugar rises. The faster it rises, the more insulin is released. Insulin is a hormone that regulates the breakdown of carbohydrates. Once broken down, the calories will be used as energy or stored for later utilization. The more insulin released, the quicker carbohydrates are broken down and sent to muscle cells to be utilized as energy. Consequently, any unused glucose is then transported to become stored energy, better known as body fat. Consistent high blood sugar, known as hyperglycemia, is associated with many long-term health problems including obesity and diabetes.

I am really tired and hungry! How do I know if I am eating enough?

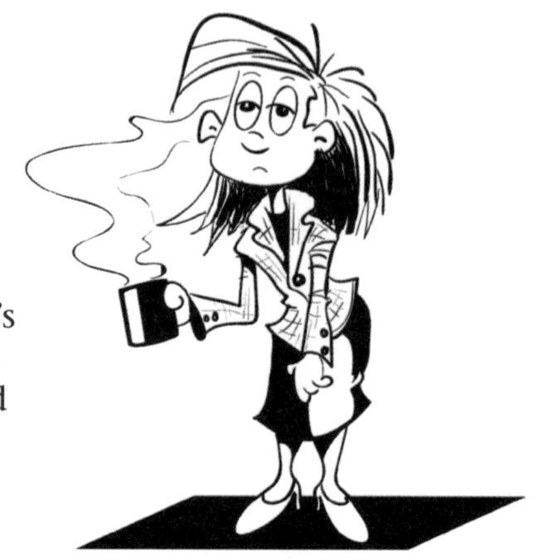

If your energy level has dropped and you're feeling hungry before the three hour mark, you may not be eating enough. If you eat too few calories at one time period and feel hungry, your blood sugar eventually dips. The fewer calories you eat, the lower it dips. As a defense mechanism, the body's metabolism naturally slows down to match the levels of calories consumed. Consistent blood sugar lows result in mental and physical fatigue, decreased mental alertness and functioning, and sleepiness and irritability. In order to avoid a blood sugar low, you will want to increase your portion size just enough to satisfy your hunger for three hours.

Eating every three hours is too much for me! Can I eat every four hours?

Eating every three hours is all about blood sugar balance. Remember, when you don't eat anything for four hours (or longer) your body believes that it is experiencing a period of famine and reacts as if you are starving! As a result, your body begins to slow down to preserve energy, your metabolism naturally slows, and your energy level drops to the floor. You are experiencing a blood sugar low. Blood sugar is the level of glucose in the blood, the body's primary source of energy. When you eat infrequently, it results in blood sugar fluctuations. In order to avoid these fluctuations in your blood sugar, and to maintain high energy and optimal metabolism, you need to eat every three hours.

What happens if I am late for a meal?

The body has an amazing defense mechanism. If you consume too little, your body reacts as if you are starving and will begin to shut down. If you're an hour late for your meal, you become extremely hungry and will naturally feel the need to overeat. When you do overeat, the body's hormones scramble to store as many calories as fat to prepare for the next "famine" period. It is OK to go three-and-a-half hours without eating but any longer causes the famine response to start.

Sometimes I go all day without eating because I quit feeling hungry. Why do I stop feeling hungry?

It is not surprising when you go several hours without eating and then feel really hungry, but you continue to prolong your "famine" period, all of a sudden, you don't feel hungry anymore. It is very common in our busy world, but it is not good for you and it doesn't help you lose weight or gain strength. You can actually lose your appetite after you've pushed through your hunger pangs. When this happens, your muscles and hormones become the primary fuel for your body and you will feel weaker. It wreaks havoc on your metabolism. Over time, this behavior can lead to eating disorders.

Why is it OK to eat an unhealthy food if there are no healthy foods around?

Eating something truly is better than eating nothing. As you already know, if you wait too long to eat, you will experience a blood sugar low and your metabolism will slow down. You want to keep your metabolism revving all day long, so it is better to eat a *little bit* of something unhealthy than to eat nothing at all.

So what does eating every three hours do for me?

As you noticed, eating frequently throughout the day is the key to proper nutrition. This will help balance blood sugar, increase your metabolism, lead to optimal energy, and establish a solid foundation for accomplishing your goals.

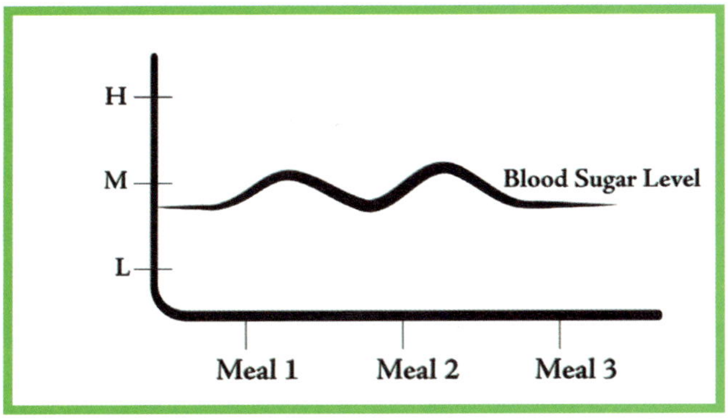

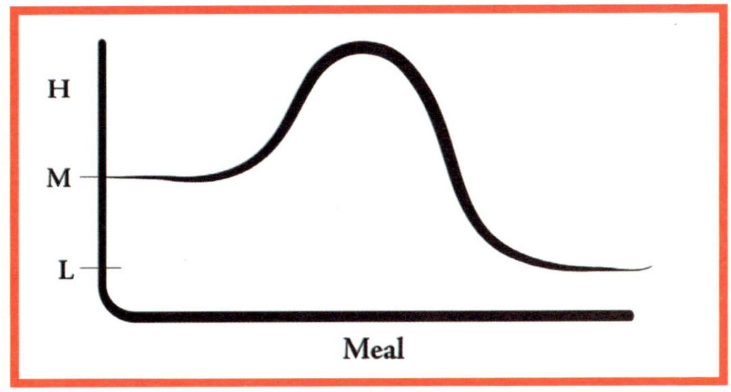

When is it too late to eat?

If you are not hungry three hours later, then you probably overate in your previous meal. You shouldn't eat if you are not hungry at 8:00 p.m. or 9:00 p.m. If you are hungry at 8:00 P.M. or 9:00 P.M. before bed, you should eat a light snack–otherwise, you may wake up hungry in the middle of the night. Your REM sleep is vital to maintain. Continue to read this chapter to learn more about your sleep.

What if it's time to work out and it is already three hours later, which is time to eat?

Your workout takes place of a meal or snack. As long as you're not very hungry, then you should be fine to work out on an empty stomach. Eating right before your workout will not feel very good on your stomach or energy.

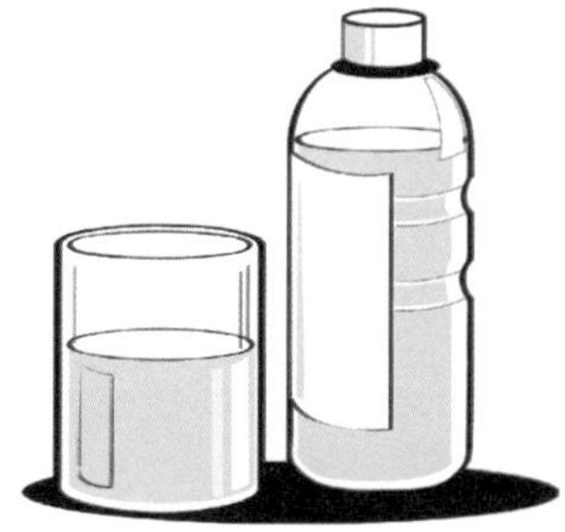

Goal:

Drink at least 1 cup (8 oz.) of water with each meal and snack and at least one cup before, during, and after your workouts.

Why?

Drinking water every three hours helps you to maintain optimal hydration. Consistent water intake regulates hormones and chemicals within your body. Water is essential to maintaining your metabolism and energy. Surprisingly, people commonly confuse thirst with hunger, when in reality, their body is simply dehydrated. When your body is dehydrated, it needs water.

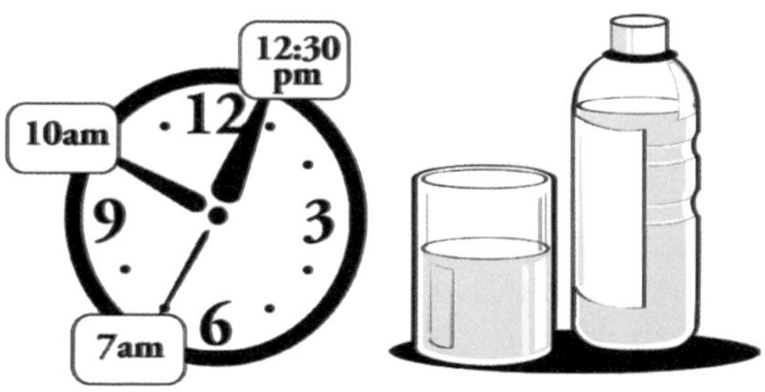

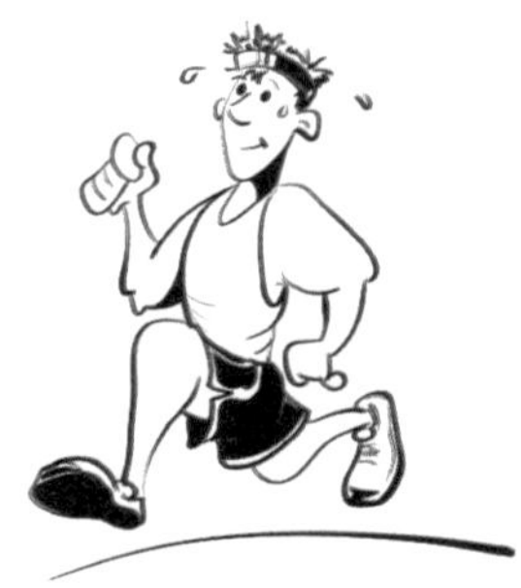

Consistant Hydration = **Optimal Metabolism and Energy**

How?

The best time to begin this habit is with your first meal of the day, breakfast. If you're not thirsty, drink water anyway. It is important to drink a minimum of 8 oz. of water with every meal, as well as an additional cup before, during, and after your workouts. However, the amount of water you need is unique to you. Your best indicator of how much you need is simply the dryness of your mouth. If your mouth is dry, you need to drink water. If you're thirsty, your body has actually been dehydrated for at least an hour. Water requirements are affected by weather temperature, humidity, the type of food you've eaten, exercise intensity, exercise duration, exercise frequency, and muscle mass. To estimate your water needs, you just need to listen to your body.

For Example:

Time	Food and Amount
7:00 AM	Bowl of Cheerios® w/ **1 glass water**
10:00 AM	String Cheese, Apple w/ **1 glass water**
12:30 PM	String Cheese, Apple w/ **1 glass water**
3:00 PM	String Cheese, Apple w/ **1 glass water**
5:45 PM	**1 glass water**
6:00 PM	Workout w/ **1 glass water**
7:00 PM	**1 glass water**
8:00 PM	Chicken, Salad, Vegetables, **1 glass water**

Questions and Answers

Why is water so important?

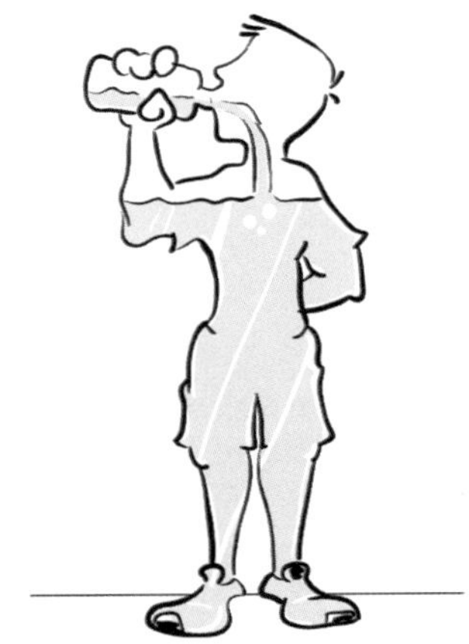

Water makes up nearly 75% of your body, and is, of course, necessary for survival. The human body requires water to support your metabolism, build muscle, burn fat and produce energy. Without water, your body cannot function properly. A lack of water disrupts all of the complex chemical reactions that your body performs on a daily basis. Water regulates your internal temperature, detoxifies the body, and lubricates your joints. A 3% to 4% water loss–which, in many cases is only one or two cups of water–can lead to energy and strength loss, lower metabolism, and decreased mental functioning.

I drink water throughout the day, but I still feel like I am thirsty!

If you feel thirsty, your body is still dehydrated. In order to function properly, your body needs to be hydrated moderately and frequently. Water requirements vary widely based on weather temperature, humidity, food intake, exercise intensity, duration, frequency, muscle mass, and medical conditions such as diabetes. There is no scientific formula to determine exactly how much water you may need; however, the best rule of thumb is to drink enough water to avoid a dry mouth. Keep it simple! Even if you're not thirsty, drink eight glasses of water. No arguing!

Why do I feel bloated drinking water in the morning?

You may be chugging down the water too quickly. Try slowing down and sipping your water in between bites during your breakfast.

Can I drink too much water?

Yes. Surprisingly enough, you can drink too much water! This is a condition called hyponatremia. Symptoms may be bloating, nausea, headaches, and vomiting. Severe symptoms can include coma, brain swelling, respiratory arrest, and even death. If you are drinking A LOT of water and feel any of those symptoms, STOP. If they persist, call your doctor.

I don't have time to drink water every three hours. Can I drink all of my water at the end of the day?

No! Your body needs to be hydrated moderately and frequently. Your body uses water throughout the day, so it makes sense to replace the water as it is used. Your body is constantly utilizing your water supply and it needs to be replenished. Besides, if you did drink all of your water at the end of the day, you may disturb your REM (Rapid Eye Movement) sleep. You will, most likely, urinate all night and many of your nutrients will be flushed away, which will leave you dehydrated for the rest of your next day

I'm on the job and don't have access to water. What should I do?

Carry a water bottle!

Goal:

Keep a nutrition log.

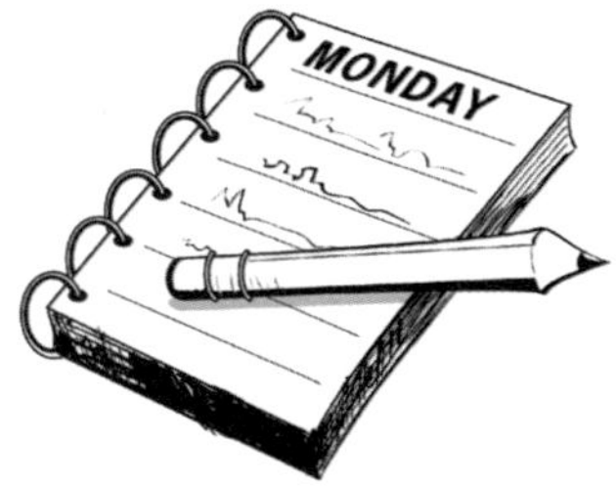

Why?

Your nutrition log is your new best friend. It will provide you with feedback to help change your nutritional habits and keep you accountable to yourself. It will also help you monitor progress towards your goals.

Accountability = Higher Success Rate

How?

On a separate sheet of paper, in a journal, or binder, write down what time you wake up consistently. (You can also make copies of the Nutrition Logon page 248). Next, write down the time you plan to eat your first meal of the day. This should be within an hour of when you wake up. Choose a time that fits into your morning routine so you can stay consistent. **Remember, you need to consume a meal or snack on an average of every three hours.** Write down EXACTLY what you eat and drink at each meal. Conversely, if you're not ready to eat three hours later, you'll need to decrease your portions enough to be slightly hungry and ready for your next meal every three hours. If you're very hungry, you'll need to increase your portions to be ready to eat three hours later. It is OK to workout two to three hours after eating a meal and then eat your next meal. This is the only exception to eating past the three hour mark. Planning ahead will teach you how to listen to your body, balance your hunger, blood sugar, and energy.

For Example:

Time	Food and Amount
6:30 AM	1 water
7:00 AM	1 cup Cheerios®, 1/2 cup milk, w/ 1 water
10:00 AM	1 string vheese, 1 Apple, w/ 1 water
12:30 PM	1 sandwich (2 slices whole wheat bread, 4 oz turkey, 1 oz cheese, mustard), w/1 water
3:00 PM	1 cup cottage cheese, 1 med. banana, w/1 water
6:00 PM	4 oz chicken, 2 cups salad and vegetables, w/1 water
9:00 PM	1 apple, w/1 water
10:00 PM	1 water

Questions and Answers

I don't have time. Do I have to maintain a nutrition log?

Yes! Keeping a nutrition log gives you useful feedback. It allows you to monitor what you eat, when you eat it, and how you feel between meals, which helps you to understand what foods and what amounts keep you satisfied. Monitoring your food habits will help make positive changes that will give you sufficient energy to meet your goals.

A simple change from three meals to five to six meals a day allowed me to have energy to exercise again. I started to run and it took me only three weeks to get my mile time down to 5:15. I couldn't believe how frequently I needed to eat, but it made all the difference in my energy and performance

- Adam Stratton

Goal:

Get at least seven to eight hours of sleep!

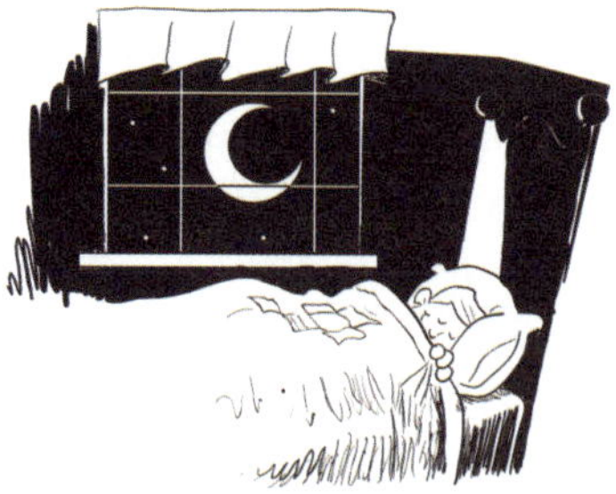

Why?

Sleep is vital! Your mind and body require seven to nine hours of sleep every night to function well. Getting enough sleep seems to be a challenge for many people in today's hectic world. With increasing demands and limited hours each day, getting adequate sleep becomes our last priority. Sleep deprivation is linked to several health consequences such as an increased risk of hypertension, heart attack, and strokes. Lack of sleep is also linked to the breakdown of your immune system. Your hormone production relies on sleep. Hormones play one of the biggest roles in allowing your body to function correctly. They signal your wake up and bed time, adjust body temperature and blood pressure, and release cortisol and testosterone at appropriate levels. When you are sleep-deprived, your hormones get out of rhythm. Ensuring you have adequate sleep is essential for good health and for establishing positive nutrition and exercise habits. Go to bed and wake up at the same time. Your circadian rhythm will automatically kick in to naturally help you fall asleep and wake up at the same time.

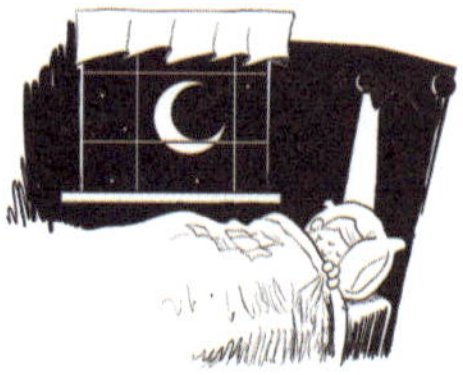

Optimal Sleep = Balance

How?

Here are some helpful tips to help you build your positive sleeping habit:

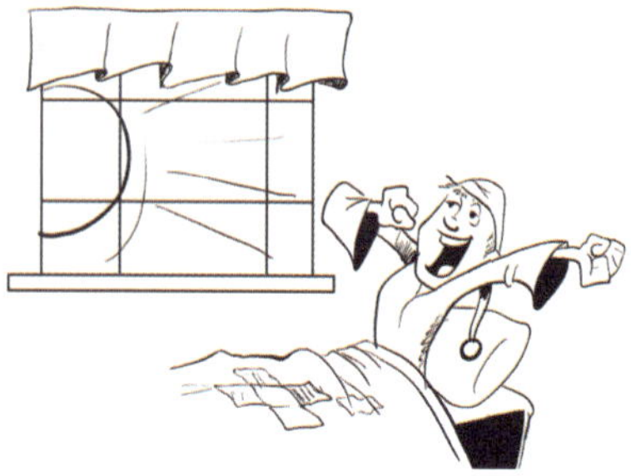

Postive daytime habits

- Wake up to bright light or sunlight. This tells your body's natural biological clock that it's time to wake up.
- Exercise every day, preferably in the morning or afternoon. Exercise can help you sleep and put the mind and body at rest.
- A power nap is good for you if you have had a sleepless night. Otherwise, avoid naps as much as you can. Naps can interfere with your circadian rhythm in establishing a healthy sleep pattern.

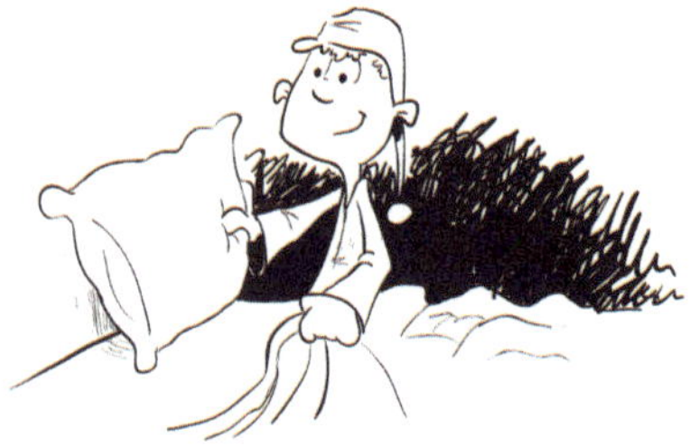

Postive sleep environment

- Make sure your bed and sheets are comfortable.
- Make sure your bedroom and bed are reserved for sleeping – not reading, eating, or watching TV.
- Make sure your bedroom is peaceful, comfortable, and well-ventilated. Keeping it quiet always help.

Postive bedtime habits

- Go to bed when you feel tired enough to go to sleep.
- Prepare for bed with 15-30 minutes in dim light, in a quiet atmosphere, letting go of your stress or worries, and clearing your mind. Jot down your concerns and list your solutions, so you don't have to think about them while lying in bed. You have to slow down before you stop.
- Before bed, listen to soft music, get a massage, take a warm bath, visualize something peaceful, or even try yoga exercises.
- Avoid light from clocks, hallway lights, or night lights. These can interfere with your sleep.
- Television and computer time too close to your bedtime can keep your mind too active. Again, you have to slow down before you stop.
- Avoid stimulants such as caffeine and energy drinks four to six hours before your bedtime.
- Avoid alcohol and tobacco four to six hours before your bedtime. Alcohol is a depressant and can interfere with your ability to harness your REM sleep. Better yet, quit smoking.
- Try to sleep in on weekends. Your goal is to avoid chronic sleep deprivation. A demanding schedule or daily life challenges require recharging your body.

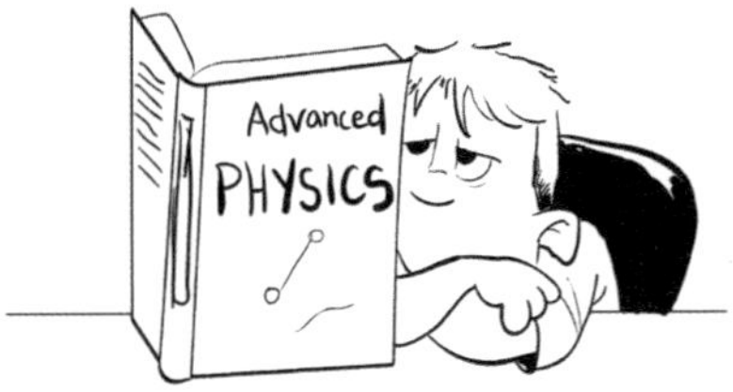

- Study or read before you go to bed. Have you ever noticed picking up a text book and trying to learn something new puts you to sleep immediately? This is one of the greatest techniques for many.
- Eat a light dinner and drink lightly a few hours before bed. Eating a large, heavy meal keeps your digestive system active and drinking too much fluid can wake you up, both of which can interfere with getting rest.

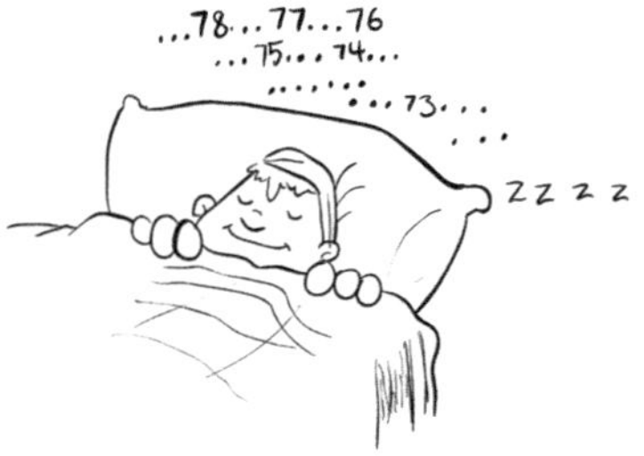

Going Back to Sleep

- Count backward from 100 to 1 very slowly. Counting is repetitive and will help your brain to shut down and sleep.
- Being unable to fall asleep can create anxiety, which keeps you awake. Go into another room and do something relaxing until you're sleepy.

As soon as you determine that one of the above sleeping tips is working for you, continue to practice the technique until it becomes a part of your positive sleeping habit.

Goal:

Take a daily multivitamin.

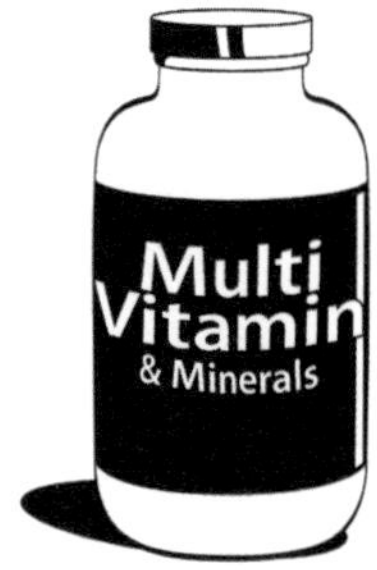

Why?

Food is the best source of vitamins and nutrients, but sometimes it is difficult to get all the nutrients you need from food alone. The nutrients found in a standard multivitamin play several key roles in preventing chronic diseases such as heart disease, cancer, and osteoporosis while fighting free radicals. A multivitamin fills in the gaps and ensures the adequate intake of all nutrients.

How?

Choose a multivitamin.

One proven method for trusting a brand is to look for one that shows the United States Pharmacopeia (USP) mark. USP is an organization that has a voluntary testing program called the Dietary Supplement Verification Program. This sets standards for drugs and supplements to ensure they contain the quality and purity of ingredients in the amount listed on the label, that they dissolve effectively, contain no harmful contaminants, and their manufacturing was safe and sanitary. Don't forget to check the expiration date. Like any food, multivitamins are sensitive to heat and humidity sensitive and can lose potency and quality.

DIETARY SUPPLEMENT USP VERIFIED™

Kevin always comes out on top. Kevin's advice has kept me from getting hurt during training. He keeps me updated with the latest techniques for bodybuilding and shows me secrets that optimize my workouts while preventing injury.

- Al Epperson

It wasn't that I became thin; it was that I was encouraged to become stronger than I had hoped. And, yes, I lost weight; but mostly, I gained confidence in myself, and lost my fear of hurting myself. Thanks to Kevin from this now 65 year old woman.

- Ann Stillman

Nutrition Log

Date:___________	Sun Mon Tues Wed Thurs Fri Sat	
	Plan	**Actual**
Meal 1	*Food & Amount*	*Food & Amount*
Time:_____		
Meal 2		
Time:_____		
Meal 3		
Time:_____		
Meal 4		
Time:_____		
Meal 5		
Time:_____		
Meal 6		
Time:_____		

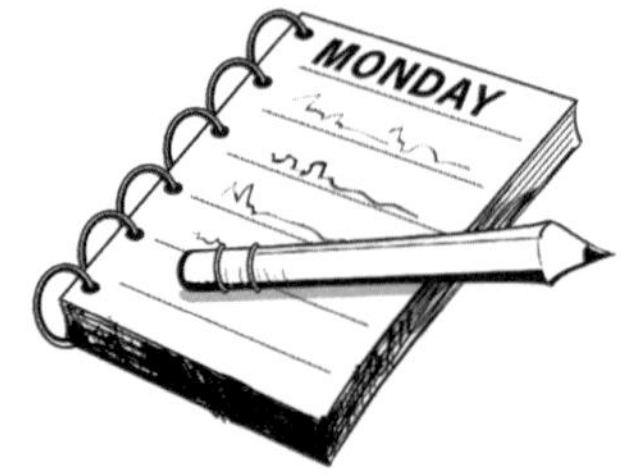

Checklist

Achieved:

- ✓ **Consume meal or snack every 3 hours**
- ✓ **Water every 3 hours**
- ✓ **Sleep optimal hours**
- ✓ **Intake multivitamin**
- ✓ **Cardio**

Key Points

Week 1

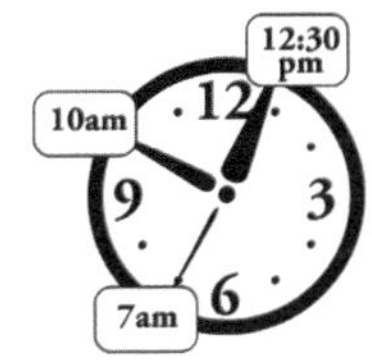

- **Eat a small meal or snack once every three hours – five to six meals per day.** Consuming some form of calories is better than consuming no calories. Frequent calorie intake is necessary for maintaining your metabolism and energy.

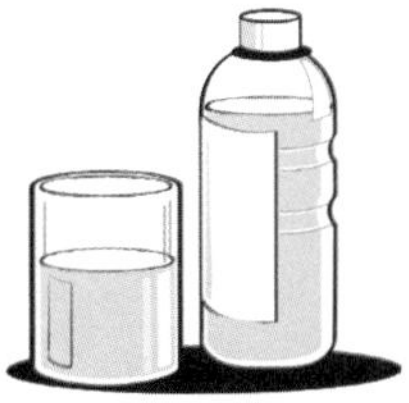

- **Drink at least 1 cup (8 ounces) of water per meal and at least one cup before, during, and after your workouts.** Water is essential in maintaining your metabolism and energy.

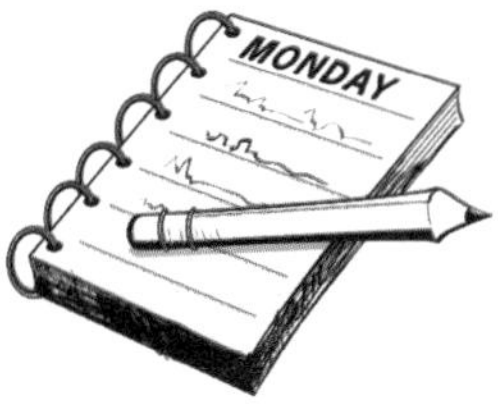

- **Keep a nutrition log.** Your nutrition log provides you with feedback to help change nutritional habits. It helps to keep you accountable to yourself and to monitor progress toward your goals.

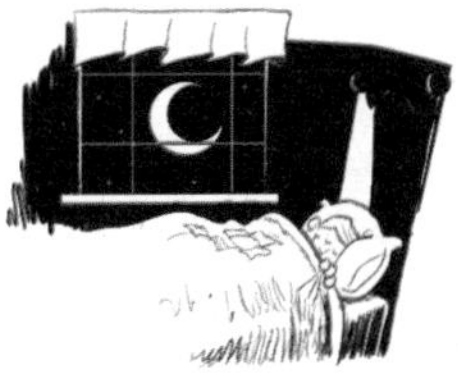

- **Sleep is vital!** Your mind and body require sleep to function well.

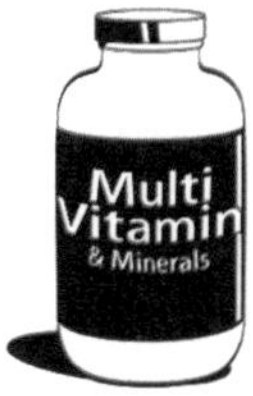

- **Take a daily multivitamin.** A multivitamin fills in the gaps and ensures the adequate intake of all nutrients.

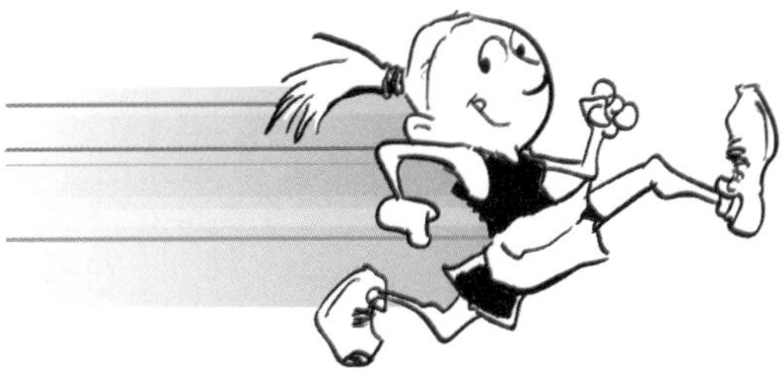

Cardio

Goal:

Complete five to ten minutes on the **Elliptical Fitness Crosstrainer (EFX)**.

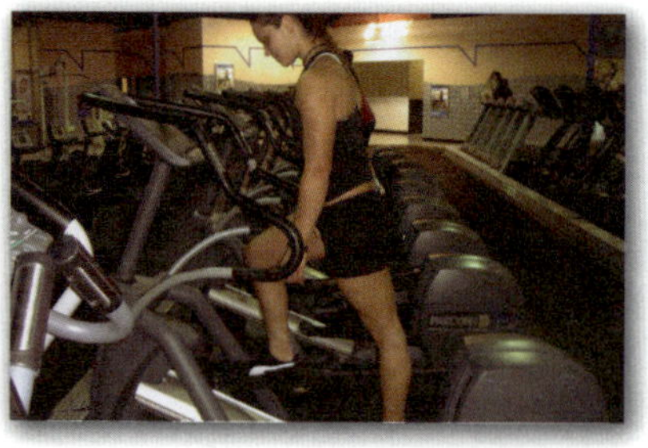

Primary
Quads
Glutes

Stabilizers
Lower back
Hamstrings
Calves

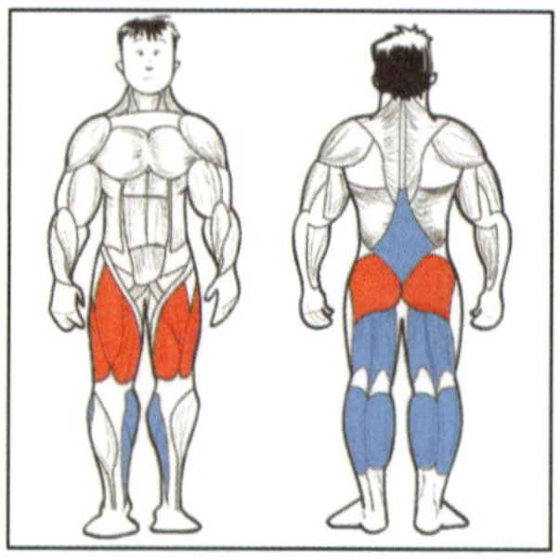

Why?

The elliptical fitness crosstrainer, EFX, is a non-impact, all-in-one cardio machine that incorporates the motions of running, cycling, and stair climbing. It simulates your natural movement while targeting the muscles of your lower body, which is the key to effective aerobic exercise and cardiovascular conditioning.

How?

Step 1 - Choose a program that resembles a hill terrain instead of a flat terrain.

Step 2 - Select 5-10 minutes for your cardio duration.

Step 3 - Your minimum speed/strides per minute (spm) should be:

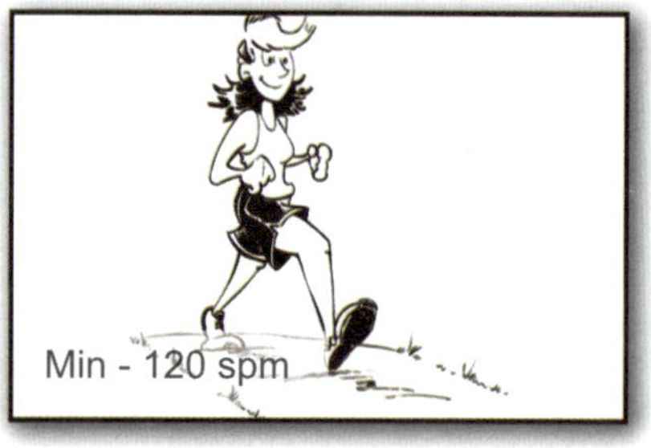

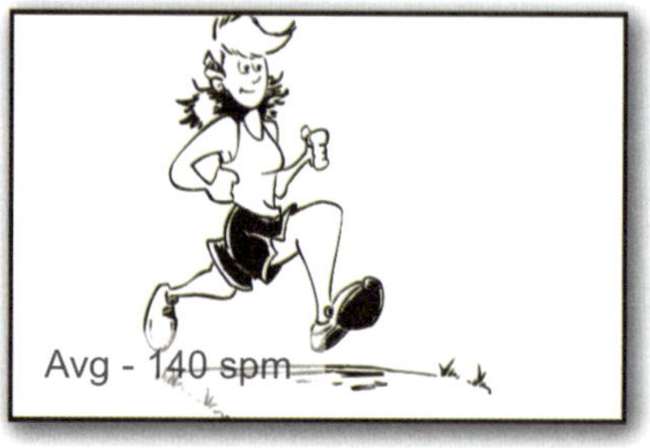

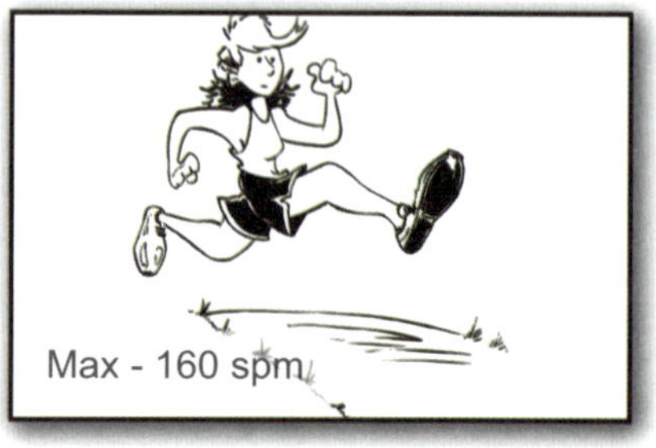

Step 4 - Intensity should be at a moderate/medium level.

The universal method to measure intensity is your breathing rate:

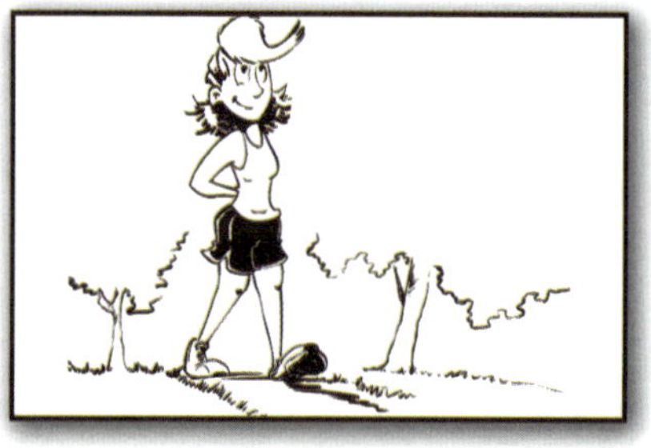

At light intensity, it resembles a walk in the park.

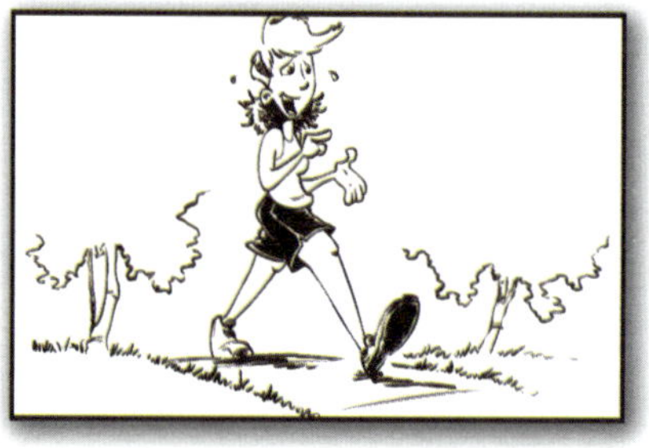

At medium intensity, it is a little hard to hold a conversation.

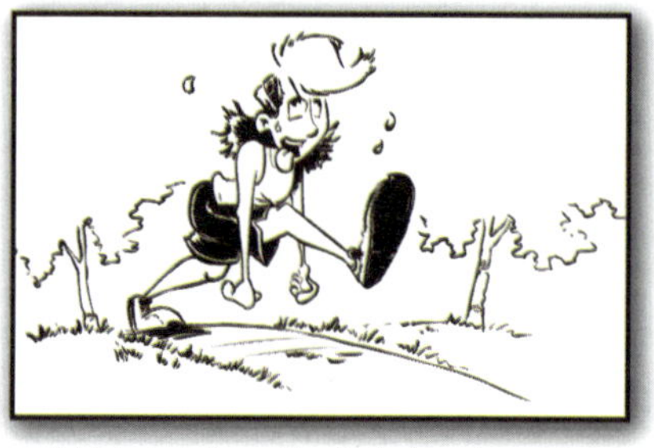

At high intensity, it is too hard to maintain a conversation.

There will be other factors that effect intensity such as muscular burning and fatigue.
Stick to the basics and use the following equation:

Cardio Intensity = Breathing Rate

Range of Motion Techniques

To Maximize Muscle Tension and Minimize Overcompensation

Dos

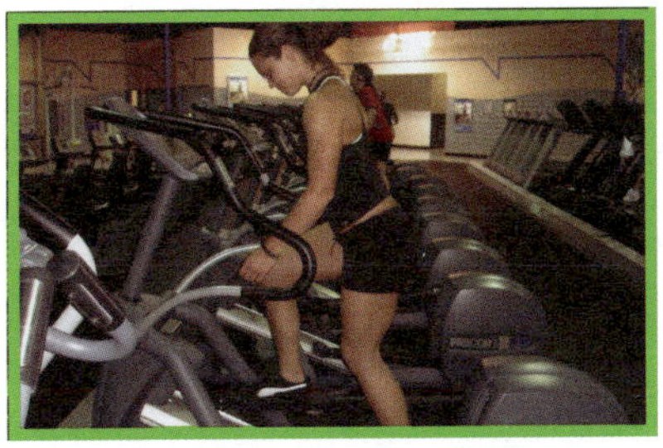

Upper Body Leans Forward,
Glutes are Pushed Back,
Weight on Heals

Don'ts

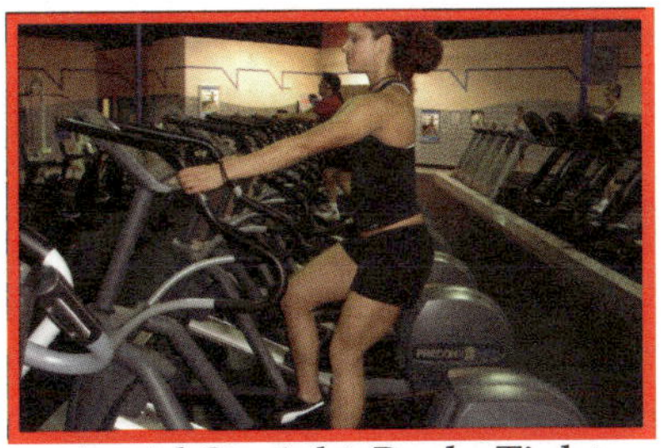

Avoid Straight Back, Tight
Hand Grip, Bouncing too
Much

Visualize

"Hill and Balloon Effect"

Position yourself on the EFX with your feet as far back as possible. Now, imagine yourself on the EFX gliding forward with ease while visualizing running uphill. This will naturally place your body in proper posture with your upper body leaning slightly forward and your glutes pushed back. These techniques relieve pressure on your lower back and knees.

Now, imagine gliding uphill as softly as possible with a balloon underneath each of your shoes. This relieves even more pressure on your lower back and knees by placing the least amount of impact on the floor of your pedals.

Visualizing correctly ensures that your leg muscles are doing the work, which helps you avoid overcompensating with other muscles and joints.

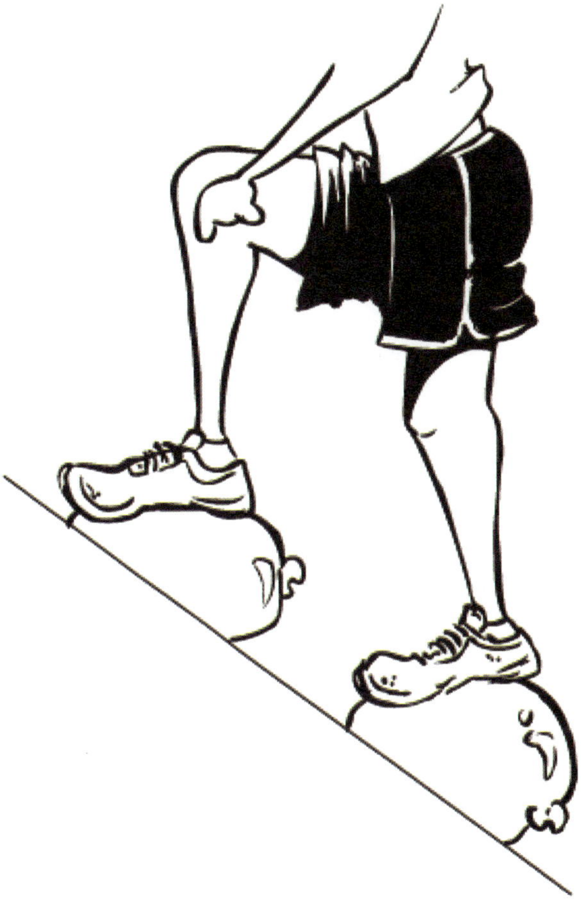

Questions and Answers

What's the purpose of staying at medium intensity for cardio?

A low intensity workout, like a walk in the park, is just that. A walk in the park, holding a conversation easily, doesn't increase the heart rate enough to burn the maximum amount of calories. If your body is not challenged, it doesn't have a reason to change its cardiorespiratory capacity or physical conditioning. When performing at a high intensity level, it is difficult to maintain a conversation. Your body burns the maximum amount of calories in the form of sugars and carbohydrates, while increasing your cardiorespiratory capacity and physical conditioning. Your goal in building a foundation is to avoid undertraining and to avoid overtraining by maintaining medium intensity: not too low and not too high. It should be a little difficult to hold a conversation and you should feel a slight burning sensation in your legs. This allows your body to stay balanced and to burn body fat calories more efficiently while safely building a solid foundation of conditioning.

What if maintaining the minimum speed of 120 SPM on the EFX is too difficult physically and/or cardiovascularly?

If you are having a hard time maintaining the minimum speed of 120 SPM on the EFX you will need to decrease your speed and/or your level of resistance. Remember, you should be working at medium intensity. It is important to accomplish your duration goal for cardio. In the beginning, you may need to break up five-minute durations into one to two minute segments. For example, use the EFX for one to two minutes, rest for 30 seconds, complete another one to two minute segment, and rest for 30 seconds. Repeat this routine until you have achieved your goal. This should help with your pace. After you have successfully completed your chosen duration, you will be able to focus on your speed. In just a few workouts, you will have the ability to maintain the minimum speed of 120 SPM.

What's the purpose of visualization?

Visualization is the process of forming mental pictures and images. It allows you to strengthen your targeted muscles. Mental focus and concentration require practice. After practicing visualization, you may feel your chest contract and reach the "pump" effect. Building muscle helps to physically contract the targeted muscle group, so you may have to wait until you've increased your strength. For now, continue practicing visualization. It will come together as you continue to work out.

Is it important to stretch after using the EFX?

Yes, stretching after, rather than before, your workout is definitely important. It allows your muscles to relax and recover faster. If your muscles are tight and you do not stretch, you increase your risk of cramping or straining. Cramps and strains are a precursor to muscle pulls and tears. A pulled muscle can take up to four weeks to heal properly and muscle tears generally take six months or longer to heal. Choose one of the following places to perform hamstring stretches for your first stretch:

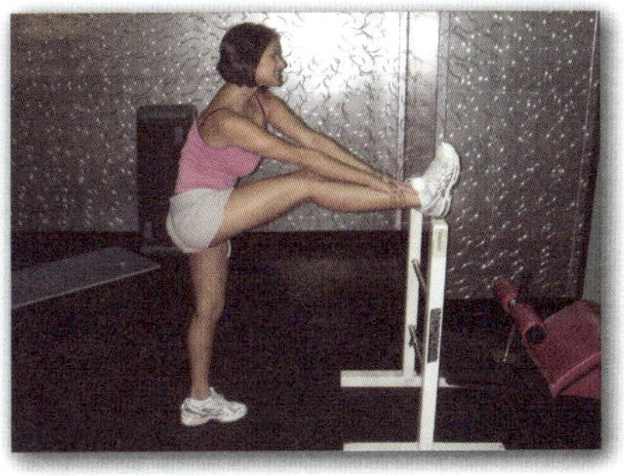

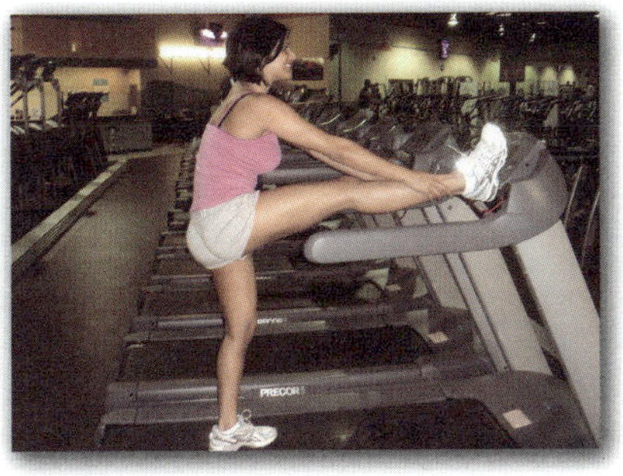

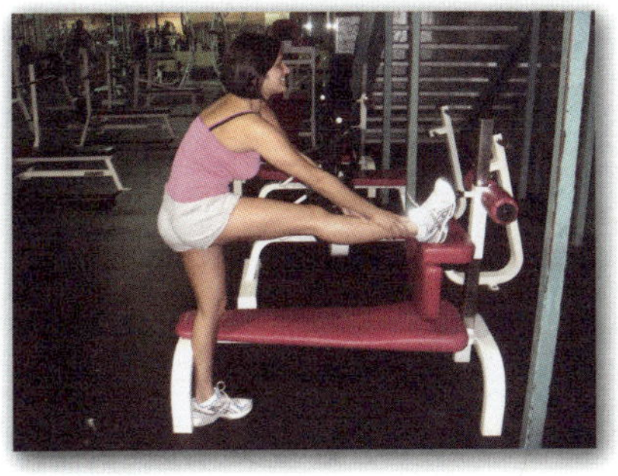

1. Stand with knees slightly bent
2. Toes and foot should be pointed straight up
3. Lean forward enough to feel a light stretch in your hamstrings
4. Stretch and hold lightly for two sets of 15 seconds each

The Secrets to Success!

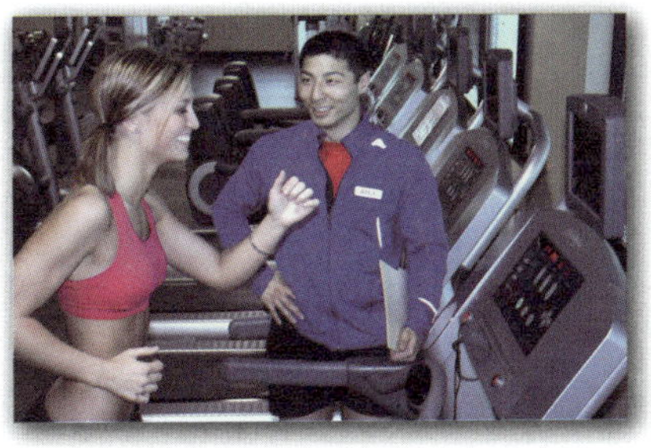

From Your Personal Trainer, Kevin Orr

Are you ready to hear this secret breakthrough to the body you want? Brace yourself. There is no special supplement or magic pill to jump start your results! There are no quick fixes! It is OK. Calm down. I know what you were feeling. You had high hopes for instant results. You may be disappointed, frustrated, and ready to give up, but wait!

You already know the secret to getting the body you want. You have been practicing it! The secret is all about pacing yourself. It's really that simple. Pacing your nutrition and exercise, staying consistent, and sticking to the basics is the secret to health and fitness. Yes, it will take some time, persistence, and patience, but I guarantee you will achieve real results much faster than the so-called "quick fixes." And your results will last! Consistency is the secret!

Example Cardio Routines

At the conclusion of every week, there will be three good examples of a workout schedule below. Use the blank schedule, on page 249, to help you design a realistic schedule for you.

Choose a workout routine based on your level of fitness and your schedule before progressing to Week Two. Write it down in your blank schedule, on page 249. If none of the example routines work for you, configure a routine that fits your needs, and write it down.

3-Day Cardio Routine

Sunday	Monday	Tuesday	Wednesday	Thursday	Friday	Saturday
	EFX: 10	EFX: 2x10		EFX: 20		

4-Day Cardio Routine

Sunday	Monday	Tuesday	Wednesday	Thursday	Friday	Saturday
		EFX: 5	EFX: 2x5	EFX: 3x5		EFX: 2x10

5-Day Cardio Routine

Sunday	Monday	Tuesday	Wednesday	Thursday	Friday	Saturday
	EFX: 5	EFX: 10	EFX: 15	EFX: 20	EFX: 20	

Note: EFX: 2x10 means: perform two sets of ten minutes on the EFX. After the first set, especially if you're too tired, take a short one to five minute break. Then continue for another ten minutes. This allows you to pace yourself if a full twenty minutes is too difficult to complete.

On another note, you'll notice Monday or Tuesday is highlighted with the color blue. This simply states the day the workout routine begins. Obviously, your schedule may differ, so adjust your first day accordingly when you're filling out your workout schedule, on page 249.

Example Schedule

This is an example of a five-day workout routine and planning ahead. On your blank schedule, page 249, write down which cardio machines along with the duration you plan to complete this week.

	Sunday	Monday	Tuesday	Wednesday	Thursday	Friday	Saturday	
Week 1 Cardio: Duration:		*EFX: 5*	*EFX: 10*	*EFX: 15*	*EFX: 20*	*EFX: 20*		

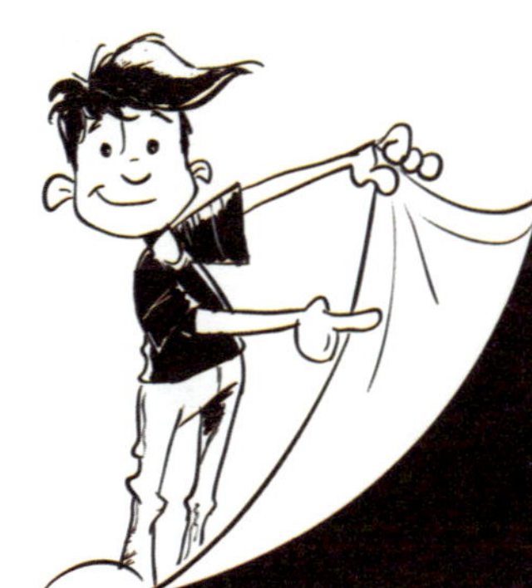

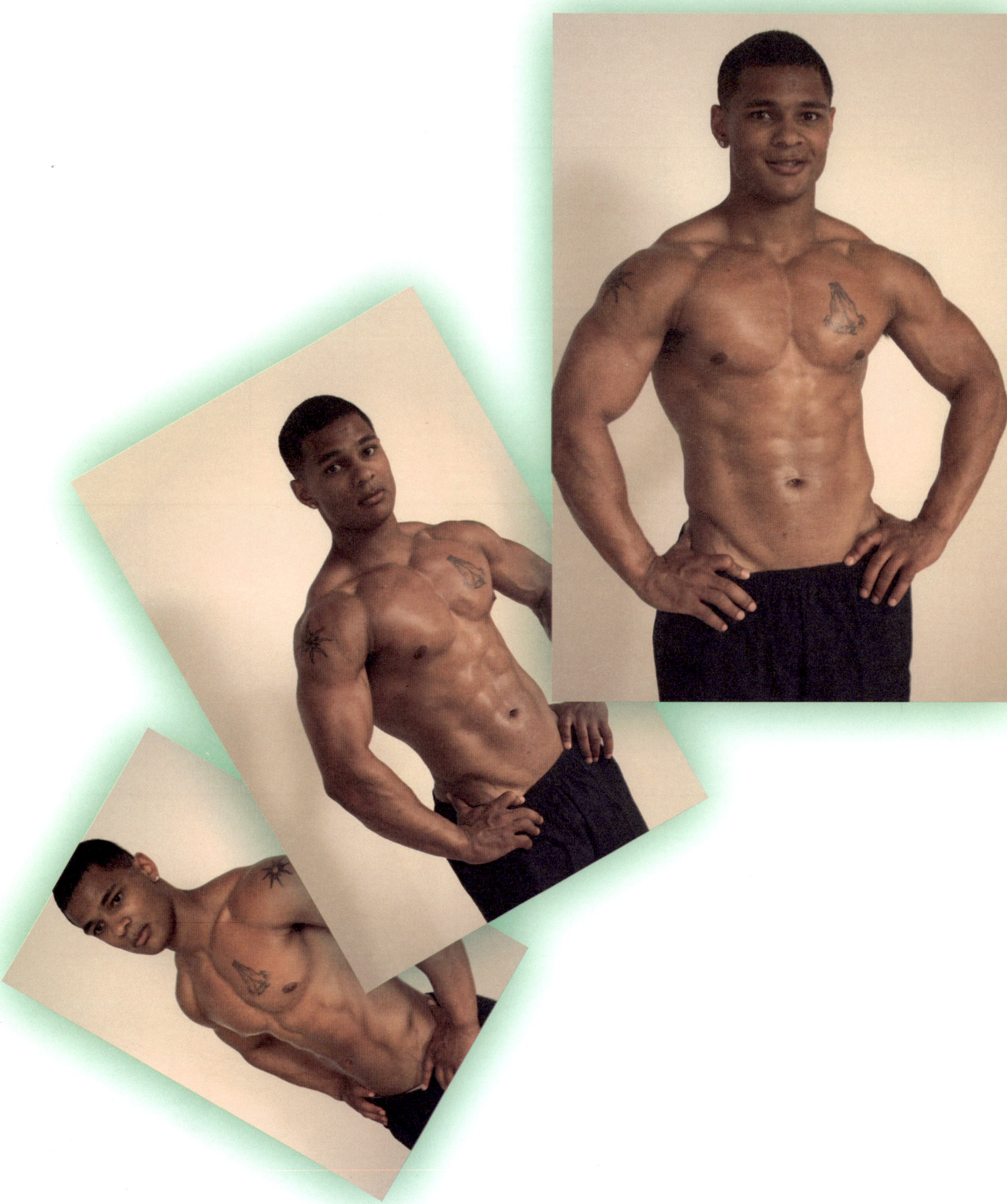

Week 2

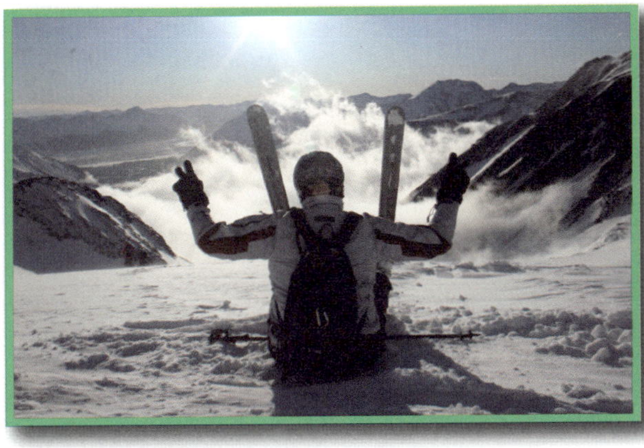

I have been successful in my endeavors through desire, effort, and proper coaching from Kevin. My success is not about numbers, it is about a feeling that I cannot put on paper. Improved performance? Absolutely. Twenty-nine ski days under my belt this season improved stamina and without injury. Improved appearance? Absolutely! A size 42 waist to a size 36. Improved energy levels? Absolutely. Equalized blood sugar through proper dietary guidance? Decreased stress levels? Absolutely. There is no measurement of my "happiness units." All that said, numbers do matter, but they really don't help the client feel better about themselves. Is the client satisfied with these values? Sure, they find value in the measurable gains, but what you can't measure is how the client feels with a new life. Simply stated, my happiness units are peaking and it is because of the effort I put forth, with the direction of the best physical trainer I have ever worked with.

Kevin's guidance has empowered me to make changes to my lifestyle that will affect my family, my business, and all those that I make contact for my remaining days.

-Dan Mitchell

Goal:

Avoid "bad" sugars.

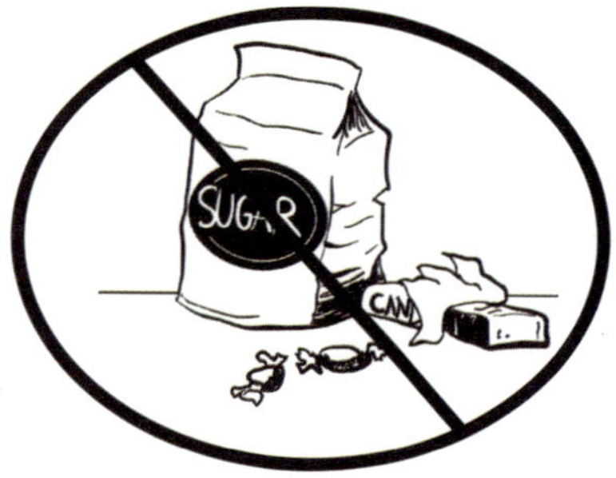

Why?

Sugars are simple carbohydrates. They are full of empty calories, provide minimal nutrients, and they digest quickly. Your goal is to substitute bad sugars with good sugars – and there ARE good sugars. Good sugars will help you satisfy your sweet tooth without sacrificing your health benefits. More importantly, they will help you better balance your blood sugar levels.

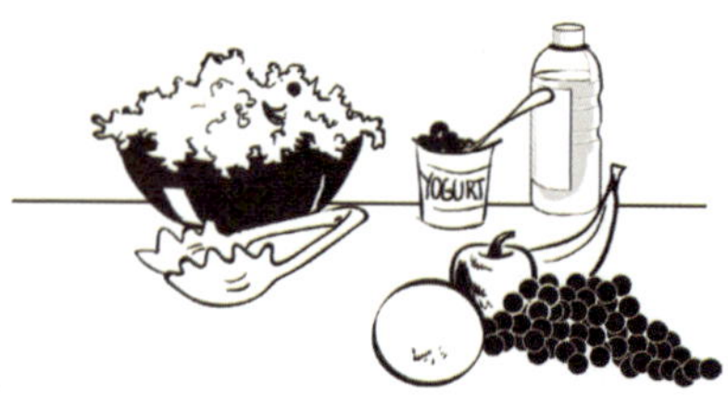

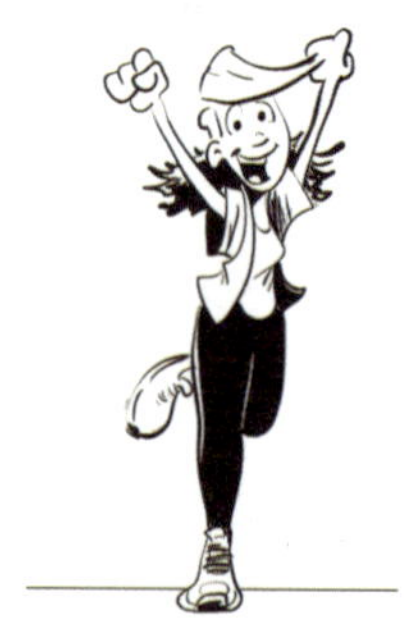

Balanced Blood Sugar = Optimal Metabolism and Energy

How?

Unlike bad sugars, good sugars, in the form of nutrient-dense foods, digest slowly and stabilize your blood sugar level. They are more satisfying and have fewer "empty" calories.

Try some of the following healthy food substitutions for the sugars you may have been eating*:

Yogurt is sweet and contains good proteins, vitamins, calcium, and most importantly, probiotics. Jams and jellies are high in bad sugars and dense in calories with no nutrients or major health benefits.
Recommendation: One serving (1 cup) of yogurt a day.

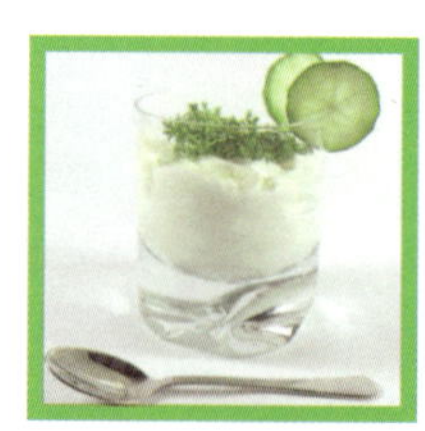

VS

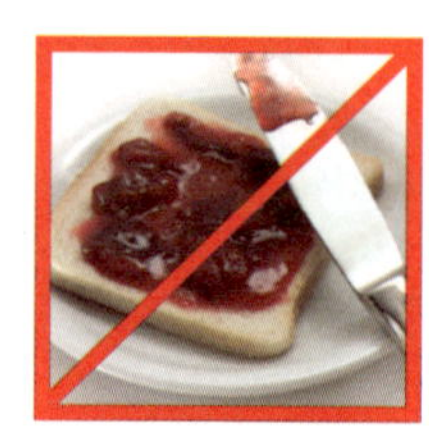

Fruit contains fructose, water, vitamins, nutrients, essential amino acids, antioxidants and, most importantly, fiber. They are nature's candy and easy to take with you most anywhere. Candy bars, on the other hand, are high in bad sugars, fats, and calories with very few, if any, nutrients.
Recommendation: Two to four servings of fruit a day (½ cup is one serving). All fruits are good choices; however, fruits brighter in color are typically more nutrient-dense.

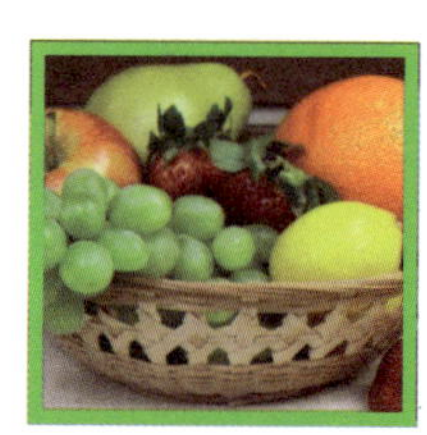

VS

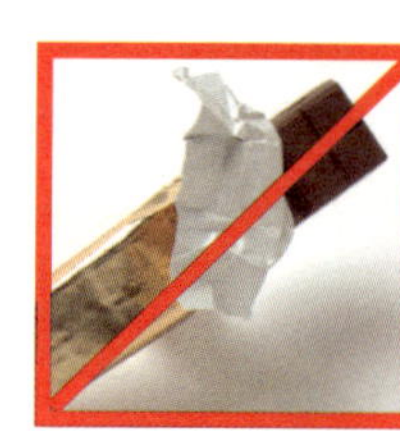

*Substitutions are based on calories per serving

Vegetables contain sugars, vitamins, minerals and, most importantly, fiber. Like fruits, vegetables brighter or darker in color are more nutrient-dense. Since vegetables are also lower in calories, you can eat more of them to help control your hunger. Granola bars, in contrast, are high in bad sugars. They provide very little nutritional value and are calorie-dense.
Recommendation: Three to five servings a day (½ cup is one serving).

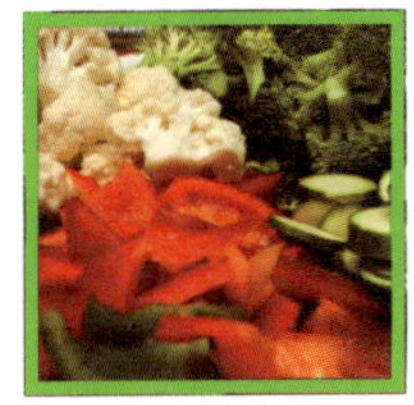

VS

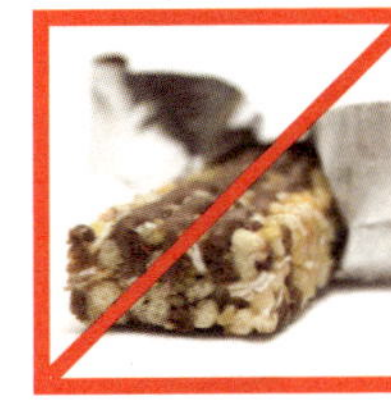

Water is essential! You learned in session one that water regulates hormones and chemicals, helps to maintain your metabolism and energy, and is required for your body to function. Pop, juice, and performance drinks contain water plus lots of extra sugar. Avoid them!
Recommendation: Drink a minimum of 64 oz (eight cups) of water a day.

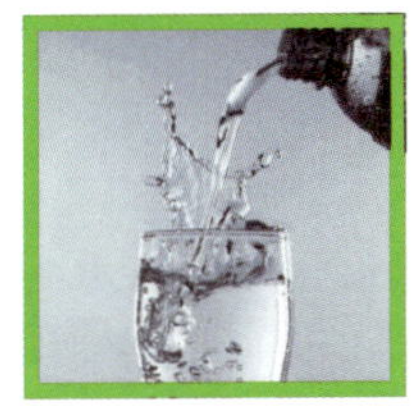

VS

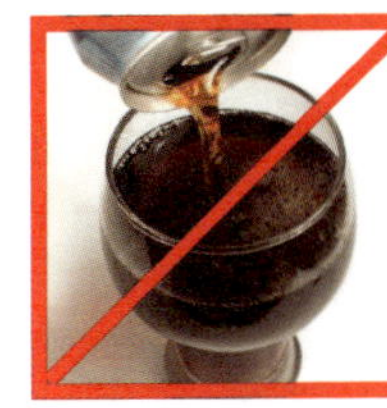

Now, turn to the first page of your nutrition log.

1. Cross out foods that contain sugar. In the substitute column, write down what you can eat to replace the empty calories.

2. Continue to write down everything you eat and drink in your nutrition log daily.

This is the first step in putting together your nutrition plan. Keep your "better choice" food selections simple. Too many food decisions at this point can lead to indecisive eating habits and can lead to overeating.

For Example:

Time	Food and Amount	Substitute
7:00 AM	Juice, pancakes, syrup	**Milk, WW Toast, Adam's® pb**
10:00 AM	Latte	Water
12:30 PM	White rice, chicken, veggies	**Brown rice**, chicken, veggies
3:00 PM	Smoothie	**Wheat bagel with lowfat cream cheese**
6:00 PM	Workout	Workout
8:00 PM	Chicken, salad, ice cream	Chicken, salad, **fruit**

WW = 100% whole wheat

Questions and Answers

Can sugars really make you fat?

Sugars digest quickly, store in your muscle cells immediately, and are ready for use as glycogen (ready-to-use fuel). If you are not active, then the excess sugar that was converted to glycogen will be transported to your body's fat cells for energy storage. In other words: THEY TURN INTO BODY FAT!

Why do I feel so tired after eating a lot of sugar?

The faster sugar digests, the faster the blood sugar rises. The faster blood sugar rises, the faster it falls. This can lead to blood sugar lows, which can make you feel tired, lethargic, depressed, or sleepy. Therefore, you want to minimize the effect of your blood sugar level for balance and long lasting energy. Try eating fruits and vegetables to help you maintain a balanced blood sugar.

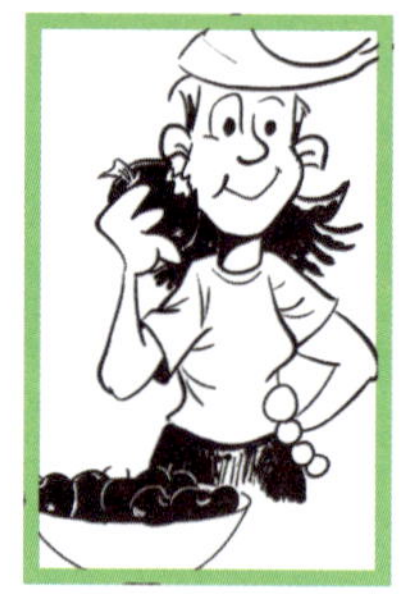

VS

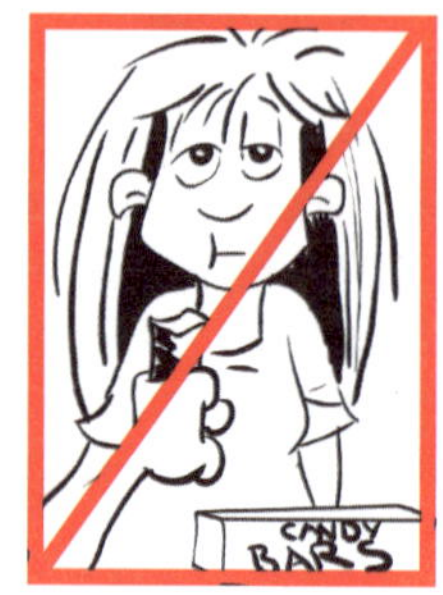

What are empty calories?

Empty calories are calories that contain few, if any, nutrients. Basically, "empty calories" is another term for junk food. Your body utilizes nutrients to digest calories. Empty calories do not provide much in the way of nutrient replenishment. They are low in nutritional value and provide little or no health benefits.

What are probiotics and where can you find them?

Probiotics are live bacteria found in yogurt that can be very beneficial to your health. These little powerhouses are good bacteria that assist your body's naturally occurring bacteria and microorganisms in providing the optimal digestive balance. They help your body absorb minerals and boost your immune system. They help decrease lactose intolerance, reduce infections, inflammation, cholesterol, blood pressure, allergies, and the risks of colon cancer. Unfortunately, not all yogurts contain probiotics, so make sure you look for "live & active cultures" on the label.

What is fiber and is it really an important part of my daily nutrition?

Fiber is basically carbohydrates that cannot be digested. The enzymes in our bodies are not able to break them down, and as a result they are not absorbed into the blood stream, and cannot be used as energy. Instead they are excreted from your body and simultaneously perform a great service for your digestive system. They bind with fatty acids, remove toxic waste, and promote regular bowel movements. Goodbye constipation! Fiber can also reduce the risks of colon cancer, heart disease, high cholesterol, diabetes, diverticular disease, and hypertension. Most of all, fiber helps slow the digestive process by stabilizing blood sugar effectively to promote optimal energy.

What are the best sources of fiber?

Load up on fruits and veggies! They are low in calories and rich in nutrients. This means you can eat more food without taking in extra calories! Additionally, they are jam-packed with nutrients, vitamins, and other chemicals which boost your energy and reduce your risk of chronic diseases. Other fiber-rich foods are legumes, whole-wheat and whole-grain products like brown rice, oat bran, barley, nuts, and flax seed.

Kevin brings to his job a great deal of technical knowledge about training the body, which is essential, and with that he adds the success components in his training manuals. Kevin adds himself to the equation. Kevin brings his personal enthusiasm, "can do" attitude, patience, creativity, empathy, sense of humor, and the greatest ingredient "heart" to each and every training session. Add this all up and you can't help but be inspired by Kevin to be the best that you can be. I owe a lot to Kevin because even on those occasional times when I'm frustrated or I've hit the plateau, he is there to encourage and inspire me to keep going.

- Beth Johnson

Nutrition Log

Date:__________	Sun Mon Tues Wed Thurs Fri Sat	
	Plan	**Actual**
Meal 1	*Food & Amount*	*Food & Amount*
Time:_____		
Meal 2		
Time:_____		
Meal 3		
Time:_____		
Meal 4		
Time:_____		
Meal 5		
Time:_____		
Meal 6		
Time:_____		

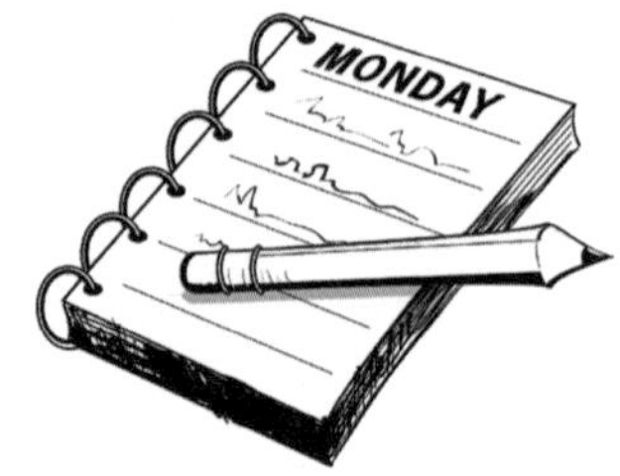

Checklist

Achieved:

- ✓ Consume meal or snack every 3 hours
- ✓ Water every 3 hours
- ✓ Sleep optimal hours
- ✓ Intake multivitamin
- ✓ Weights and cardio

Avoided:

- ✓ **Sugars**

Key Points

Week 1

- Eat a small meal or snack once every three hours – five to six meals per day.

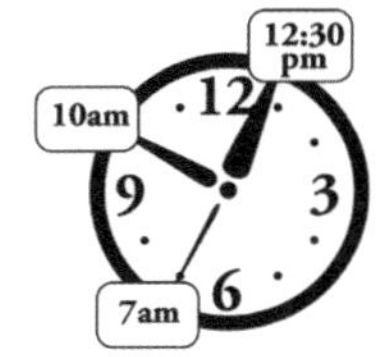

- Drink at least 1 cup (8 ounces) of water per meal and at least one cup before, during, and after your workouts.

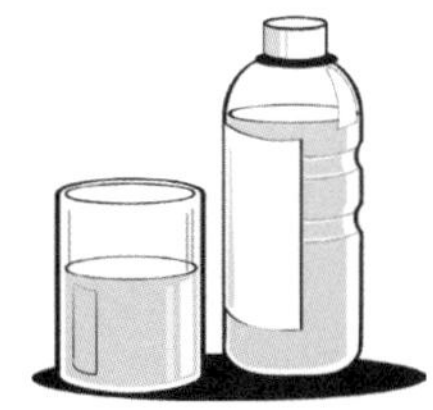

- Keep a nutrition log.

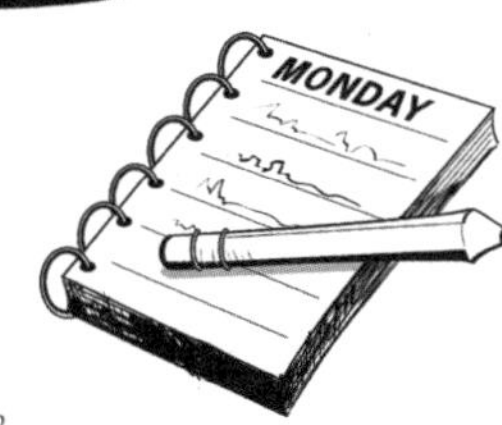

- Sleep is vital!

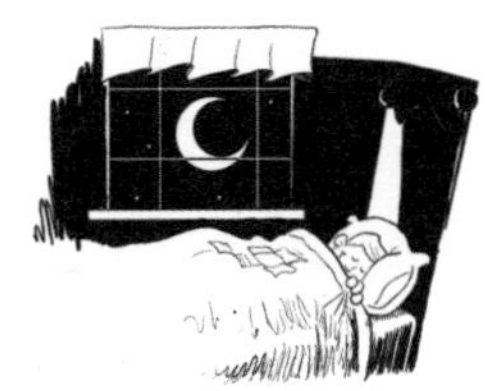

- Take a daily multivitamin.

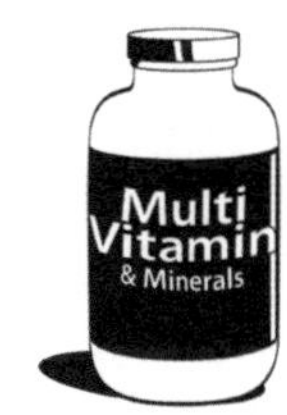

Week 2

- **Avoid bad sugars.** They are unnecessary calories that do not replenish nutrients lost in the digestion process. Substitute bad sugars with good sugars such as yogurt, fruit, and vegetables.

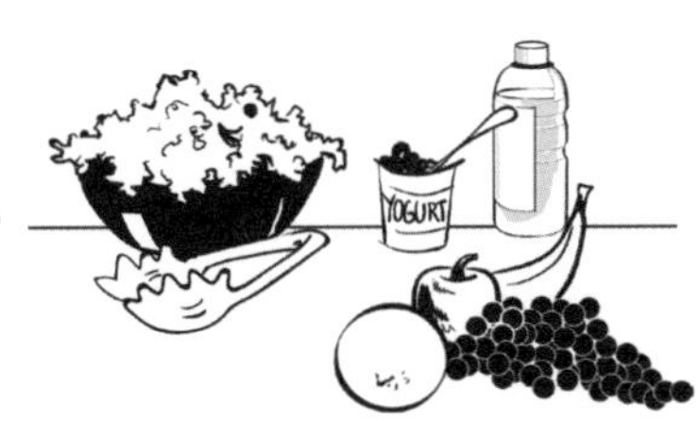

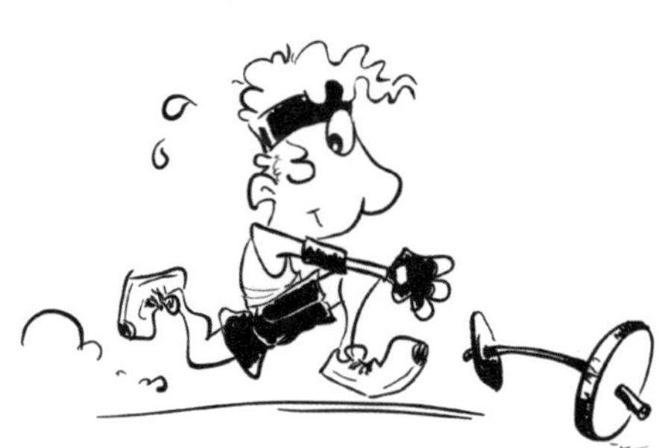

Chest

Goal:

Complete two sets of 15 reps on the **bench press**.

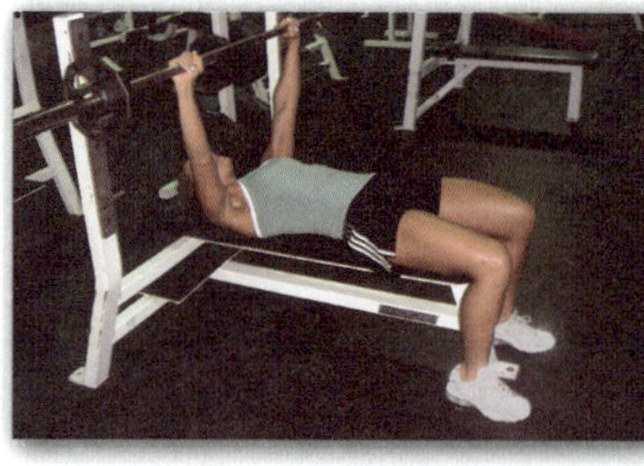

Primary
Chest

Stabilizers
Shoulders
Triceps
Forearms
Core

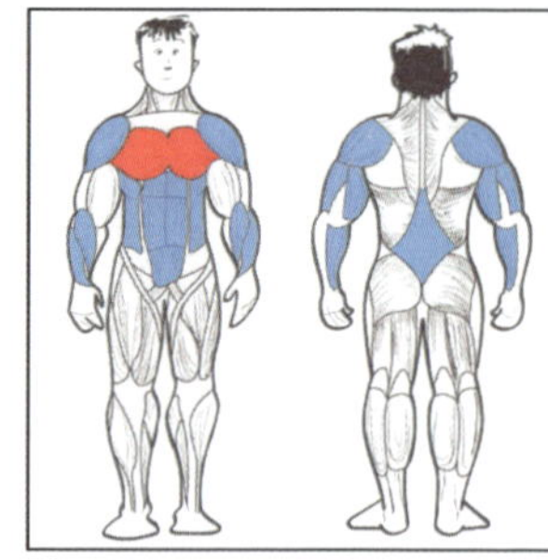

Why?

The bench press is a free weight, compound exercise targeting your chest. The muscle stabilizers include your shoulders, triceps, and forearms, as well as the rest of your core. Bench press is the first of three exercises you will perform in this week to establish a solid foundation of physical conditioning.

How?

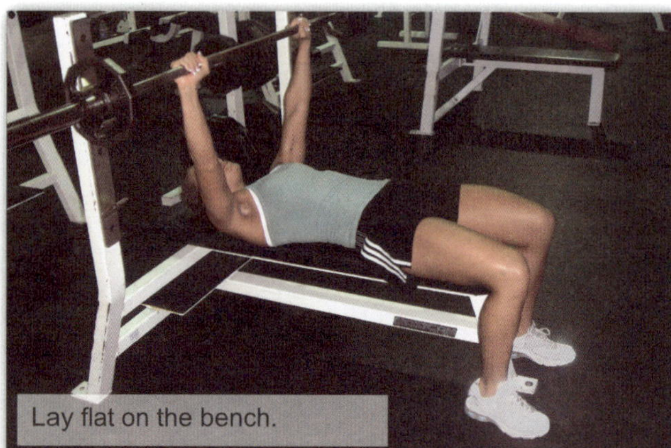
Lay flat on the bench.

Step 1 - Always squeeze your abs to assist the lower back's neutral position.

Step 2 - Scoot up or down along bench to keep your chin below bar.

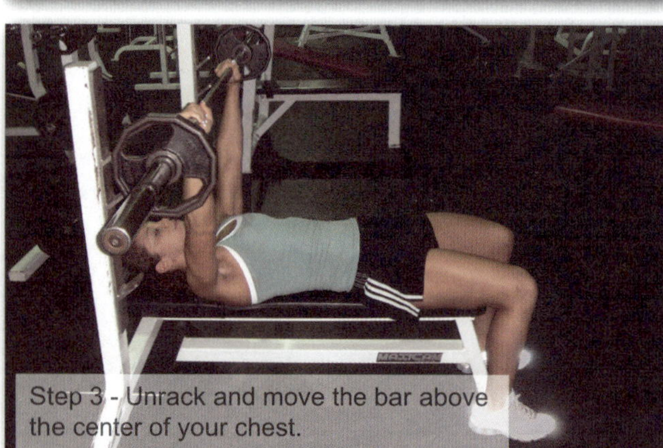
Step 3 - Unrack and move the bar above the center of your chest.

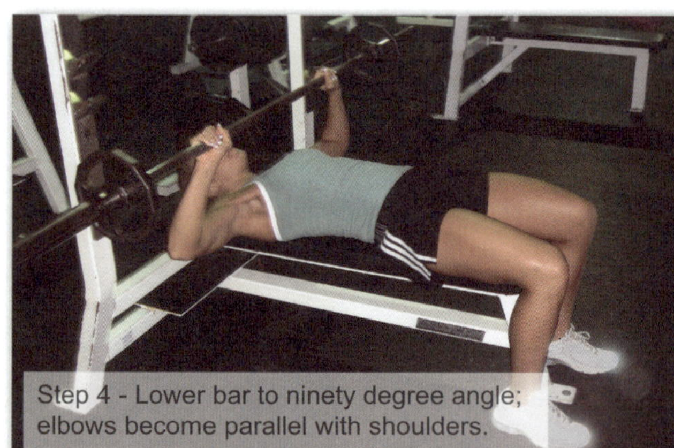
Step 4 - Lower bar to ninety degree angle; elbows become parallel with shoulders.

Step 5 - Push up and repeat.

Your goal is to complete two sets of fifteen (2 x 15).

Week 2

Range of Motion Techniques

To Maximize Muscle Tension and Minimize Overcompensation

Dos

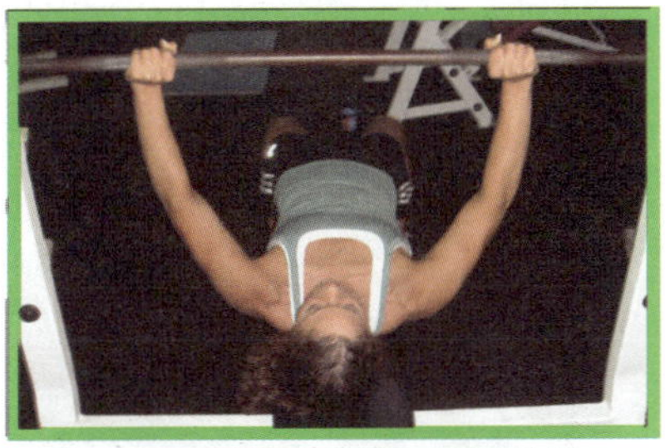

Squeeze Your Chest While Keeping Elbows Slightly Bent

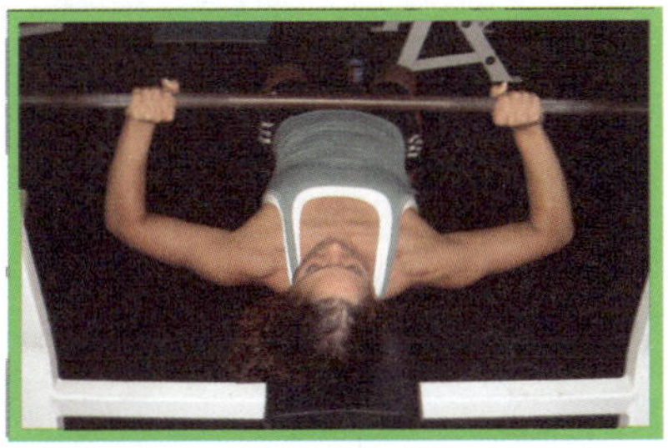

Feel Light Stretch in Chest While Elbows are in Line with Shoulders

Don'ts

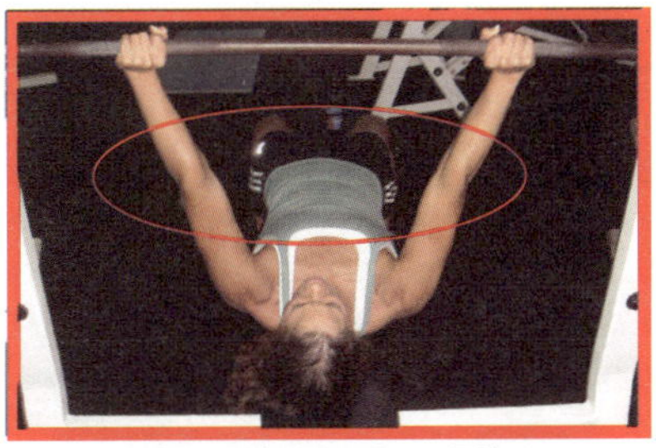

Avoid Locking Out Elbows

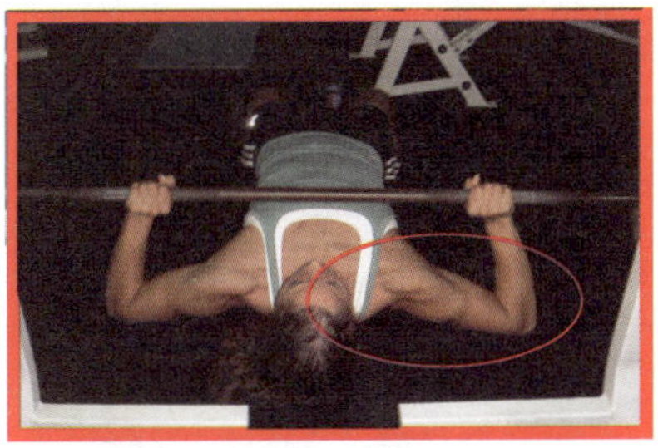

Avoid Dropping Elbows Below Shoulders

Visualize

"Semicircle and Stretch Effect"

Lay on the bench. Resist the bar as you lower it. Visualize pulling your arms apart in a semicircular motion and focus on feeling the stretch in your chest by pulling and stretching the bar apart before pushing it back up.

As you push the bar up in a semicircular motion, visualize bending the ends of the bar together as if your hands are about to touch.

As you discover your visualization technique working, your goal is to stay within the proper range of motion to maximize chest tension. This will decrease the risk of injury associated with poor technique.

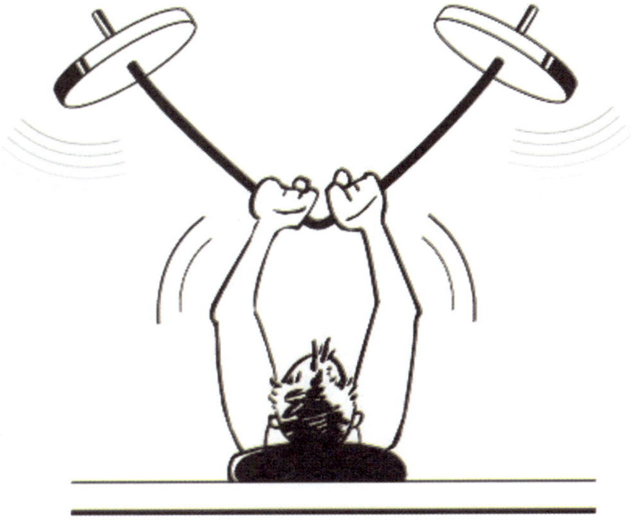

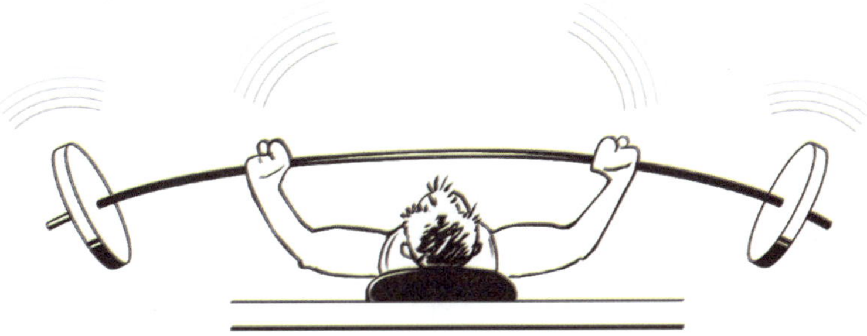

Questions and Answers

I have a hard time pressing my lower back on the bench. Is this necessary?

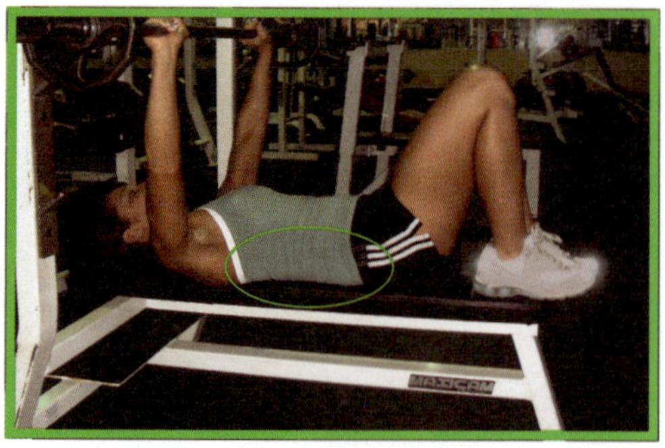

Yes, pressing your back against the bench decreases the pressure in your lower back. If you have trouble flattening the arch of the lower back, try squeezing your abs to press your back flat against the bench. You can also rest your feet on top of the bench to assist in keeping your back flat.

I feel too close to the bar when my chin is directly below. Can I scoot down on the bench?

No, it is best to place your chin directly below the bar. This position places your shoulders in the correct position to avoid too little or too much range of motion, without adding pressure in your rotator cuffs. A major goal when weight training is to minimize the risk of injury.

How fast should I perform my reps?

Your tempo should be two seconds down and two seconds up using a smooth and controlled motion. Expect to be a little unbalanced and unsteady until your stabilizers strengthen more. This slower tempo will help you to maintain form and control, which minimizes your risk of injury.

Can I hold the bar with a closer hand-grip?

No, at this point in your training, it's best to hold the bar with your arms at a 90-degree angle. Holding the bar with a closer hand-grip involves using more of the triceps. Holding the bar with a wider hand-grip involves using more of the shoulder muscle and shoulder joint. To maximize the chest tension and contraction, you'll want your hand-grip to be at a 90-degree angle as much as possible.

How much weight should I lift?

Start with the lightest weight possible. When it comes to weight lifting there is no magic number. The amount of weight will vary from person to person, and from exercise to exercise. You have to remember that some days you will be stronger than others. Building a foundation of strength and conditioning is not about how much weight you can lift, it is all about how effectively you work the muscles to fatigue. You should lift enough weight to be fully fatigued by the end of your set. For example:

Your goal is to complete two sets of 15 reps.

• First set should be a warm-up. Choose a weight light enough to easily achieve your first set of 15 reps. This warm-up lubricates your joints, ligaments, and tendons in preparation for higher intensity sets. Remember, you can increase the intensity by increasing the number of reps or the amount of weight you lift.

• Second set should be higher intensity. You should be lifting enough weight to fatigue by the fifteenth rep. If you can continue with one or more reps beyond 15 reps, then you're not fully fatigued. You'll need to increase the weight in your next workout.

As an idea, keep a record of how much weight it took to fatigue your muscles so that you'll have a good starting point for your next workout session.

How long of a rest should I take in between each set?

The average rest period for building a foundation of conditioning is 30 seconds. Sometimes rest periods can vary significantly based on the goal of the athlete. Endurance athletes require less rest, while athletes focusing on strength and power require more rest. You should apply the 30-second rest period to all exercises.

Can I do more than two sets of fifteen reps my first time?

It depends. If you have not weight trained for a few months, you'll need to begin with two sets of 15 to avoid overtraining. If you have been weight training on and off for the past month, you can begin with three to four sets of 15. Your goal is to avoid getting too sore from your initial workouts so that you can continue to workout. If you are still sore from your first workout when it's time to weight train again, you will need to wait to work out those muscle groups until you're not sore. Weight training the sore muscle groups does not make you stronger. In fact, it makes you weaker. Working out breaks down your muscles. If you are still sore from your last workout, your muscles have not recovered. If you were to work out, you would weaken your muscles by breaking them down even further. Muscles need time to repair and recover to grow and become stronger.

Do I need someone to spot me?

If this is your first time on the bench press, you may need someone to stand behind you and assist in lifting and racking the bar until you become more comfortable with the bench press.

When should I breathe?

You should always inhale at your starting position and exhale as you complete your range of motion. For example, when performing the bench press exercise, inhale as you lower the bar and exhale as you push the bar up to your starting position.

Back

Goal:

Complete two sets of 15 reps on the **lat pulldown**.

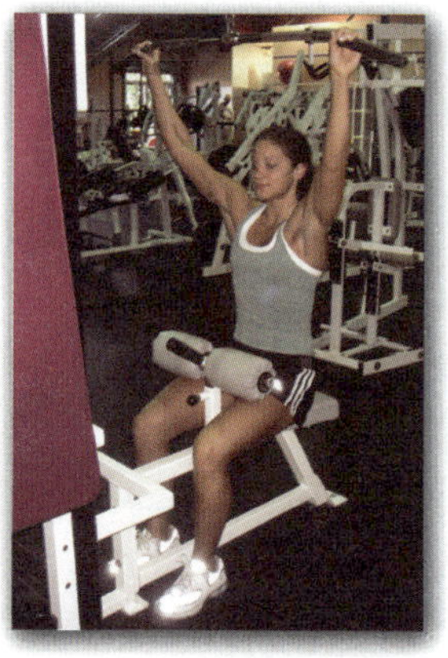

Primary
Lats

Stabilizers
Shoulders
Biceps
Forearms
Core

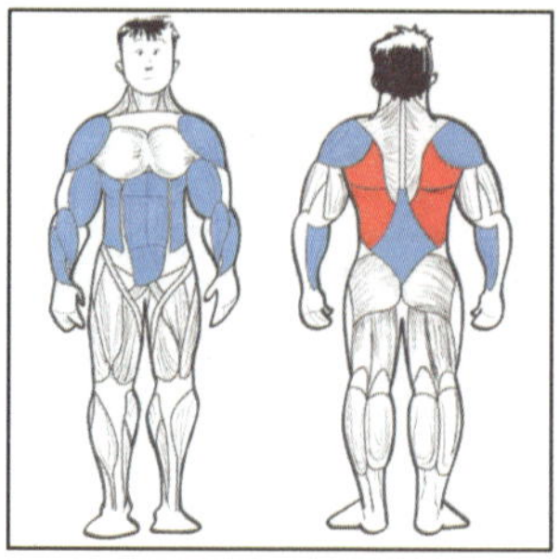

Why?

The lat pulldown is a machine exercise that is similar to performing a pull up. This exercise targets your lats, the "wings" of your back. The muscle stabilizers include your shoulders, biceps, and forearms, as well as the rest of your core. The lat pulldown is the second of three exercises you will perform in this session to establish a solid foundation of physical conditioning.

How?

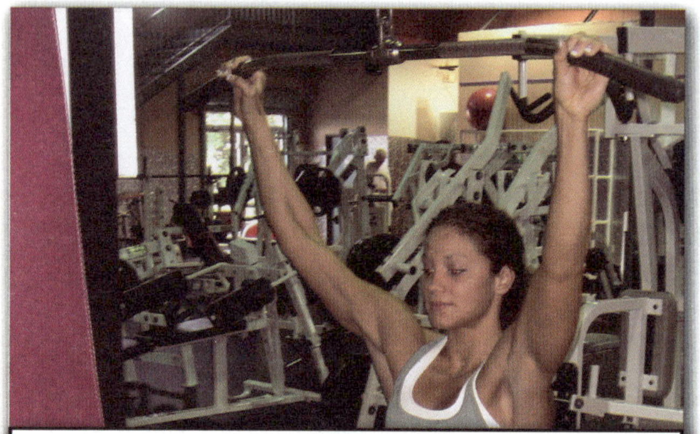

Step 1 - Grab the bar with a ninety degree angle grip, sit down, and lean back slightly.

Step 2 - Squeeze your abs to push your lower back into a neutral position.

Step 3 - Pull the bar down to your nose or eye level to reach the peak contraction of your lats.

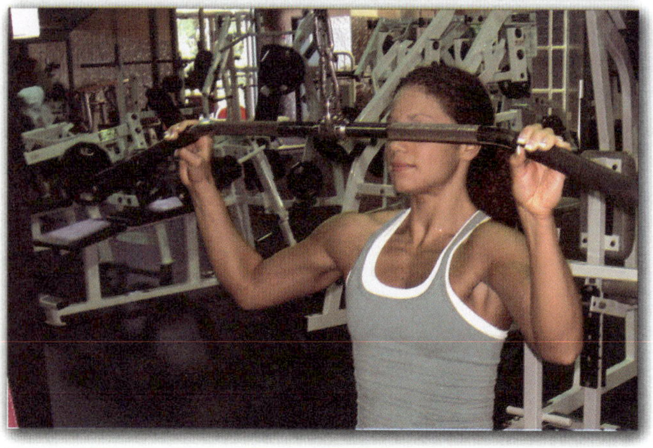

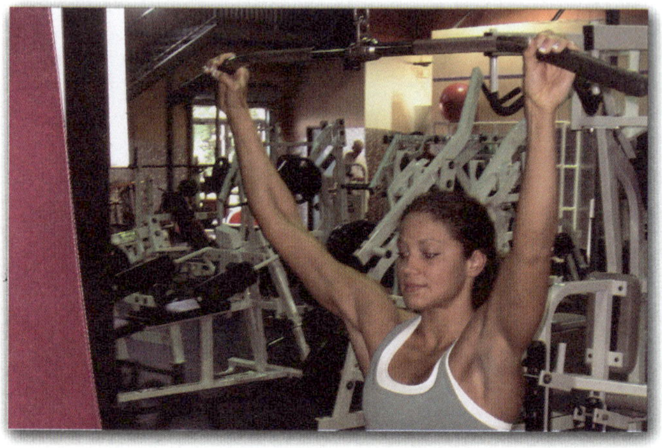

Step 4 - Allow the bar to rise up to the point of feeling a small stretch in your lats with your elbows unlocked and slightly bent.

Step 5 - Repeat with a smooth and fluid motion to maximize your lat tension.

Your goal is to complete two sets of 15 (2 x 15).

Range of Motion Techniques

To Maximize Muscle Tension and Minimize Overcompensation

Dos | **Don'ts**

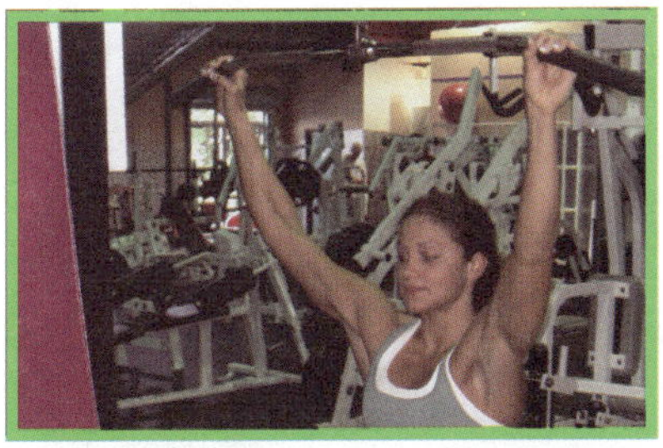

Stretch Lats While Keeping Elbows Slightly Bent

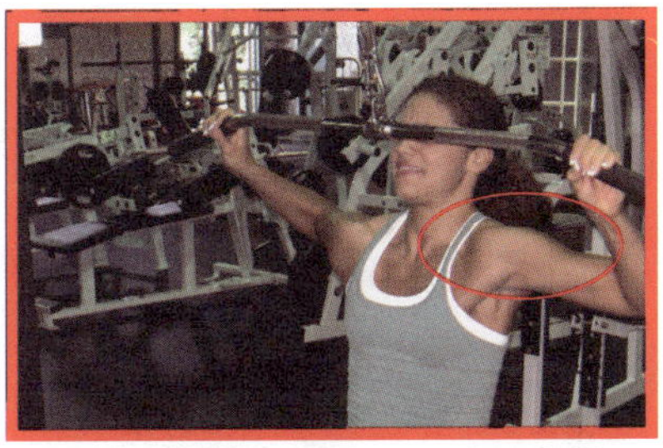

Avoid Pulling Elbows Back Too Far

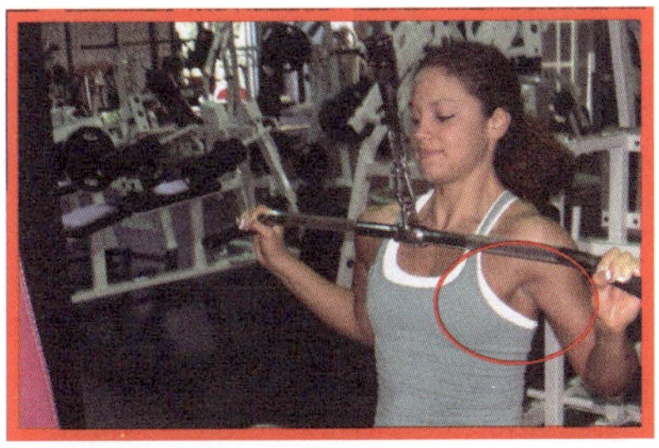

Avoid Pulling the Bar Down Too Low

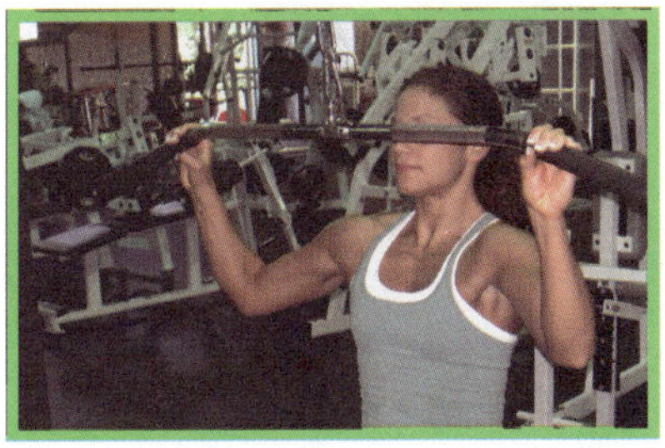

Elbows Almost Lined up with Shoulders

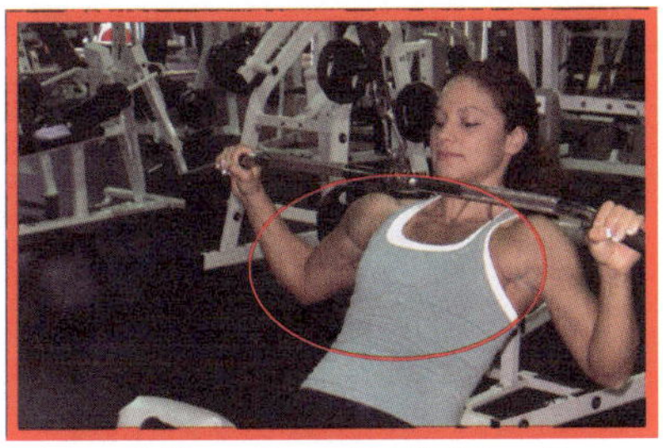

Avoid Leaning Back Too Far

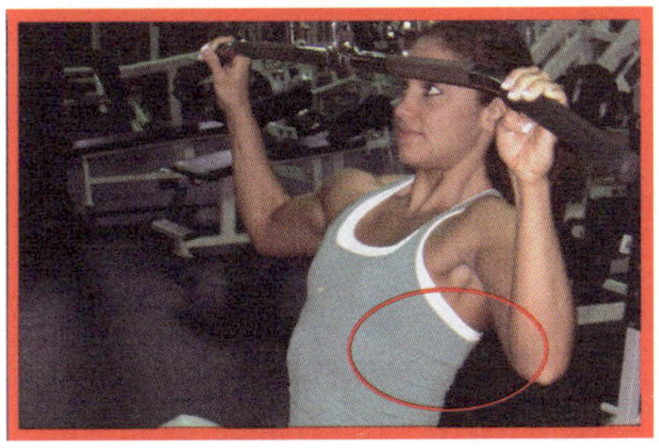

Avoid Arching Lower Back

Visualize

"Flare and Stretch Effect"

When seated, pull the straight bar down and resist it while coming up. Visualize flaring your lats out at your starting position by pulling your elbows slightly forward and rounding your upper back. Pull down to your maximum muscle contraction while maintaining your lat flare and visualization.

Continue to visualize your lats flared out to feel a stretch in your lats at the top of your starting position.

Visualize each rep to maximize your lat tension. This will minimize shoulder, biceps, and forearm overcompensation.

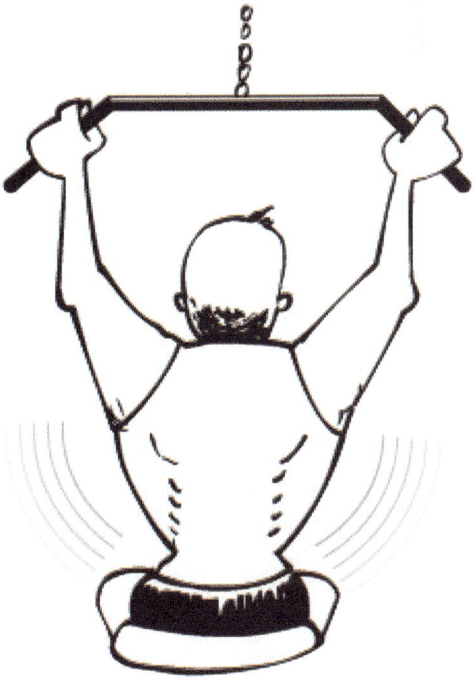

Questions and Answers

I thought I was supposed to have an arch in my lower back. Isn't that correct form?

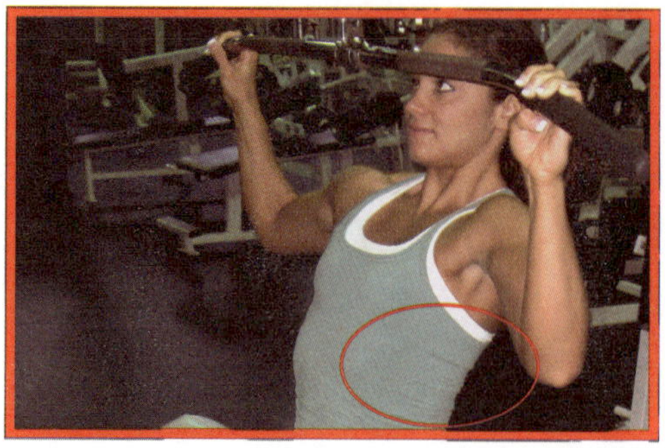

No. Correct form decreases joint tension to maximize muscle tension. When focusing on building a foundation of conditioning, you should squeeze your abs to push your lower back into a neutral position. This relieves the pressure in your lower back, helps to avoid overcompensating, and forces your lats to do the work. Anytime you decrease joint tension, you will always increase muscle tension.

Can I pull the bar down further than eye level?

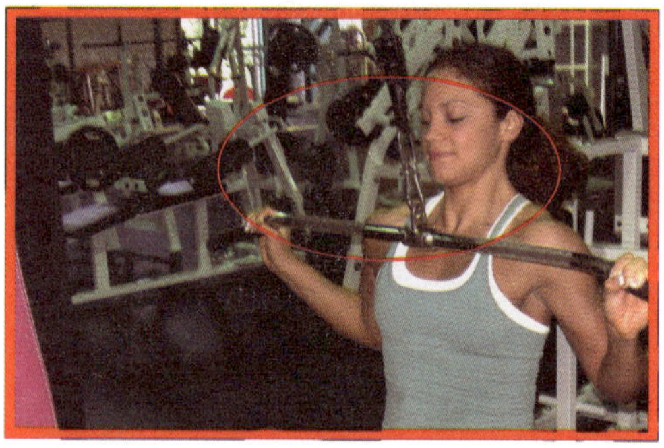

No, it is best to pull the bar down to eye level. If you pull down any further, you will lose the peak contraction of your lats. This forces your shoulders and biceps to overcompensate. Overcompensating reduces the effectiveness of your lat muscle contraction.

Why do I need to feel the lats stretch?

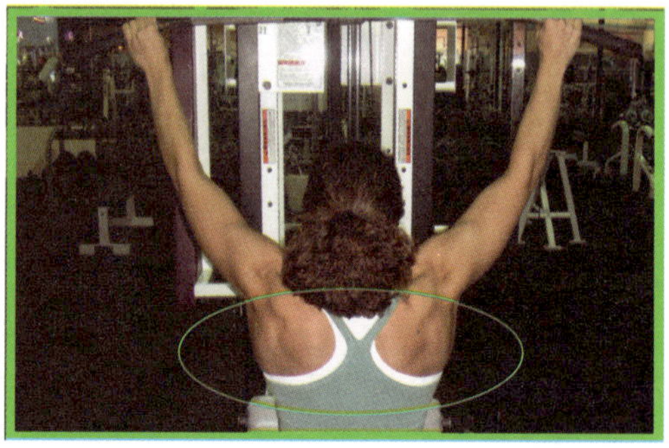

Feeling a small stretch in your lats is the key in knowing whether your lat muscles are resisting. This can take practice and some strengthening. If you don't feel the stretch, your shoulders and forearms are doing the work.

Why is leaning back and swinging to pull the bar down incorrect?

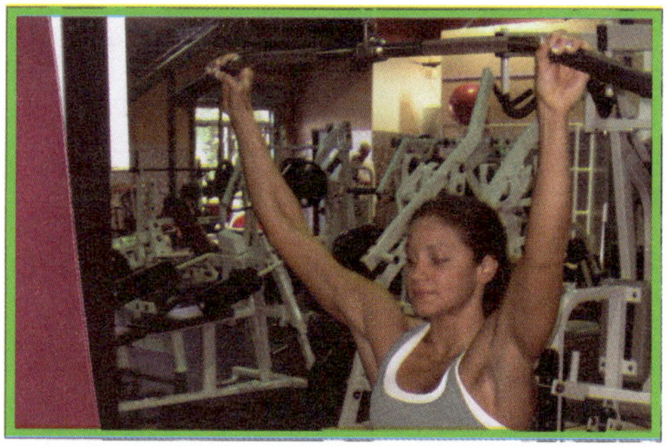

It depends on which muscle groups you want to train. Leaning back can emphasize your rhomboids while requiring your stabilizers to do more work. Swinging can emphasize your lower back tension and momentum. To maximize the tension in your lat muscles, you need to have your lower back in a neutral position. This reduces lower back tension, momentum, and stabilizer utilization, which forces your lats to do the work.

I feel my forearms. Am I doing something wrong?

If you are feeling your forearms, your grip is probably too tight. You should maintain a light hand grip to allow your lats to do the work; otherwise, your forearms and biceps, the stabilizers, will overcompensate. Also, gripping too hard increases wrist joint tension, which you need to avoid as much as possible to reduce the risk of injury.

How do I hold onto the bar?

Your thumbs should wrap around the bar to secure your wrists. Securing your wrists provides wrist stability and helps to keep your wrists strong. Your grip should be as light as possible. Gripping too tightly increases wrist joint tension and overcompensation of the forearms. Every once in awhile, it is OK to keep your thumbs on the outside of the bar. However, as a general rule, you should secure your wrists by wrapping your thumbs around the bar to avoid overcompensation and possible injuries.

When should I breathe?

You should always inhale at your starting position and exhale as you complete your range of motion. In lat pulldown, inhale as you pull the bar down and exhale as you let the bar up to your starting position.

I was taught to breathe out!

As an analogy, would you exhale before or on your way up in pull ups and inhale as your lower yourself? Probably not. You would definitely lose your strength quickly.

Shoulders

Goal:

Complete two sets of 15 reps on the **machine shoulder press**.

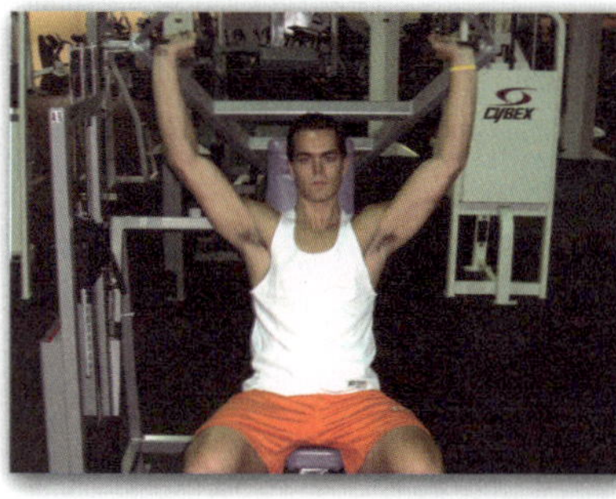

Primary
Shoulders

Stabilizers
Triceps
Forearms
Core

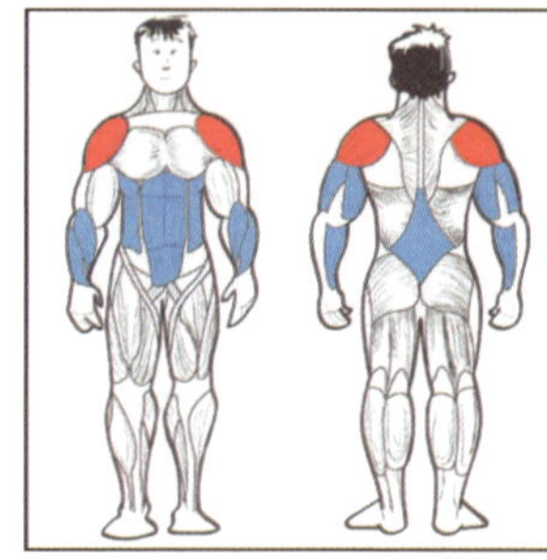

Why?

The machine shoulder press is a machine exercise targeting your shoulders. The muscle stabilizers include your triceps and forearms, as well as the rest of your core. The machine shoulder press is the third exercise you will perform in this session to establish a solid foundation of physical conditioning.

How?

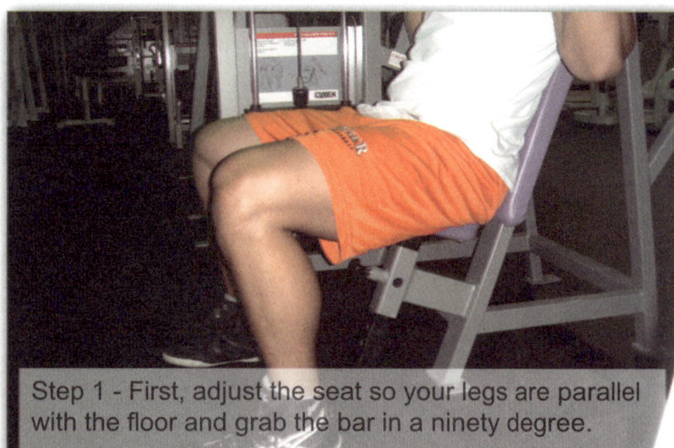

Step 1 - First, adjust the seat so your legs are parallel with the floor and grab the bar in a ninety degree.

Step 2 - Squeeze your abs to push your lower back into a neutral position against the pad.

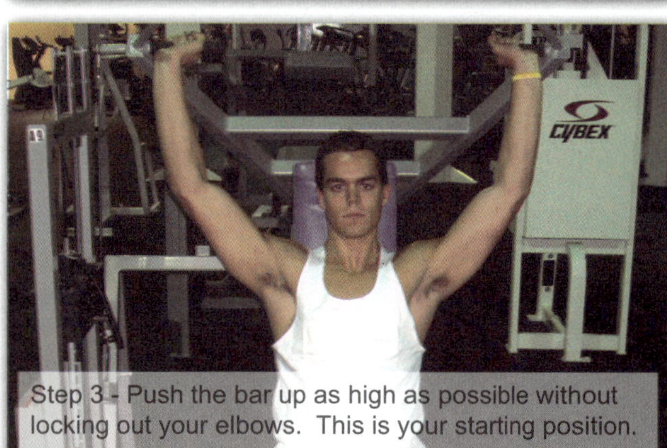

Step 3 - Push the bar up as high as possible without locking out your elbows. This is your starting position.

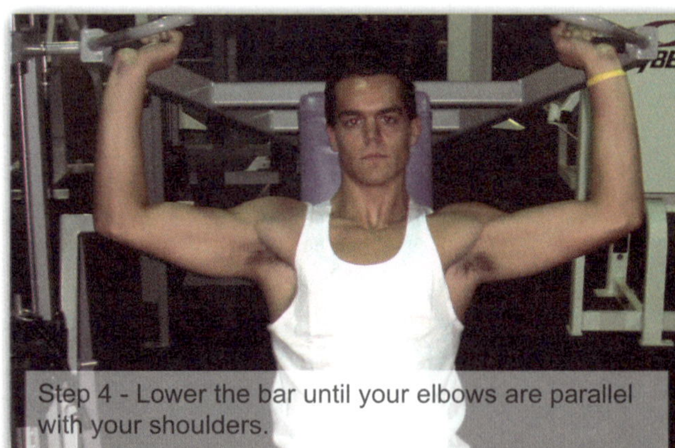

Step 4 - Lower the bar until your elbows are parallel with your shoulders.

Step 5 - Push up in a controlled, smooth motion to complete one rep.

Your goal is to complete two sets of 15 (2 x 15).

Range of Motion Techniques

To Maximize Muscle Tension and Minimize Overcompensation

Dos

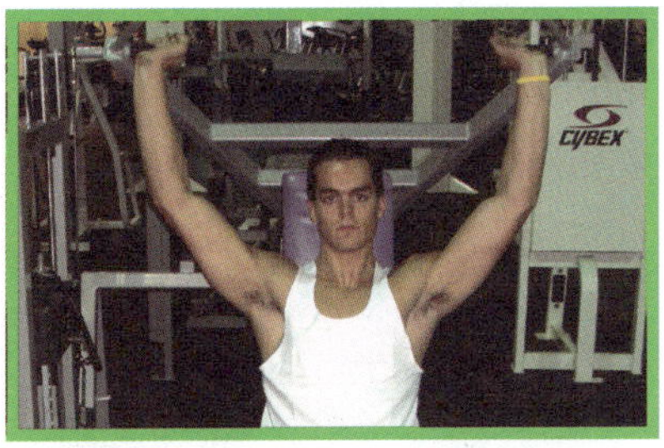

Begin with Elbows Slightly Bent

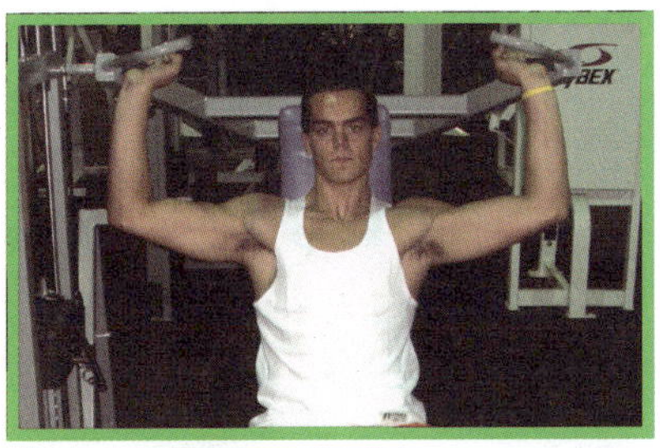

Lower Elbows to Line up with Shoulders

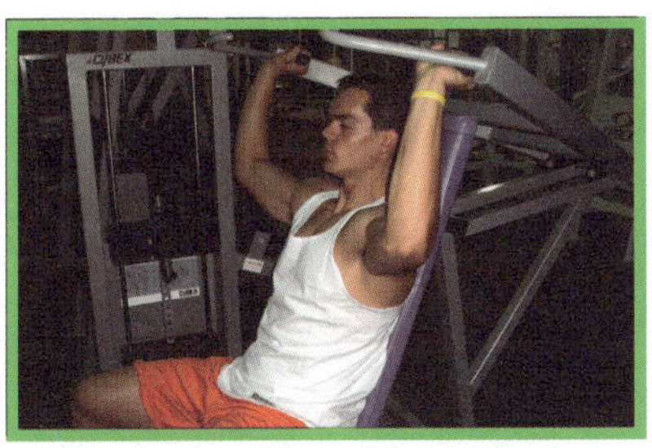

Maximize Shoulder Tension When Elbows are Vertical and Lower Back is Flat

Don'ts

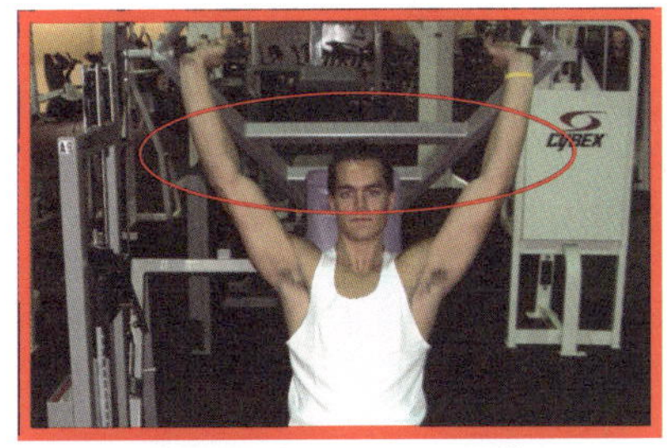

Avoid Locking Out Elbows

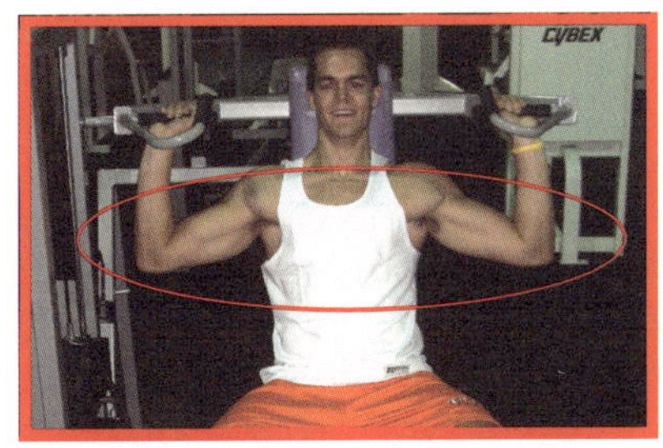

Avoid Dropping Elbows Below Shoulders

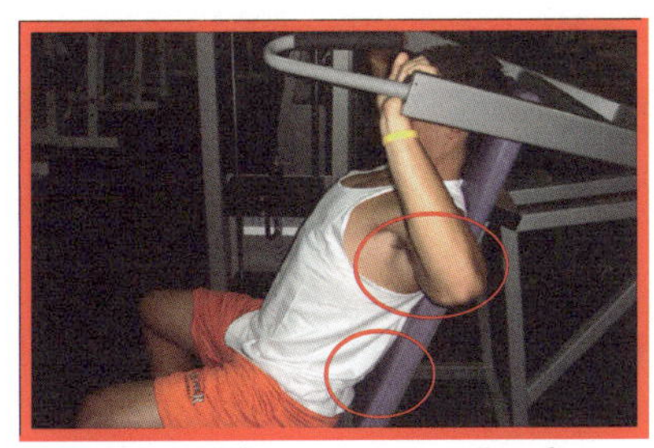

Avoid Arching Lower Back or Pulling Elbows Too Far Back

Visualize

"Semicircle and Stretch Effect"

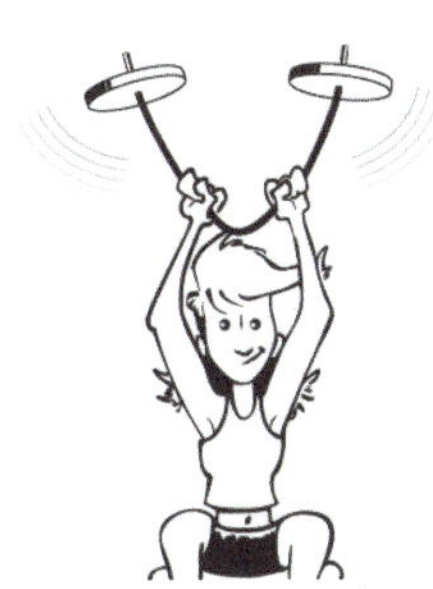

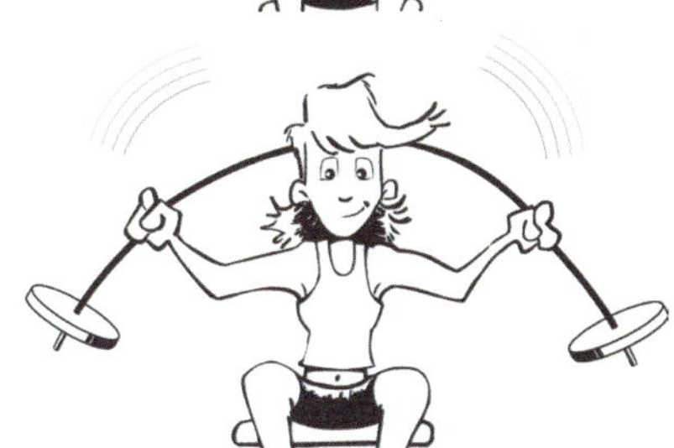

The visualization technique for the shoulder press is exactly the same as it is for the bench press; only now you are in an upright body position.

Resist the bar as you lower it and visualize stretching the bar apart in a semicircular motion. Focus on feeling the stretch in your shoulders by pulling and stretching the bar apart before pushing it up.

As you push the bar up in a semicircular motion, visualize bending the ends of the bar together as if your hands are about to touch.

Visualize every rep. Practicing visualization will allow you to maximize the use of your shoulders and minimize the tension in your shoulder joints, elbows, and wrists.

Questions and Answers

I have a hard time keeping my back flat. Is this important?

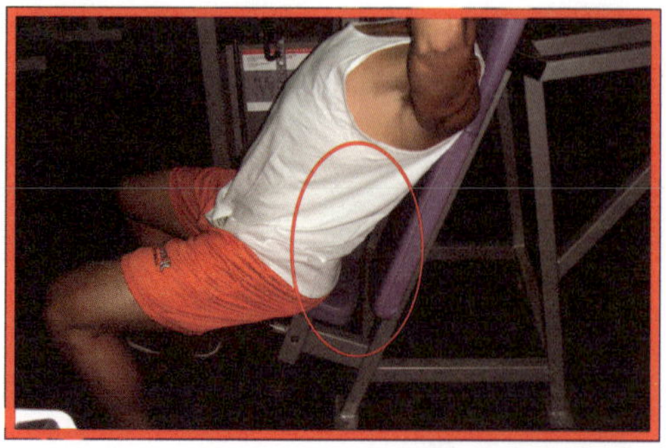

Yes, keeping your back flat relieves the pressure in your lower back. Maintaining a neutral lower back position reduces overcompensation and forces your shoulders to do the work. If you have trouble flattening the arch of the lower back, try squeezing your abs to press your back flat against the bench.

Can I perform the shoulder press with a full range of motion?

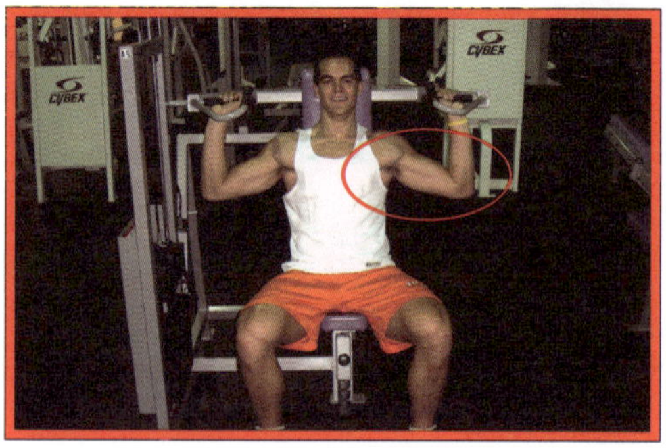

A full range of motion is not the most appropriate range of motion for building a foundation of conditioning. Your goal is to effectively work the shoulder muscles without overcompensating with other muscles or joints. A full range of motion, beyond a 90 degree angle, increases overcompensation. For example, lowering your elbows below parallel with your shoulders places unnecessary strain on the shoulder joints and allows your forearms to overcompensate, thus increasing your risk of injury.

Can I weight train with the two exercises I've learned and perform four sets each?

Weight training with just two different exercises and four sets of each is not the most effective weight training routine for your conditioning goals. Our foundation training is preparing you to progress to the next level. Once you have established a solid foundation, you can focus on body fat loss, strength, or endurance.

When should I breathe?

You should always inhale at your starting position and exhale as you complete your range of motion. In the shoulder press, inhale as you lower the bar and exhale as you push it up to your starting position.

Training with Kevin has influenced my life in many ways. Not only have I lost weight, increased muscle tone and definition, and learned how to eat properly, but I also found that I had a passion for fitness that I wasn't aware of. While training with Kevin, I found myself researching fitness and nutrition in my free time and made it a part of my everyday life. Since training with him, I have decided to become a certified personal trainer myself, which is something I had never considered before. I feel healthier physically and mentally because of Kevin. He truly has changed my life!

- Cailyn McIntosh

When I re-joined the gym, I asked for Kevin only because I had remembered that he was a good and experienced trainer. It wasn't until then when he was actually training me that I realized how good he really was. For the first time in years, I once again enjoyed my workouts and I started seeing results. And the most amazing fact of all, I was working out less; Kevin just had me working out, as he states "more effectively." That is his phrase. I finally felt productive in the gym. I soon came up with the slogan "Kevin does a body good." That soon spread throughout the gym and the training times with Kevin were the hottest commodity to get!

- Carol Davis

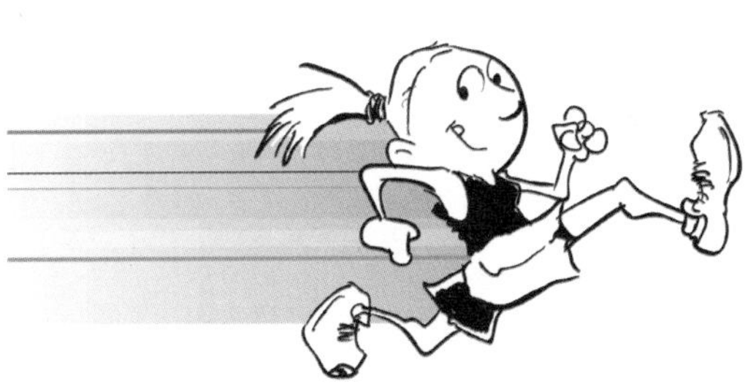

Cardio

Goal:

Complete 15 minutes on the **treadmill** and 15 minutes on the EFX.

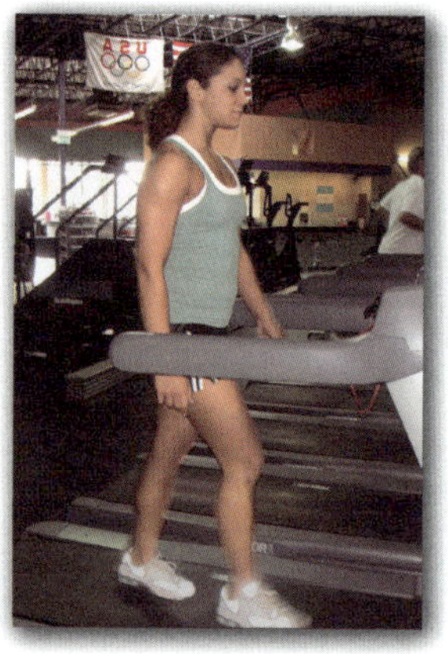

Primary
Quads
Glutes
Hamstrings

Stabilizers
Calves
Shins
Core

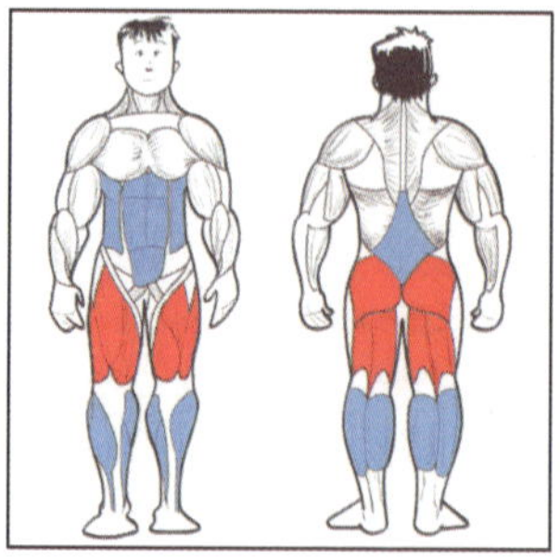

Why?

The treadmill is a cardio machine that allows you to walk, jog, or run. It absorbs more impact than outdoor surfaces such as asphalt, concrete, sand, or older tracks. Additionally, the treadmill is a step up in intensity from the EFX and other similar stationary machines because it requires more balance and stability while utilizing more of the stabilizing muscles.

How?

Step 1 - Step onto the treadmill and press **QUICK START** or select **MANUAL PROGRAM**.

Step 2 - Depending on your physical condition, set the speed to a comfortable walking pace between 2.5 to 4.0 mph. Basically, walk as fast as you can without holding on or running. You should maintain a smooth and fluid walking motion.

Step 3 - Increase your incline to one percent.

Step 4 - Your cardio goal is to walk on the treadmill for 15 minutes in addition to your 15 minutes on the EFX. Remember to work out at medium intensity, a breathing rate at which it's slightly difficult to hold a conversation.

Range of Motion Techniques

To Maximize Muscle Tension and Minimize Overcompensation

Dos

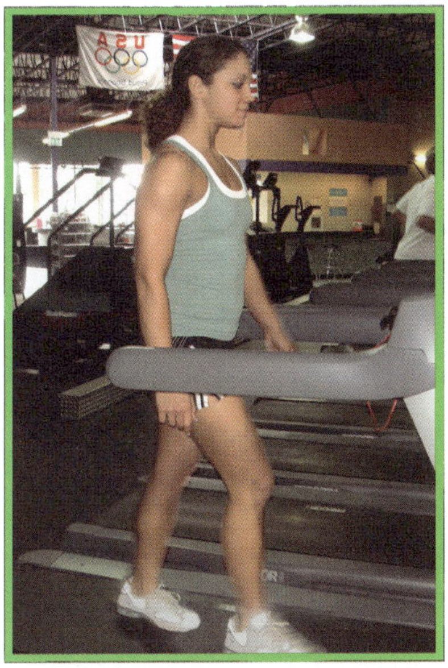

Let Arms Swing Naturally and Avoid Holding On

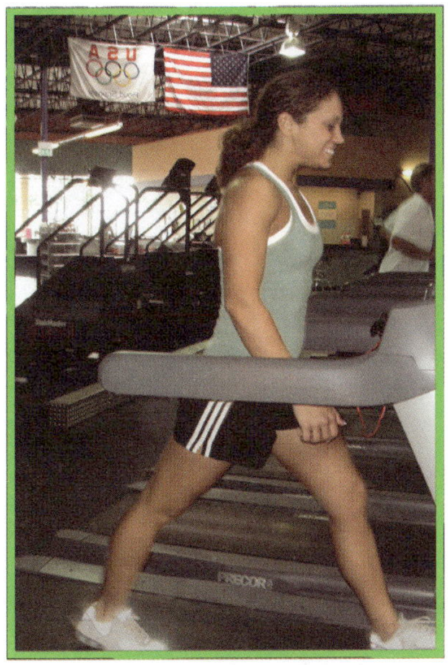

Maintain Long Strides

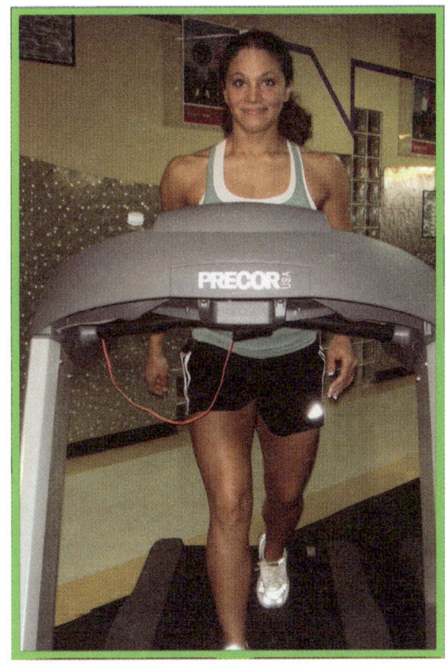

Shoulders Aligned and Even

Visualize

"Water and Sound Effect"

Walking on water and walking with the least amount of sound are the two most effective visualization techniques for walking.

Visualizing walking on water places your body into a position to walk naturally with the least amount of impact. Walking quietly assists in forcing your quads, hamstrings, and calves to absorb the impact of walking. Loud, high impact walking forces your lower back and knees to overcompensate by absorbing the pressure and tension.

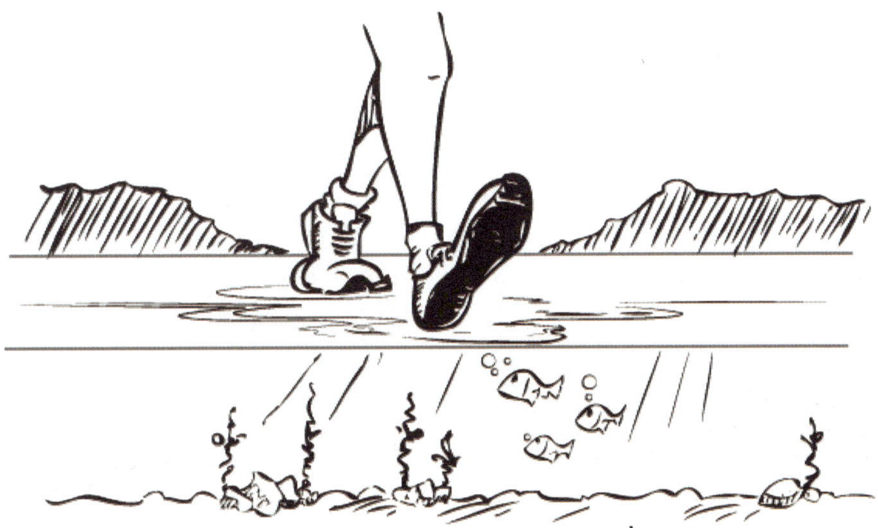

Questions and Answers

Is it OK to hold on?

No, it is best to let your arms swing naturally as you walk. If you feel the need to hold on, you're probably walking too fast. Holding on doesn't allow your natural walking form and gait to take place.

Should I weight train before or after cardio?

At this point, the order of your weight and cardio training doesn't matter. The order becomes more important as you fine tune your goals for body fat loss, strength, or endurance. For now, complete your training in whatever order is comfortable for you.

Why do I need to walk at 1% or higher on the treadmill?

You should avoid walking at zero percent. Surprisingly, walking at zero percent is similar to walking downhill. Walking downhill places excessive joint and ligament pressure on your knees, hips, and lower back. Minimizing this extra pressure will help decrease your risk of injury.

Why do I feel constricted in my walking motion while visualizing and walking on the treadmill?

Walking with proper form will take time and practice. Your arms should sway naturally. Your knees should be bent and you should take long, natural strides. This allows the body to flow in its most natural walking form and gait while minimizing impact and pressure in your joints. Over time, with practice, it will feel natural.

Should I do any other stretches besides the hamstring stretch?

Yes, you will need to stretch your calves. Before incorporating your second stretch, stretch your hamstrings for two sets of 15 seconds again. Next, stretch your calves. Stretching your calves should be relaxing and not too intense. Complete one of the following calf stretches:

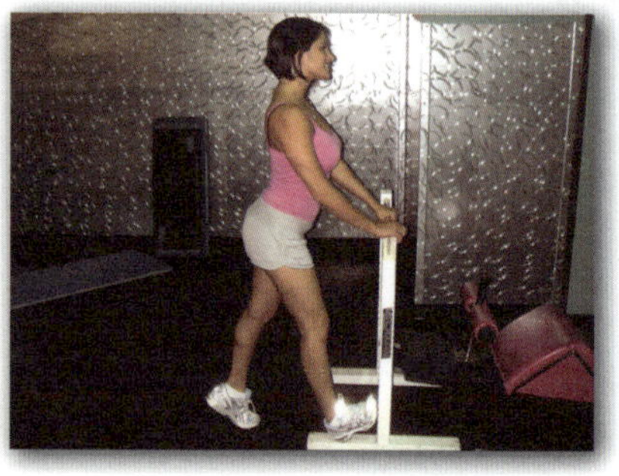

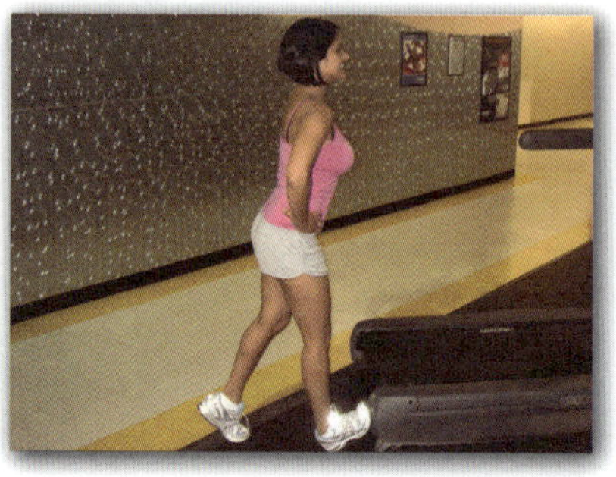

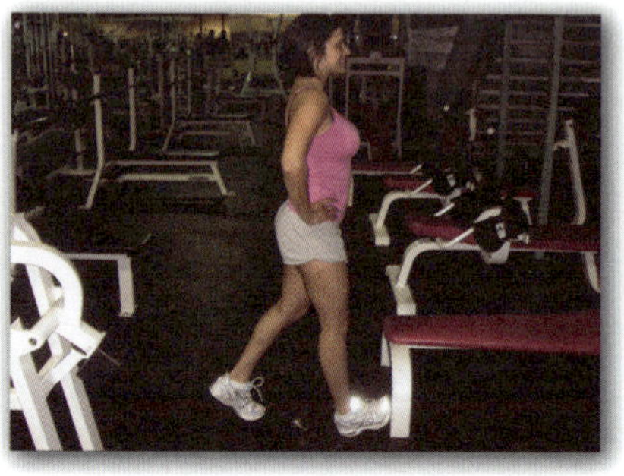

1. Extend one leg and place your foot at an angle against a wall or bench.
2. Your body should lean forward slightly.
3. Lift your back heel off the floor and slightly bend your front knee.
4. Stretch and hold lightly for two sets of fifteen seconds.

The Secrets to Success!

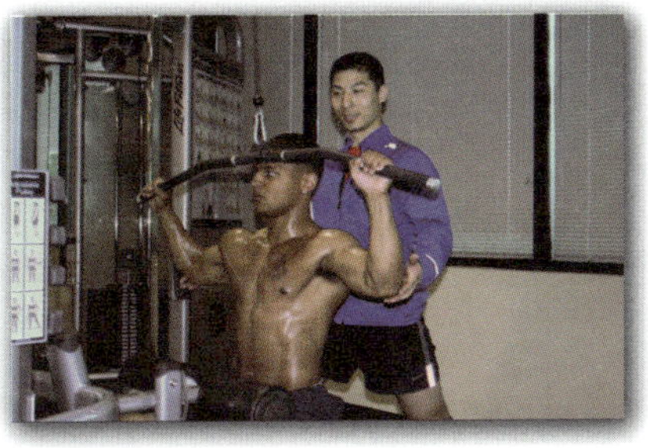

From Your Personal Trainer, Kevin Orr

I have had many clients follow my step-by-step process to achieve their own personal goals. What is so great is that they really achieved their goals and have maintained them. They did it by pacing themselves to master each step before taking the next step. That is so important to your success. Step by step.

It is exciting to truly learn how to accomplish your fitness and lifestyle goals with simple changes. Achieving one step and pacing yourself to master the next step takes commitment, dedication, and most importantly, self-motivation. You are doing this for YOU and you have what it takes to succeed. Everyone does. Focus on one step at a time. Trying to accomplish too many steps at once can be overwhelming. Pace yourself and practice what you learn with focus and determination. Remember, you are building a foundation for positive lifestyle changes. Pacing yourself is the secret to achieving your goals!

Example Weight & Cardio Routine

Choose a workout routine based on your level of fitness and your schedule before progressing to Week Three. Write it down in your schedule, page 249. If none of the example routines work for you, configure a routine that fits your needs, and write it down. Planning ahead will help you set yourself up for success.

Weight Routine 1

Sunday	Monday	Tuesday	Wednesday	Thursday	Friday	Saturday
	Chest/Back/ Shoulders 2x15			Chest/Back/ Shoulders 3x15		

Weight Routine 2

Sunday	Monday	Tuesday	Wednesday	Thursday	Friday	Saturday
		Chest/Back/ Shoulders 2x15			Chest/Back/ Shoulders 3x15	

Weight Routine 3

Sunday	Monday	Tuesday	Wednesday	Thursday	Friday	Saturday
	Chest/Back/ Shoulders 2x15		Chest/Back/ Shoulders 2x15		Chest/Back/ Shoulders 3x15	

Choose routine 1, 2, or 3 to begin your weekly cardio routine, or rearrange your cardio training to best fit you.

Cardio Routine 1

Sunday	Monday	Tuesday	Wednesday	Thursday	Friday	Saturday
	EFX: 15 Tread: 15		EFX: 15 Tread: 15		EFX: 15 Tread: 15	

Cardio Routine 2

Sunday	Monday	Tuesday	Wednesday	Thursday	Friday	Saturday
		EFX: 15 Tread: 15	EFX: 15 Tread: 15	EFX: 15 Tread: 15		EFX: 15 Tread: 15

Cardio Routine 3

Sunday	Monday	Tuesday	Wednesday	Thursday	Friday	Saturday
	EFX: 15 Tread: 15	EFX: 15 Tread: 15	EFX: 15 Tread: 15	EFX: 15 Tread: 15	EFX: 15 Tread: 15	

Example Schedule

On your schedule, page 249, continue to write down which cardio machines along with the duration you plan to complete this week.

	Sunday	Monday	Tuesday	Wednesday	Thursday	Friday	Saturday	
Week 1 Cardio: Duration:		*EFX: 5*	*EFX: 10*	*EFX: 15*	*EFX: 20*	*EFX: 20*		Why *Too Tired* Solution *Pace Yourself*
Week 2 Weights: Sets: Cardio: Duration:		*Chest/Back* *Shoulders: 2x15* *EFX: 15* *Tread: 15*	*EFX: 15* *Tread: 15*	*Chest/Back* *Shoulders: 2x15* *EFX: 15* *Tread: 15*	*EFX: 15* *Tread: 15*	*Chest/Back* *Shoulders: 3x15* *EFX: 15* *Tread: 15*		

Before moving on...

Did you follow through with your plan? If not, cross out what you did not complete on your schedule and write in what you did complete before moving on to the next week.

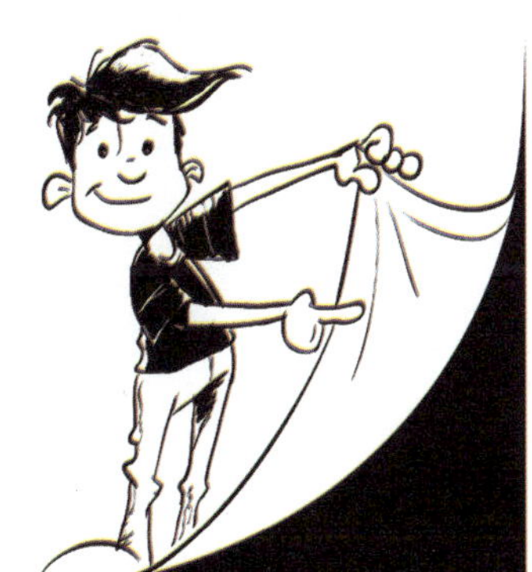

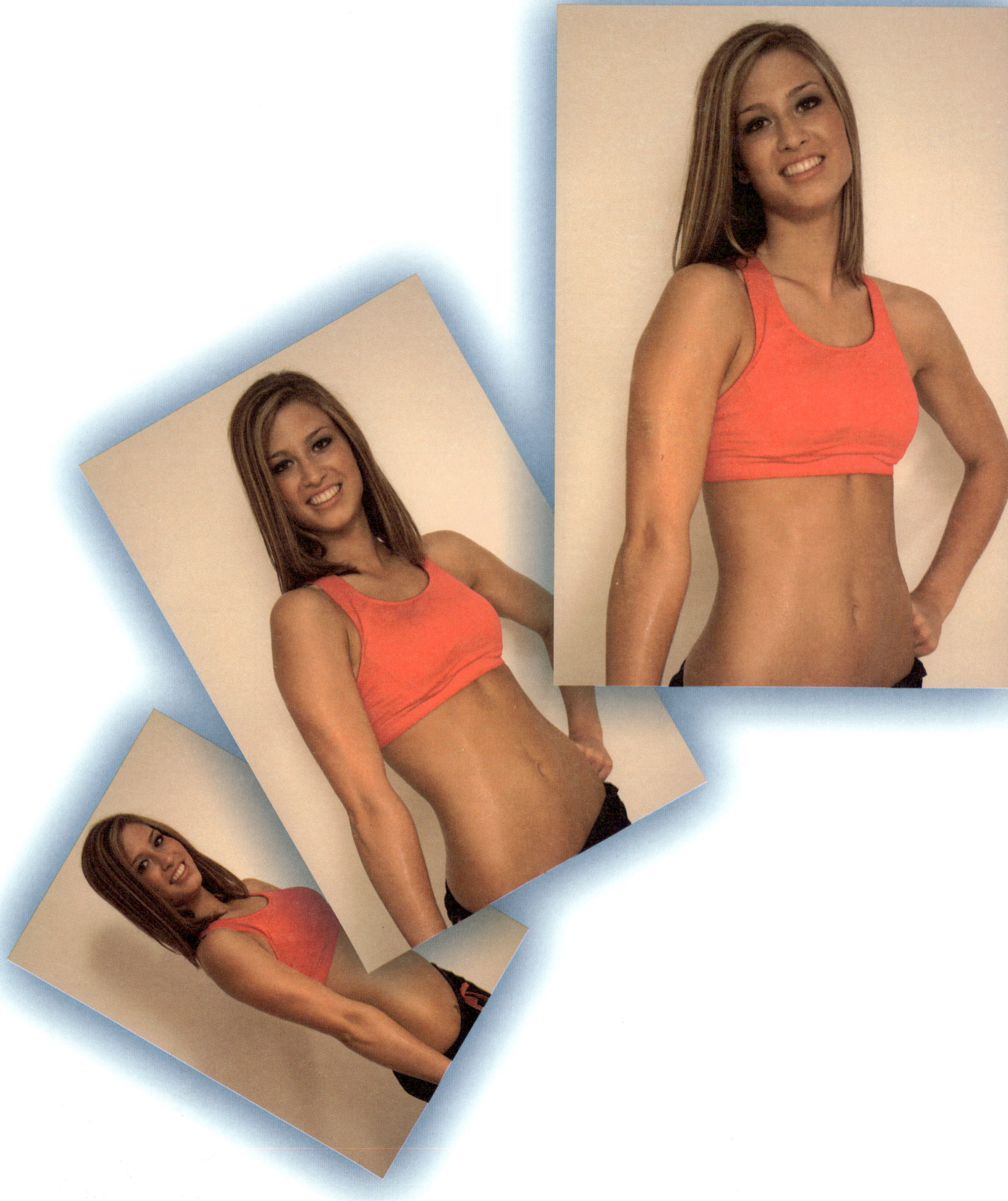

Week 3

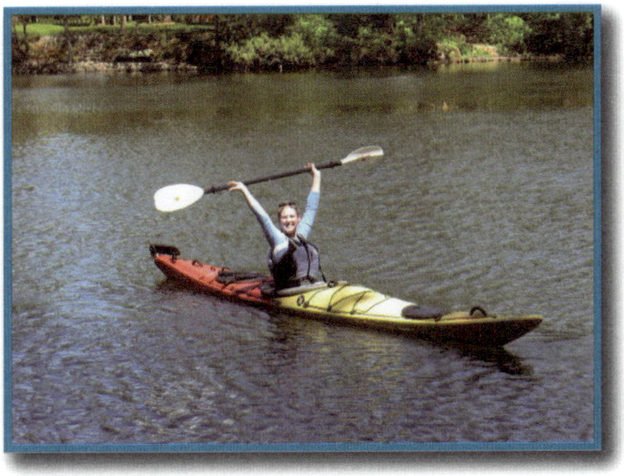

It has never been easy. Controlling weight in my family has never been easy. Motivating myself has never been easy and seeing results has never been easy. When I started working out with Kevin, it was all about weight to me, the number on the scale. But what I have learned is that it is about so much more than a number. Did I see that number change? Yes, I lost 15 pounds by changing my workout philosophy and lifestyle habits. With Kevin's guidance, I realized it was so much more than that. I was training my body not to just lift weights and do cardio on machines, but I was training my body and my mind to positively chase after my goals. By changing my workout philosophy, I was able to pick up and do a 12-mile kayak race with no kayaking experience as part of an adventure race and gained our team a 48 position jump. By training my mind, my self-confidence in the work-place heightened. I learned to step up and ask for challenges and create my own path instead of allowing other people to lead me. Because of that, I have received two promotions over the last two years. My life has not changed, but my lifestyle has.

Kevin's advice has made it easy to eat healthy and still maintain an active social life. People always ask me what diet I went on to lose the weight I've lost and my answer is, "I'm not on a diet." It is now easy to get motivated knowing that I will see results and won't have to be at the gym for half the day. And the scale is no longer an evil object that yells at me if I go out to dinner. This is an addictive way of life that my family has even started to pick up on. Kevin has made it easy. Kevin has made it achievable, and Kevin has showed me how to change my lifestyle to do the work for me.

-Amy Gurske

Goal:

Avoid white flour and white rice.

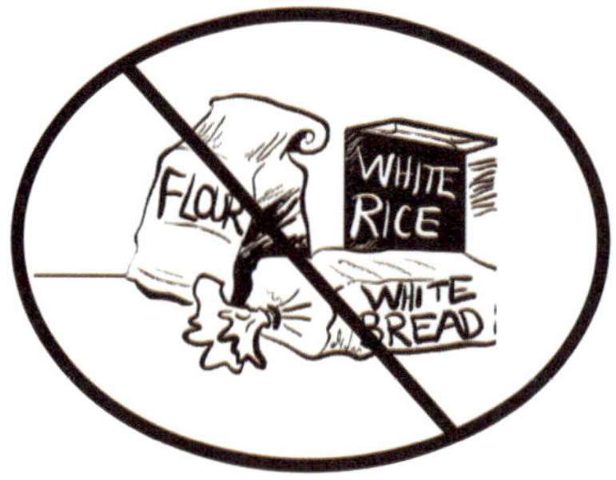

Why?

White flour is a complex carbohydrate. It is another form of empty calories that provide few, if any, nutrients. White flour is calorie-dense, digests rapidly, and does not replenish the nutrients lost in the digestion process. It is OK to eat white flour in moderation occasionally, but you should avoid it as much as possible. Do not eat it on a daily basis!

As you learned in your last weekly chapter, sugar digests very quickly. White flour digests almost as fast and plays the same role in fuel utilization and body fat storage:

- Carbohydrates are converted into glucose.
- Glucose is easily used as fuel by your body.
- Your body utilizes as much of the glucose as possible.
- Your body has a limit as to how much it can use at one time.
- When it is full, it is full and the excess glucose is stored as body fat.

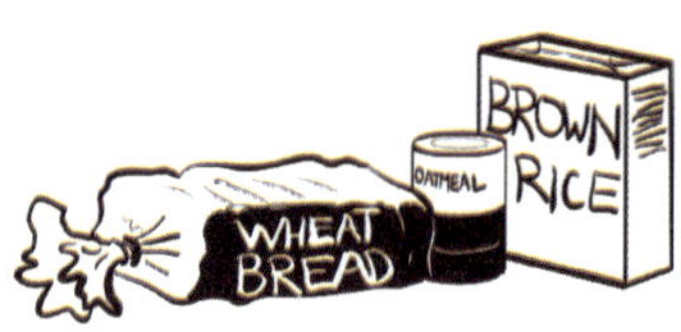

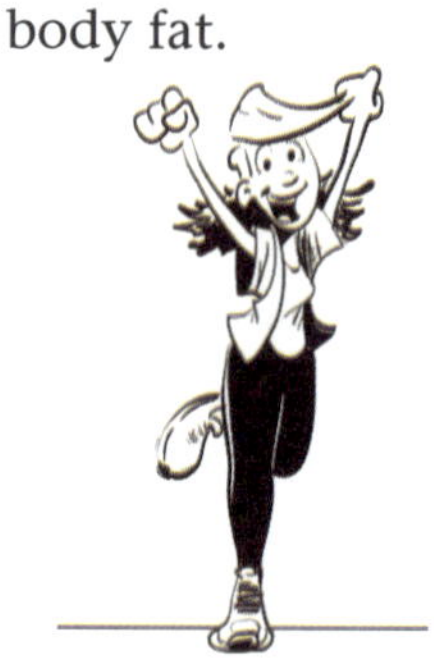

Balanced Blood Sugar = **Optimal Metabolism and Energy**

How?

Replace food products made with white flour and white rice with 100% whole grain food products. These healthy substitutions will help to balance your blood sugar levels, optimize your metabolism and boost your energy. Try some of the following healthy substitutions to help you eat whole grains:

REPLACE THIS...	WITH THIS...
White Bread	100% Whole Wheat Bread
White Pasta	Whole Wheat Pasta
White Rice	Brown Rice or Wild Rice
White Flour	Whole Wheat Flour or Oat Flour
Flour Tortillas	Whole Wheat Tortillas
Cereal	100% Whole Grain Oatmeal
Crackers	Whole Grain or Whole Wheat Crackers
Donuts	Whole Grain Bagel
Muffins	Whole Wheat English Muffin

White flour food products have been heavily processed and have very little nutritional value, even products that are "vitamin fortified." Typically, these products have significantly fewer nutrients and provide minimal health benefits. Whole grain food products, on the other hand, pack a nutritional punch. They contain protein, vitamins, minerals, phytonutrients, and most importantly, fiber. Whole grains supply many nutrients that are crucial for the health and maintenance of our bodies. They reduce the risk of some chronic diseases and have many other health benefits.

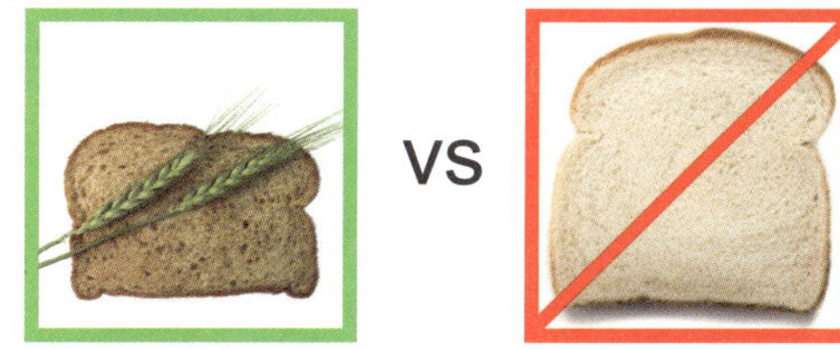

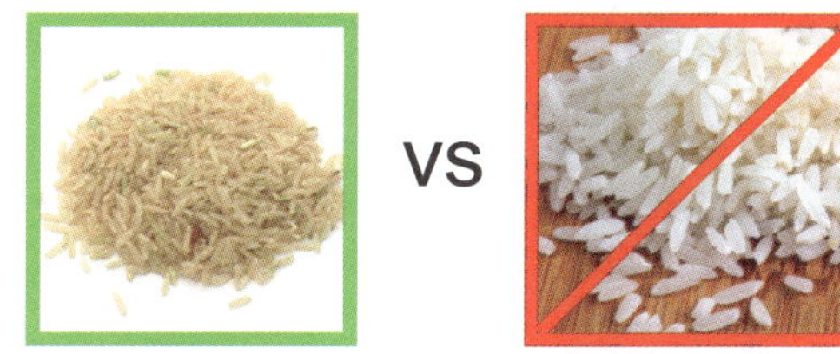

Recommendation: Eat three to six servings of whole grains a day.

Making healthy choices is not always easy. Packages can be very deceptive and you may think you are making a healthy choice, when in fact, you are not. For example, color is not necessarily an indicator of whole grains. Just because bread is brown doesn't mean it is healthy or made with whole grains. You have to read the food labels.

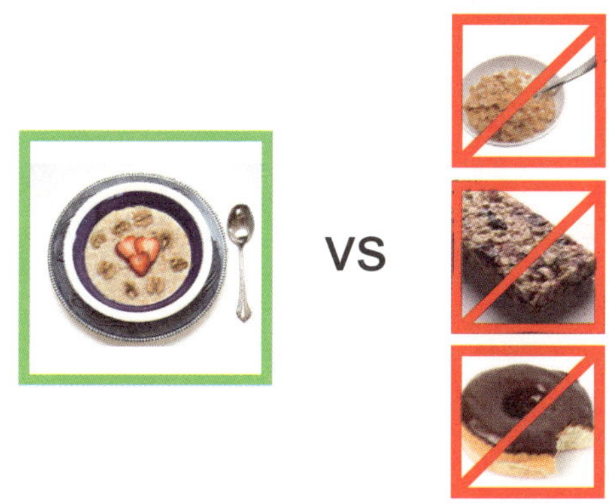

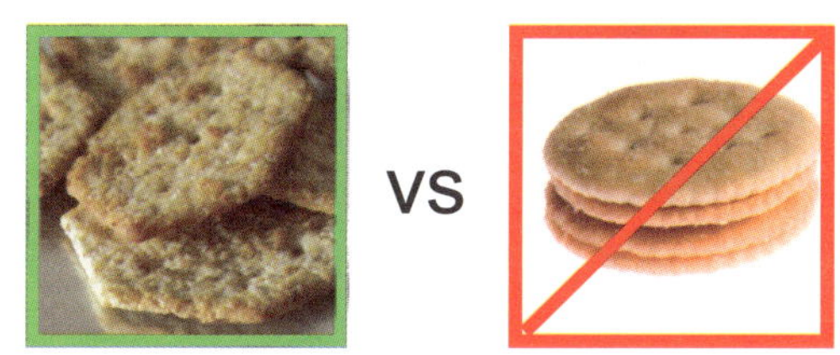

The following chart contains common ingredients on food labels:

100% Whole Grain	Partial Whole Grains	Forms of White Flour
100% whole wheat	Wheat flour	Semolina
Whole wheat flour	Stoned wheat	Durum wheat
Rolled oats	Cracked Wheat	Flour
Brown rice	Seven Grain	White flour
Wild rice	Multi-grain	Organic flour
Whole Rye	100% pure durum semolina	Enriched flour
Whole Grain (name of grain)	Bran	Unbleached flour
Whole wheat	Wheat germ	Organic unbleached flour
Durum whole wheat		Degerminated
Whole (other grain)		
Whole durum flour		
Popcorn		
Barley		

Time to review your nutrition log.

1. Cross out all foods that contain white flour.

2. Next to the foods you crossed out, write down a healthy substitution.

3. Continue to write down everything you eat and drink in your nutrition log daily.

4. Keep your "better choice" food selections simple. Too many food decisions at this point can lead to indecisive eating habits that can lead to over eating.

For Example:

Time	Food and Amount	Substitute
7:00 AM	Nutri-Grain® bar	**WW toast with Adam's® PB**
10:00 AM	Ritz® crackers, cheese	**WW crackers,** cheese
12:30 PM	White rice, chicken, veggies	**Brown rice**, chicken, veggies
3:00 PM	White bagel with cream cheese	**WW bagel with lowfat cream cheese**
6:00 PM	Workout	Workout
8:00 PM	4 oz. Chicken, salad, white pasta	4 oz. Chicken, salad, **WW pasta**

WW = 100% whole wheat

Questions and Answers

I enjoy my white flour food products. Is it that important to switch to 100% whole wheat, grain, and oats?

Absolutely. When you eat food made with refined white flour at one time, you may experience blood sugar lows, which temporarily decrease mental alertness, brain function, and motor skills. Blood sugar fluctuates based on the amount and type of carbohydrates you eat. Again, sugar digests very quickly and white flour digests almost as fast. Foods lacking in nutrients digest rapidly, raising your blood sugar and insulin levels. Insulin processes starches and sugars to keep blood sugar at an even level. The faster the blood sugar and insulin levels increase, the faster they come down. This can bring about blood sugar lows, making you feel tired, lethargic, depressed, or sleepy.

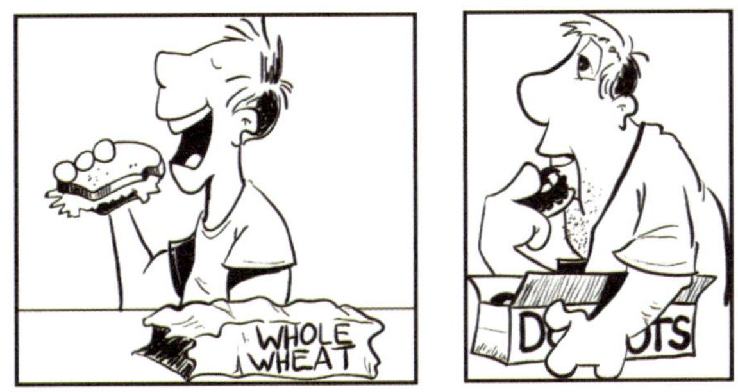

What other health benefits are derived from 100% whole wheat?

The fiber in 100% whole wheat provides the similar health benefits as fruits and vegetables. It protects against diabetes, obesity, insulin resistance, cholesterol levels, heart disease, strokes, and prevents constipation, too. Fiber in 100% whole wheat also protects against atherosclerosis, lymphomas, and other chronic diseases. Research has shown that fiber helps to reduce the risks of many types of cancer: stomach, colon, rectum, breast, uterus, mouth, throat, liver, and thyroid! Better yet, for people working to improve their nutrition to control their weight, fiber, counted as carbohydrates on nutrition labels, does not really function as a true carbohydrate because it cannot be broken down into sugar. It passes through the body undigested, which means it cannot be stored as body fat! In addition, foods made with whole wheat flour digest more slowly, causing a minimal rise in blood sugar and insulin levels. They are good for system balance and long lasting energy.

Caution: When you eat a fiber-rich diet it is important to drink plenty of fluids. Otherwise, the fiber will absorb water from your system which can cause, rather than prevent, constipation.

If white flour is not very healthy, then what is the purpose of having white flour food products available?

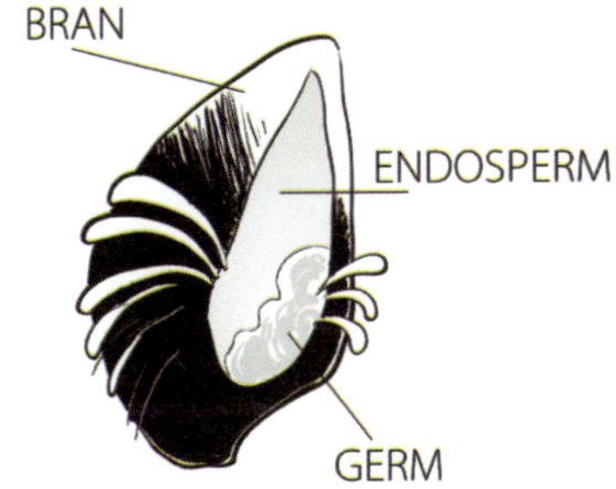

The purpose is to extend the shelf-life of food. Food processors chemically bleach, preserve, and age whole grains, which becomes white flour, to increase its shelf-life. The whole grains are whitened by adding chemicals and synthetic ingredients. Processors do enrich white flour with some vitamins and minerals; however, it's very minimal compared to the natural source from the bran and germ in whole grains. The public is typically unaware that refining whole grains to white flour normally requires the removal of the bran and germ. The bran is the outside layers and the germ contains most of the fiber, vitamins, and essential nutrients and minerals. However, whole grains are healthier, providing more protein, fiber, vitamins, and nutrients. The Vitamin E in whole grains is a natural preservative that protects it from turning rancid for several months.

How can I be certain that I am eating 100% whole grain foods?

Identifying whole grain products can be a challenge. Products that list "whole grain" may actually contain only small amounts of 100% whole grains. For example, a loaf of bread may contain a mixture of enriched white flour and whole wheat flour and far less fiber than bread that is 100% whole grain. "100% whole wheat" will be listed as the first ingredient, if indeed the loaf of bread contains 100% whole wheat. You can also look for the Whole Grain stamp. The Whole Grains Council has created this packaging symbol to identify genuine whole grain products. The Whole Grain Stamp and the 100% Whole Grain stamp both include the number of fiber grams in the product. Many whole grain food products are not yet using the Whole Grain stamp, so be sure to check the ingredient list for "**100% whole wheat**."

I'm happy to say that my weight varies between 144 and 149 lbs, and I work out usually five days a week, doing both weight training and cardio at a gym. When I think back, I know I can thank Kevin Orr for inspiring me to have the desire to continue to live a healthy life.

- Dwight Karlsen

Nutrition Log

Date:____________	Sun Mon Tues Wed Thurs Fri Sat	
	Plan	**Actual**
Meal 1	*Food & Amount*	*Food & Amount*
Time:______		
Meal 2		
Time:______		
Meal 3		
Time:______		
Meal 4		
Time:______		
Meal 5		
Time:______		
Meal 6		
Time:______		

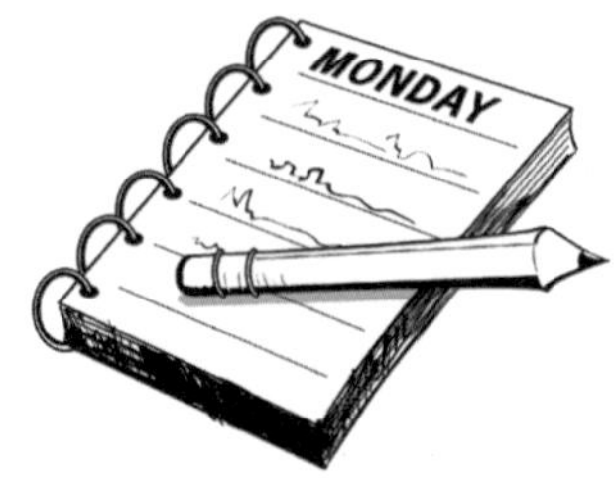

Checklist

Achieved:

- ✓ Consume meal or snack every 3 hours
- ✓ Water every 3 hours
- ✓ Sleep optimal hours
- ✓ Intake multivitamin
- ✓ Weights and cardio

Avoided:

- ✓ Sugars
- ✓ **White flour**

Key Points

Week 1

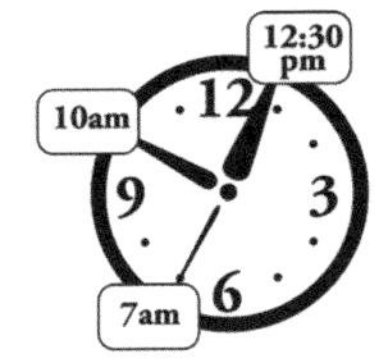

- Eat a small meal or snack once every three hours – five to six meals per day.

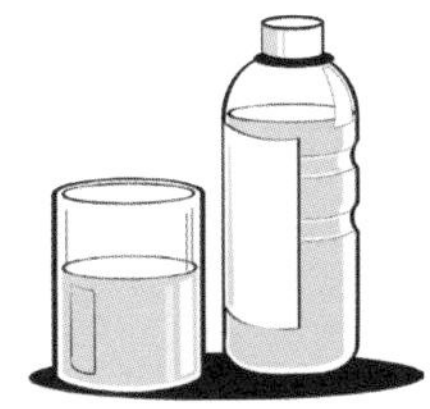

- Drink at least 1 cup (8 ounces) of water per meal and at least one cup before, during, and after your workouts.

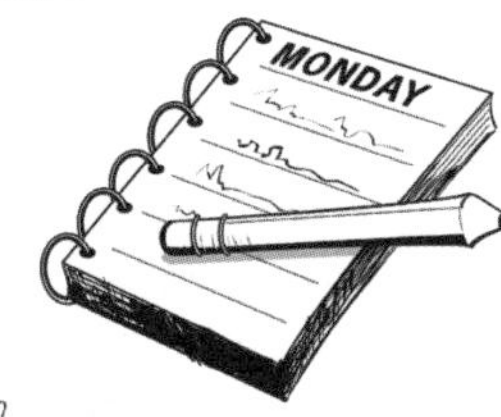

- Keep a nutrition log.

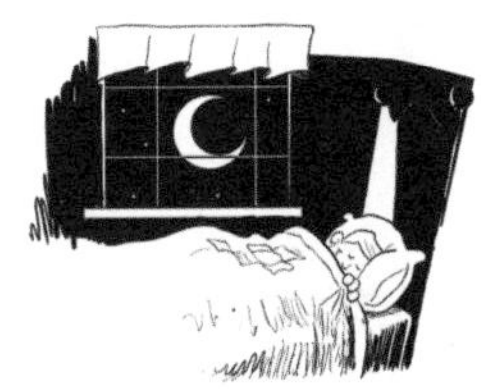

- Sleep is vital!

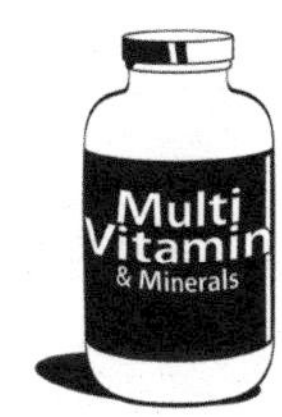

- Take a daily multivitamin.

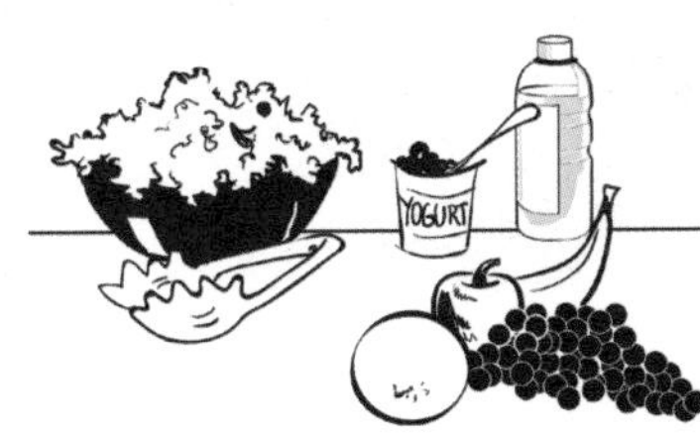

Week 2

- Avoid bad sugars.

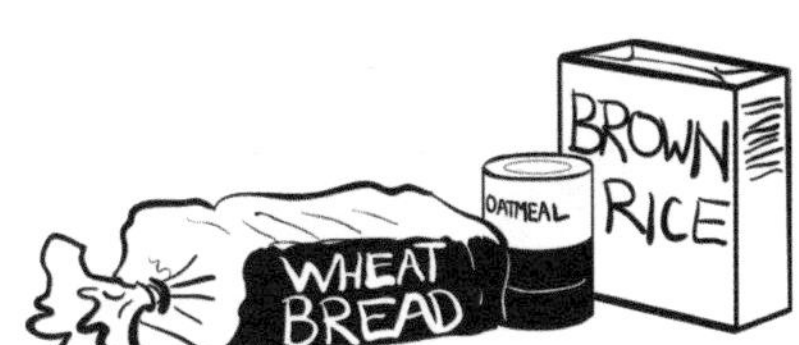

Week 3

- **Avoid white flour and white rice.** It is another form of empty calories that provides few, if any, nutrients. Replace foods made with white flour with 100% whole wheat flour, grain, and oat food products.

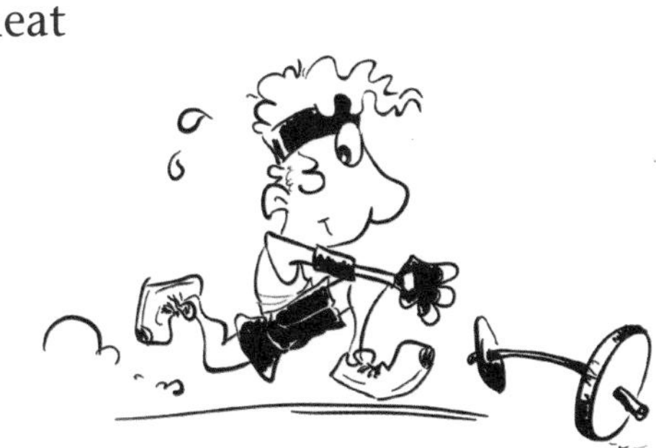

Biceps

Goal:

Complete two sets of 15 reps of the **dumbbell biceps curls**.

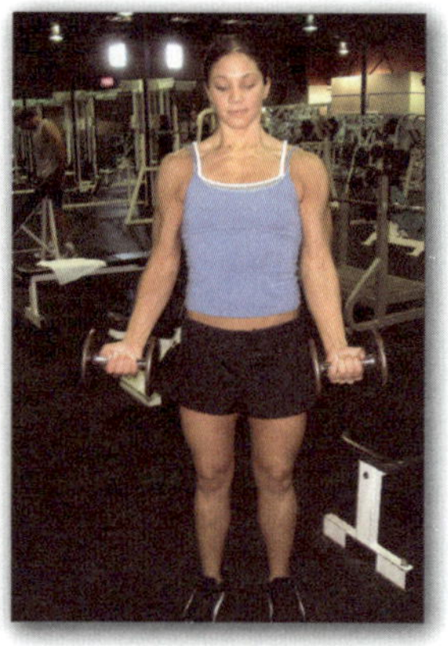

Primary
Biceps

Stabilizers
Shoulders
Forearms
Core

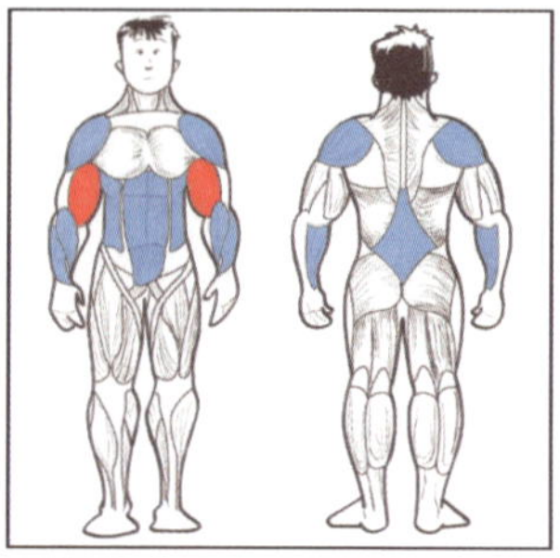

Why?

The dumbbell biceps curl is a free-weight exercise targeting the biceps. The stabilizing muscles include your shoulders and forearms, as well as the rest of your core. Free weight exercises are a step up in intensity from machine exercises. In general, free weight exercises require more strength and stability to perform. They utilize multiple stabilizers throughout your body that are not normally activated in machine exercises.

How?

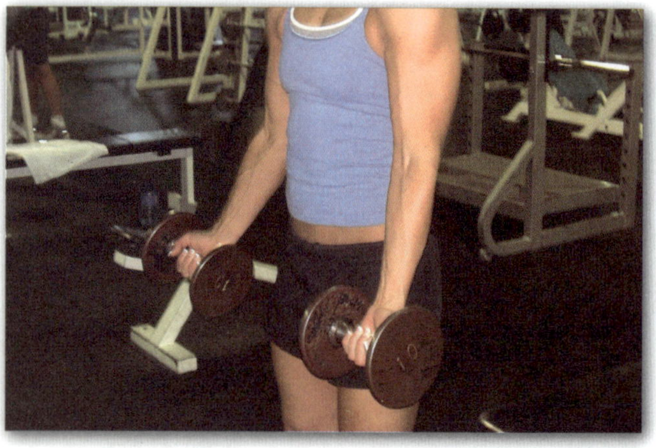

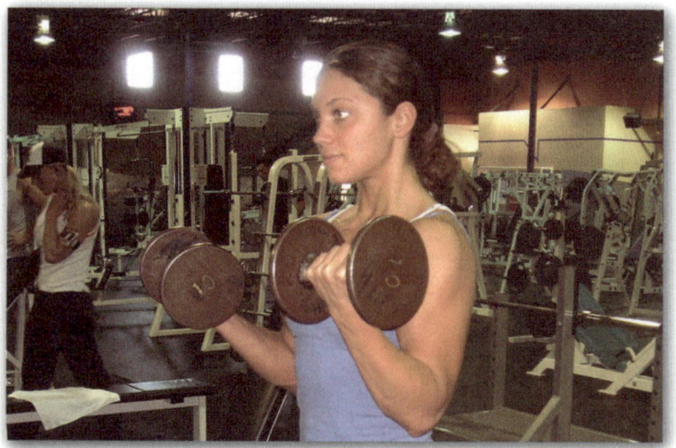

Step 1 - Begin with a shoulder-width stance, a dumbbell in each hand, palms facing forward.

Step 2 - Squeeze your abs to assist the lower back's neutral position.

Step 3 - Curl your dumbbells up, squeeze your biceps, keeping your elbows in a stationary position slightly away from your body.

Step 4 - Lower your dumbbells back to your starting position. Repeat in a smooth and controlled motion.

Your goal is to complete two sets of 15 (2 x 15).

Range of Motion Techniques

To Maximize Muscle Tension and Minimize Overcompensation

Dos | **Don'ts**

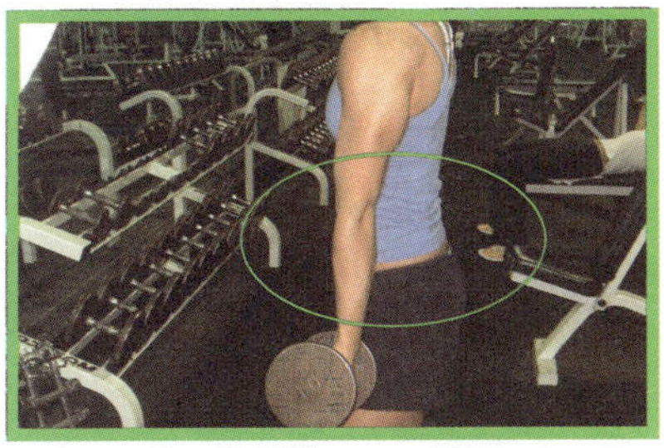

Lock Elbows Out

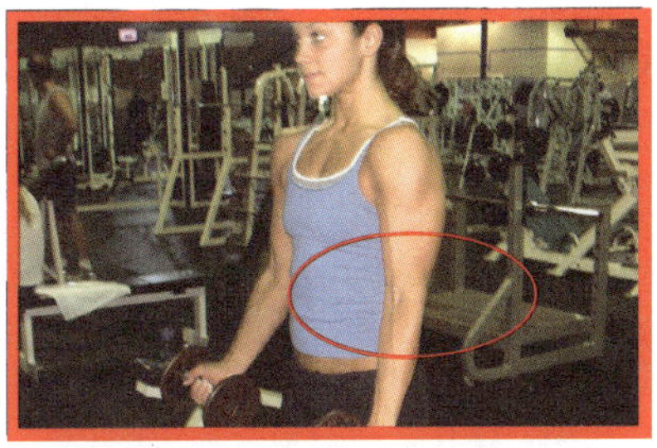

Avoid Maintaining Bent Elbows

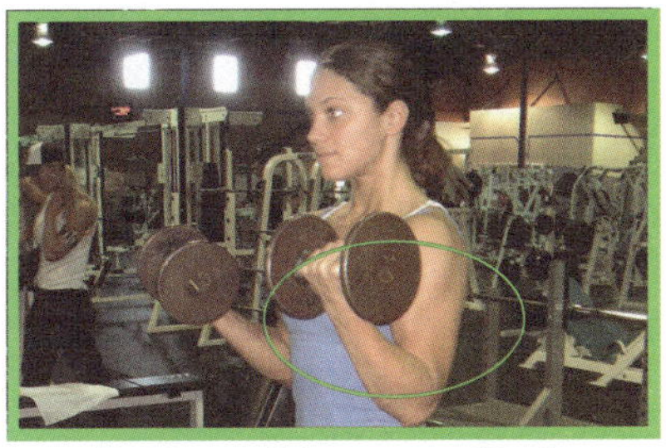

Squeeze Biceps to Peak Contraction

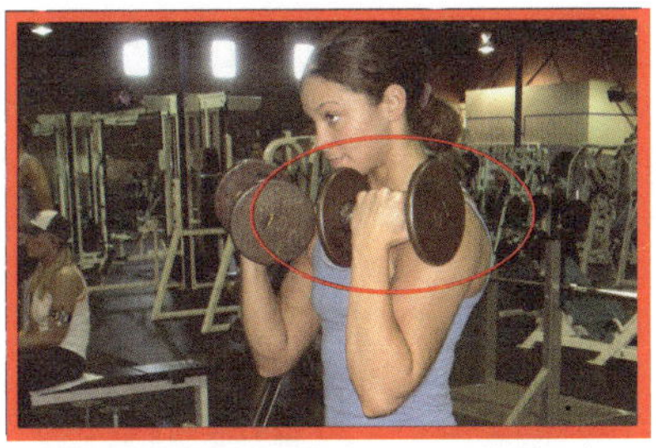

Avoid Curling Beyond Peak Biceps Contraction

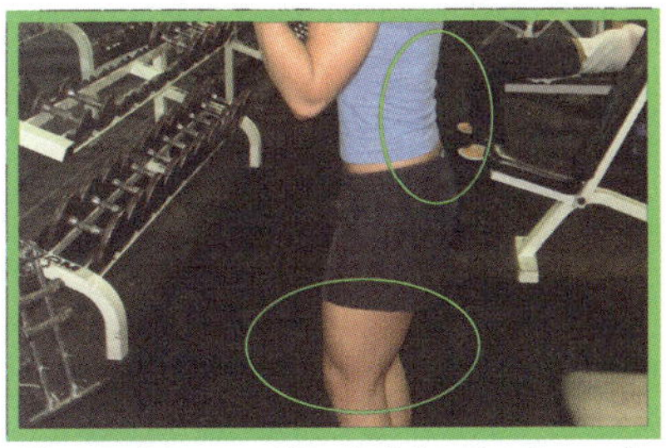

Keep Lower Back Neutral and Knees Slightly Bent

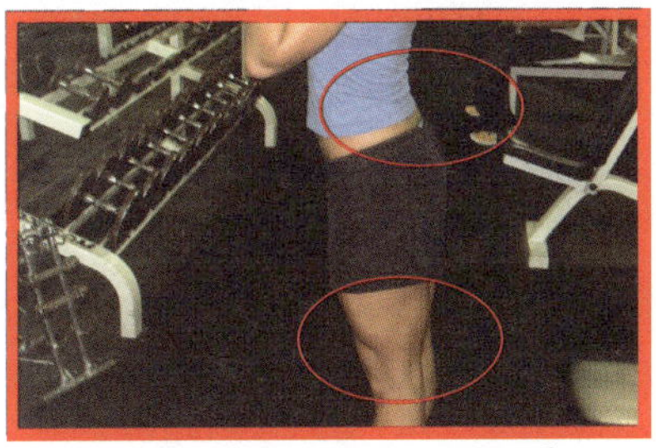

Avoid Arching Lower Back or Locking Out Knees

Visualize

"Ball and Stretch Effect"

As you curl the dumbbells up, visualize curling your biceps into the biggest balls you can curl them into. Continue to squeeze the ball in your biceps while resisting the weights as you lower the dumbbells. Focus on feeling the stretch in your biceps at the bottom of your range of motion.

Visualizing while staying within the proper range of motion will maximize the tension in your biceps and minimize the tension in your lower back, forearms, and wrists.

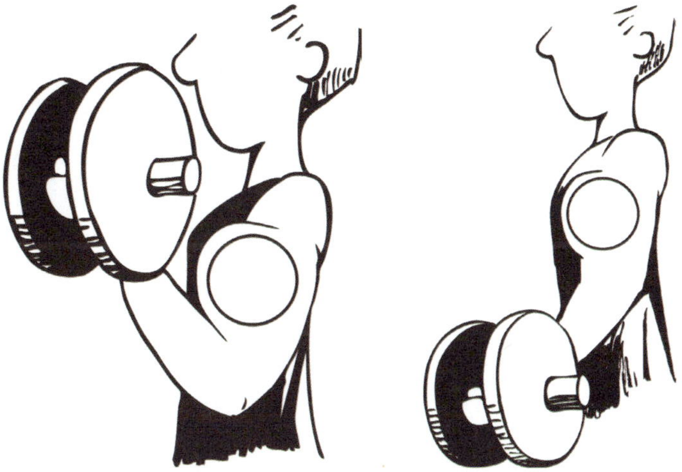

Questions and Answers

My lower back tends to arch. Is correcting it necessary?

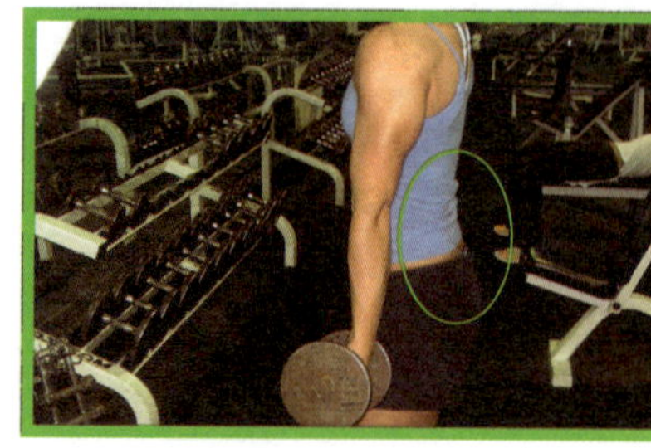

You bet. Maintaining a neutral lower back position is paramount. It relieves the pressure in your lower back and decreases joint tension. As you know, decreasing joint tension increases the tension in the targeted muscle group. Try squeezing your abs to flatten your lower back while bending your knees. This is one of the best methods for maintaining a neutral lower back. If this doesn't help, you might be lifting too much weight.

How fast should I perform my reps?

Your tempo should be two seconds down and two seconds up. Expect to be a little unstable and unbalanced until your stabilizers have strengthened. Focus on maintaining a smooth and controlled motion. Using proper form increases the effectiveness of the exercise and decreases your risk of injury.

My forearms are burning! Am I doing something wrong?

If you're not used to training your biceps, it's normal to feel your forearms burn. Your forearms act as a stabilizer when performing biceps curls. Your stabilizers must be strengthened first because they provide the foundation for strength. Be sure to keep your grip as light as possible to reduce forearm tension and overcompensation.

My wrists hurt! Should I continue to lift?

If you are in pain, **stop lifting**. Pain is feedback from your body telling you that you need to correct your form and technique. Make sure that your wrists stay in a neutral position. Allowing your wrists to bend back places excessive tension in your wrist joints. Keep your grip light. Gripping too tightly increases wrist tension.

I feel tension and pain in my elbows when lowering my dumbbells to lock out! What should I do?

When lowering your dumbbells to lock out, you should feel a stretch in your biceps. In order to feel the stretch, your elbow position must be slightly in front of your body. If your elbows are too close to your body, it can also place the pressure in your elbows, instead of your biceps. Adjust your elbow position to shift the tension from your elbows to your biceps.

How much weight should I lift?

Start with the lightest weight possible. The amount of weight will vary from person to person, and from exercise to exercise. You should lift enough weight to fully fatigue by the end of your set.

What's the purpose of feeling a stretch in my biceps?

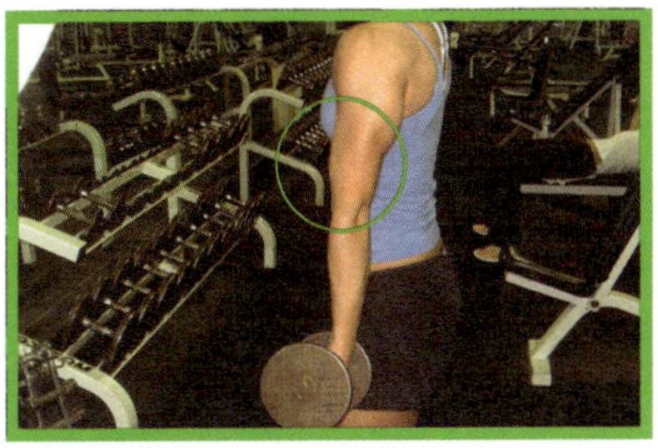

Remember, dumbbell biceps curls target your biceps. In order to get the most effective workout, your biceps need to be doing the majority of the muscle work. Your goal is to have the least amount of assistance from your stabilizers. Feeling a small stretch in your biceps as you lower the dumbbells to lock out ensures your biceps are resisting, not the shoulders, forearms, or any other stabilizers.

How do I know when I've reached my peak contraction?

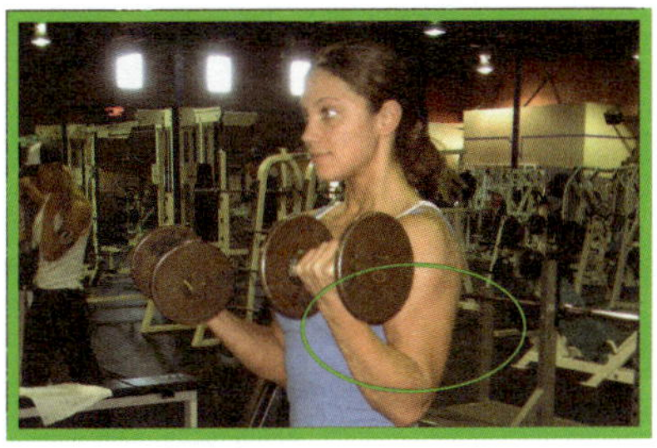

When performing dumbbell biceps curls, your elbows should be slightly forward and remain in a stationary position while curling the dumbbells up. The moment your elbows begin to move forward, you have reached your peak contraction. Curling past your peak contraction causes overcompensation. If you allow your elbows to move forward, the tension shifts from your biceps to your shoulders and lower back. Keep in mind, the most effective way to train is to isolate the targeted muscle group and to avoid allowing your stabilizers to provide assistance.

When should I breathe?

You should always inhale at your starting position and exhale as you complete the range of motion. In dumbbell biceps curls, inhale as you lift the dumbbells and exhale as you lower them to your starting position.

Triceps

Goal:

Complete two sets of 15 reps of the **cable triceps pushdown**.

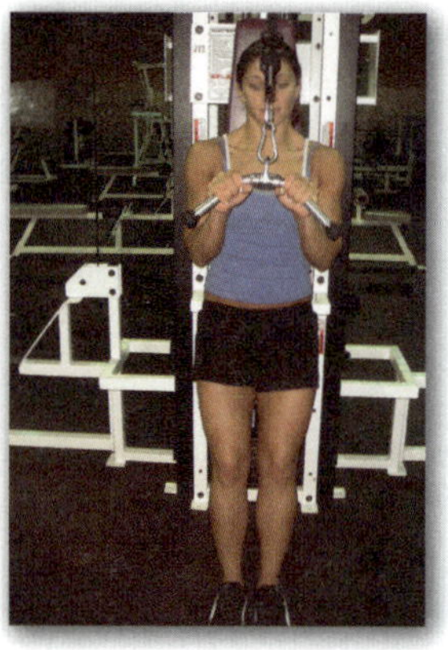

Primary
Triceps

Stabilizers
Shoulders
Forearms
Core

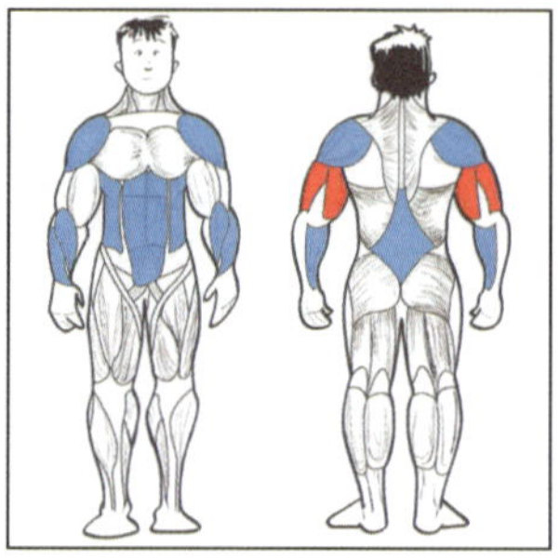

Why?

Cable pushdown is an exercise machine that targets your triceps. The stabilizing muscles include your shoulders and forearms, as well as the rest of your core. Cable pushdown is one of the most effective triceps exercises and it places the least amount of tension in the elbows.

How?

Step 1 - Grip the v-bar as close and as high as possible.

Step 2 - Squeeze your abs to push your lower back into a neutral position.

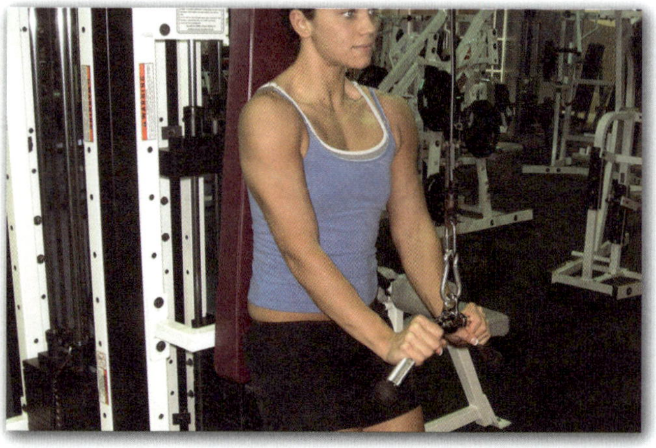

Step 3 - Begin with your bar position underneath your slightly-bent elbows.

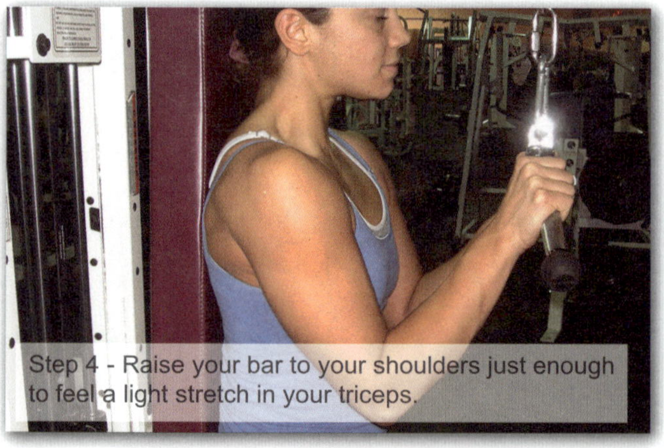

Step 4 - Raise your bar to your shoulders just enough to feel a light stretch in your triceps.

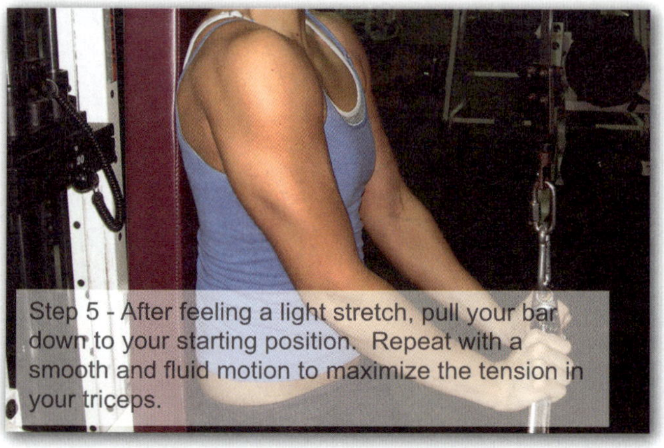

Step 5 - After feeling a light stretch, pull your bar down to your starting position. Repeat with a smooth and fluid motion to maximize the tension in your triceps.

Your goal is to complete two sets of 15 (2 x 15).

Range of Motion Techniques

To Maximize Muscle Tension and Minimize Overcompensation

Dos

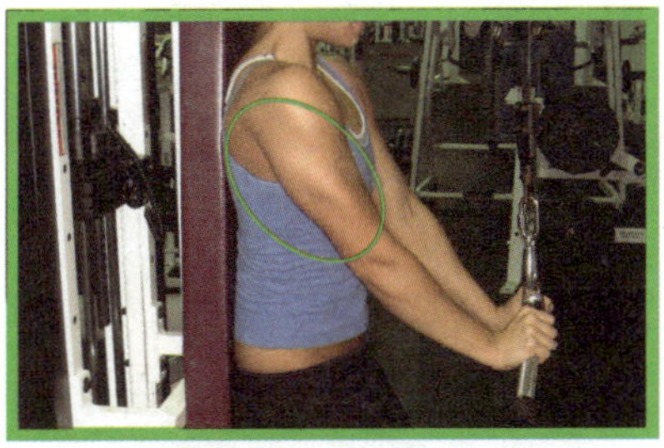

Begin with Elbows Bent

Don'ts

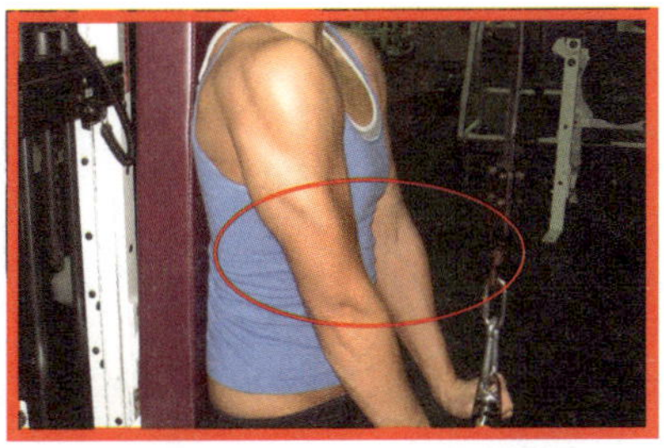

Avoid Locking Out Elbows

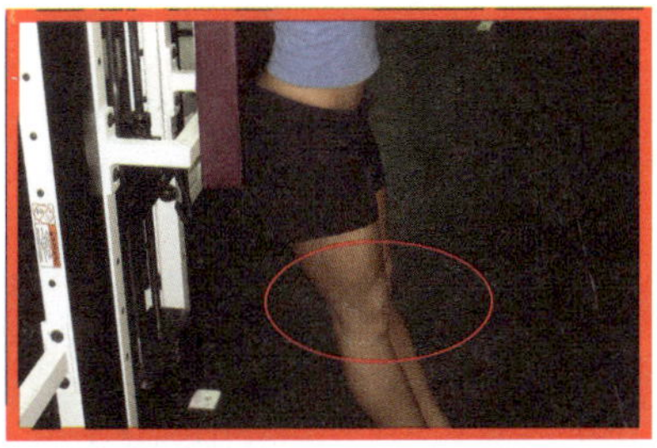

Avoid Locking Out Knees

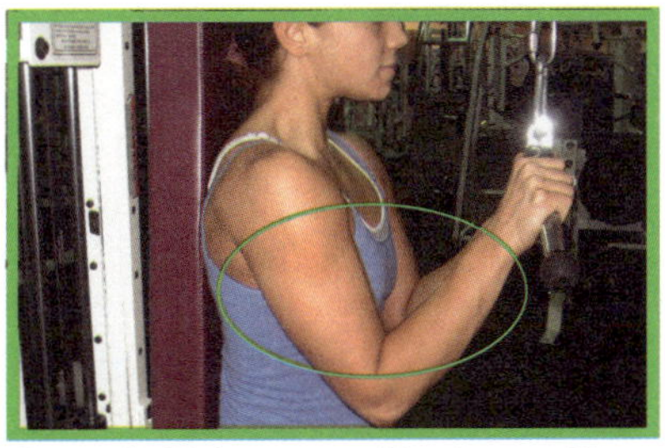

Stretch Triceps to Resist at Top

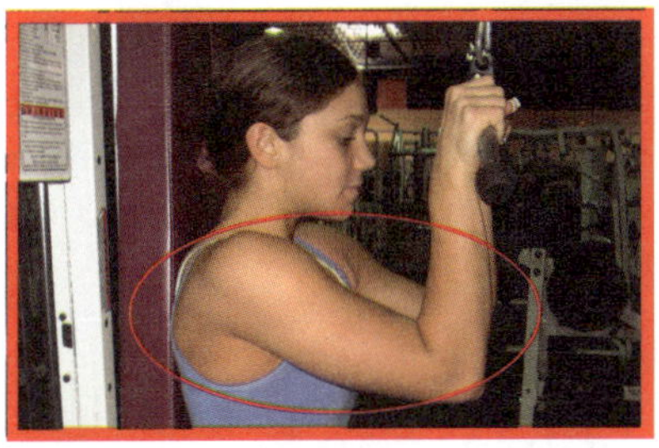

Avoid Coming Up Too High

Visualize

"Cable and Stretch Effect"

While leaning against the back support in your starting position, imagine your elbows are being pulled together by a cable. Visualize yourself resisting the v-bar as it comes up, and focus on feeling the stretch in your triceps as you're resisting the v-bar. Continue to visualize your elbows being pulled in by a cable as you contract your triceps to push down to your starting position.

Visualizing, while staying within the proper range of motion, will maximize the tension in your triceps and minimize the tension in your shoulders, elbows, and wrists.

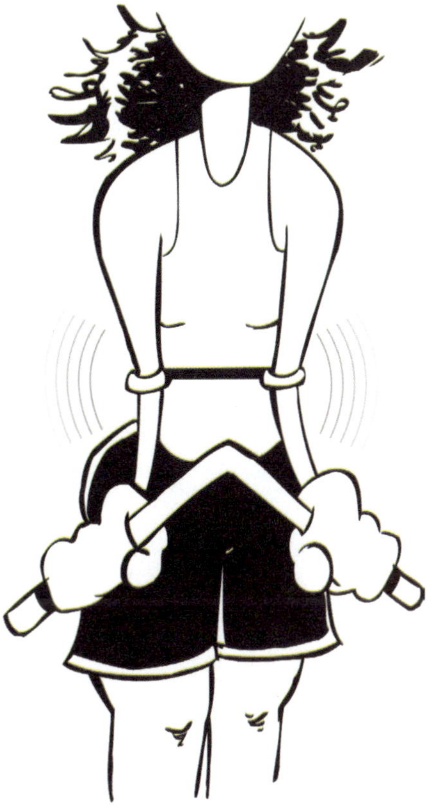

Questions and Answers

What should I do if I can't feel my triceps?

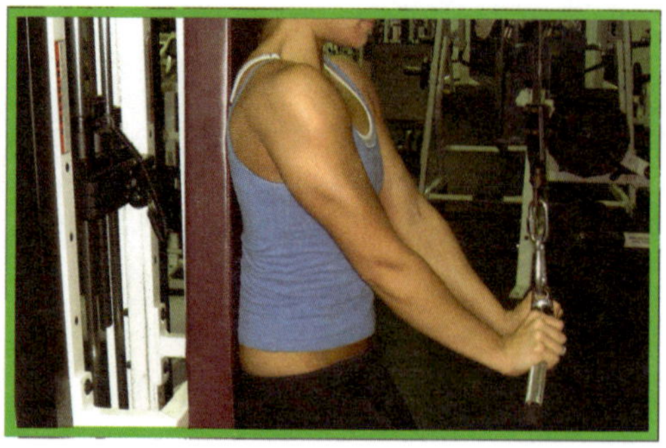

If you can't feel your triceps, you are probably overcompensating with other muscles and joints. Remember, your lower back should be in a neutral position and your knees should be slightly bent. This relieves joint pressure and forces your triceps to do the work. Keep your elbows tucked in and remember to visualize! Allow the bar to rise up just enough to feel a light stretch in your triceps. Feeling a stretch in your triceps ensures that your triceps are resisting, not your forearms or any other stabilizers.

What should I do if I feel tension in my wrists?

Feeling tension in your wrists is generally caused by overcompensation. To reduce overcompensation and secure your wrists, your thumbs should wrap around the bar and your grip should be as light as possible. Securing your wrists provides wrist stability and helps to keep your wrists strong. Maintaining a light hand grip decreases wrist joint tension.

When should I breathe?

Again, you should always inhale at your starting position and exhale as you complete the range of motion. In triceps pushdown, inhale as you raise the bar up and exhale as you push the bar down to your starting position.

While I was training with Kevin, I was easily motivated into a fitness and nutrition program that worked for me. His insight and knowledge proved valuable in helping me achieve my fitness goals. Thank You Kevin!

- Denise Manes

Abs

Goal:

Complete two sets of 20 reps of **crunches**.

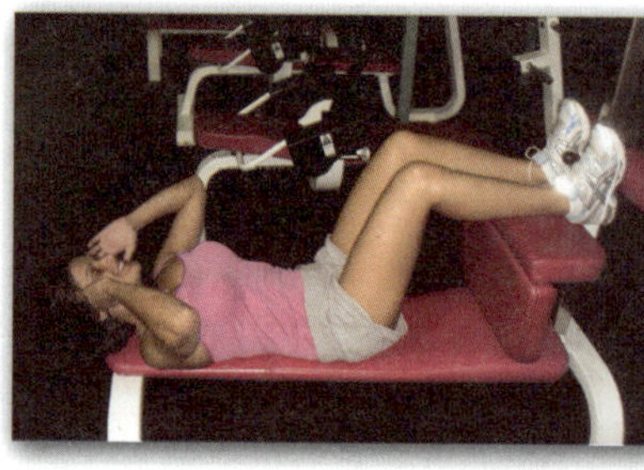

Primary
Abs

Stabilizers
Lower back
Neck
Core

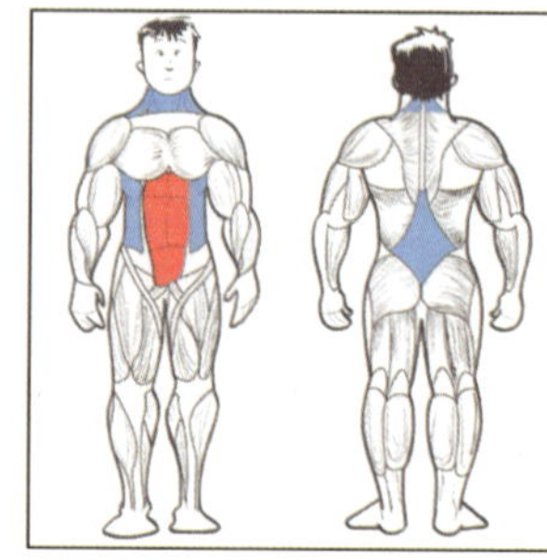

Why?

Crunches are a very effective exercise that targets the entire region of your abdominal muscles. The stabilizing muscles involved include your neck and lower back. Your abs are one of the largest stabilizers of your core. They play a key role in maintaining proper posture and technique.

How?

Step 1 - Lay flat on your back either on the floor or bench with your legs lifted up in a 90-degree angle.

Step 2 - Squeeze your abs to push your lower back into a neutral position against the bench.

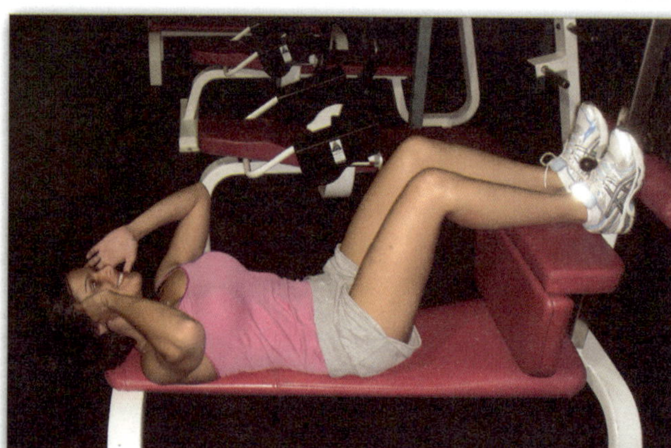

Step 3 - Place your finger tips on your temples.

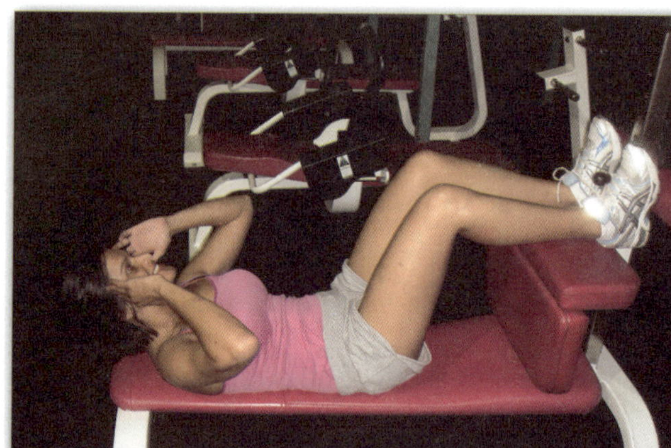

Step 4 - Curl up as high as possible while keeping your lower back flat.

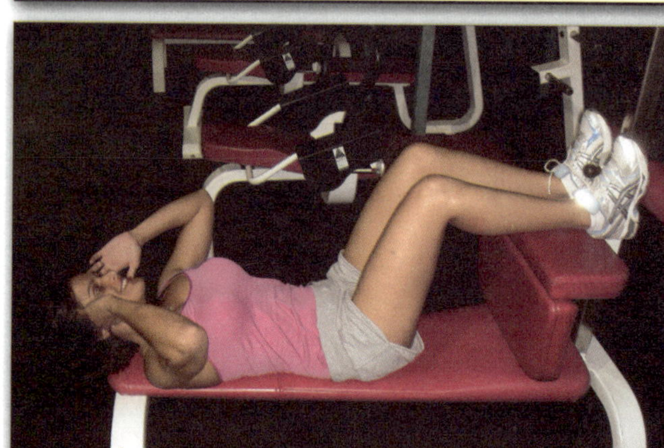

Step 5 - Lower yourself down slowly until your shoulder blades lightly touch the pad and repeat.

Your goal is to complete two sets of 20 (2 x 20).

Range of Motion Techniques

To Maximize Muscle Tension and Minimize Overcompensation

Dos

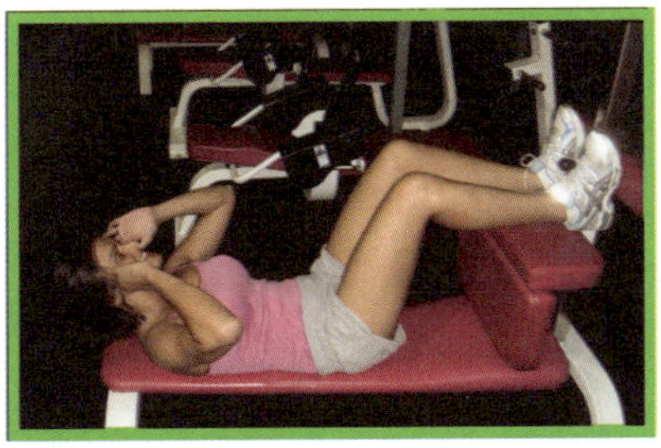

Squeeze Your Abs at the Top While Keeping Chin Up

Don'ts

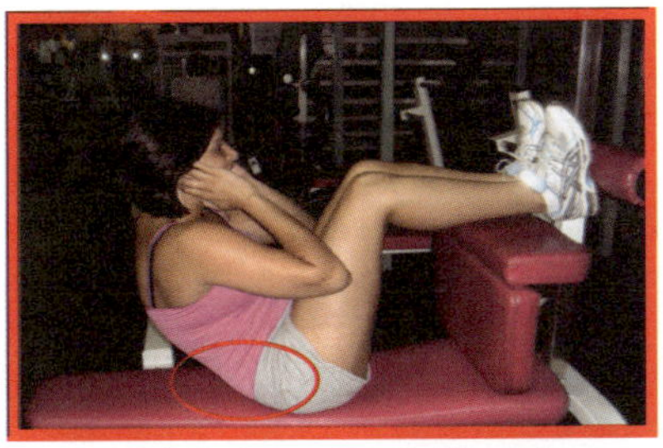

Avoid Lower Back Tension When Lifting Up Too Far

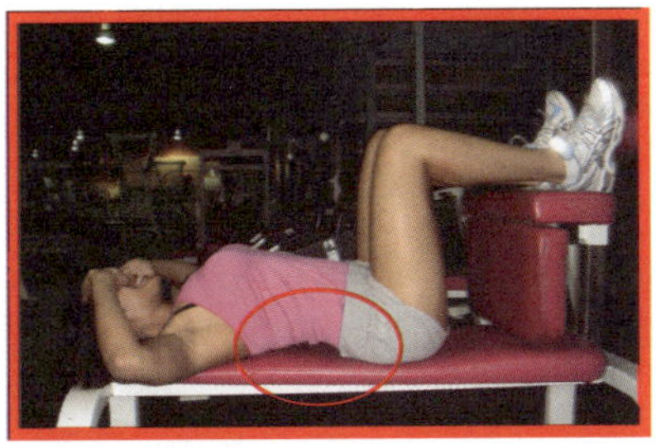

Avoid Arching Lower Back

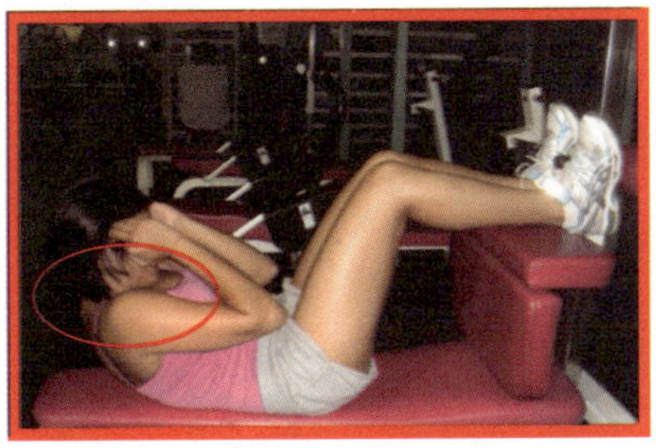

Avoid Neck Tension

Visualize

"Rubber band and Stretch Effect"

While lying on a bench, squeeze your abs as you are curling your upper body up to your peak contraction. Keeping your abs tight, resist and stretch your abs as you lower yourself down. Imagine your abs are a rubber band. As you lower yourself down, watch the rubber band stretch to its limits and as you crunch up, watch the rubber band tighten, pulling you back together.

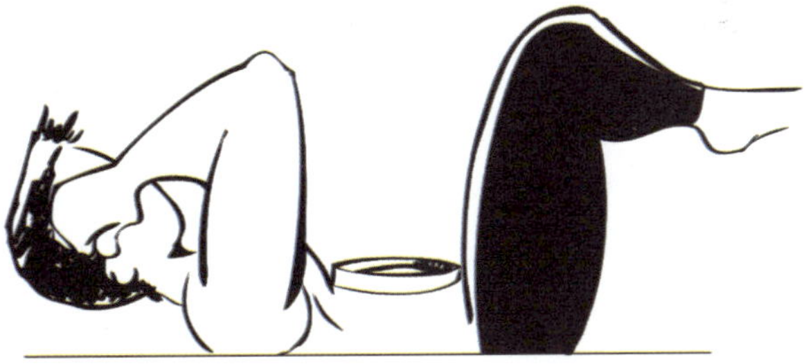

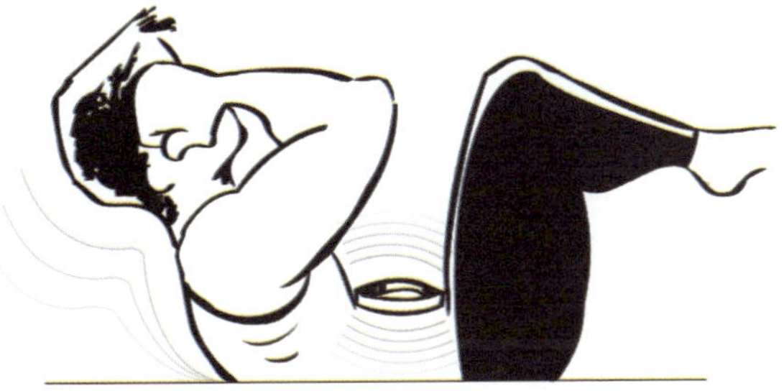

Visualizing and staying within the proper range of motion will maximize the tension in your abs and minimize overcompensation.

Questions and Answers

What should I do if my lower back is burning?

The burning sensation in your lower back indicates muscle fatigue. Muscle fatigue is a positive feeling because it leads to muscle strengthening and conditioning. However, if you're feeling pain in your lower back while performing crunches, you may be arching too much. Focus on squeezing your abs to push your lower back flat into a neutral position against the bench. This relieves the pressure in your lower back and forces your abs to do the majority of the muscle work.

When should I breathe?

You should always inhale at your starting position and exhale as you complete the range of motion. In crunches, inhale as you crunch up and exhale as you lower yourself back down. Also, when it comes to crunches, it is OK to breathe either way.

By learning the fundamentals in training, I have become more balanced and consistent as a person, which I feel has parlayed into many different avenues in my life and has changed me for the better.

- Forrest Belmont

Kevin demonstrated the correct posture to use with all of the weight equipment. He made me write a list of realistic goals, which he provided and encouraged me to meet. Because of his excellent training, motivational skills, and continued encouragement, I have been challenged to make a commitment to work out as regularly as I can and am succeeding in doing so.

- Jaime Hongel

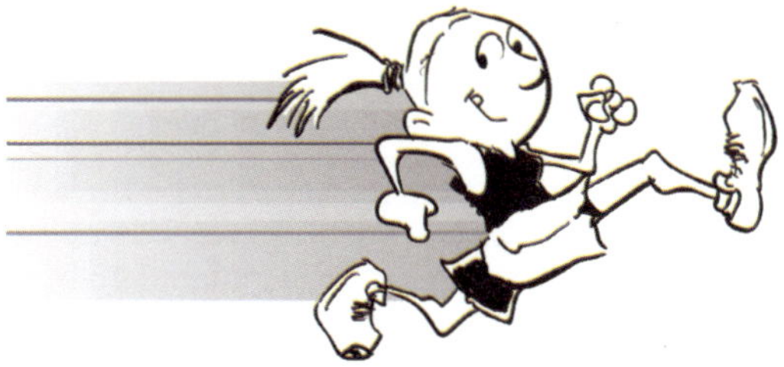

Cardio

Goal:

Complete 15 minutes on the **treadmill: ramp training** and 15 minutes on the EFX.

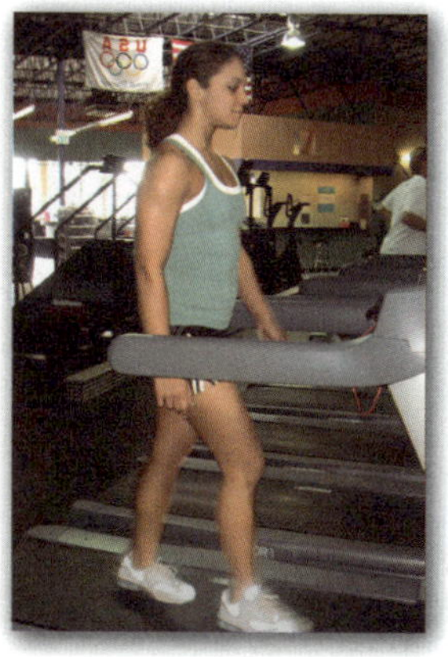

Primary
Quads
Glutes
Hamstrings

Stabilizers
Lower Back
Calves
Shins
Core

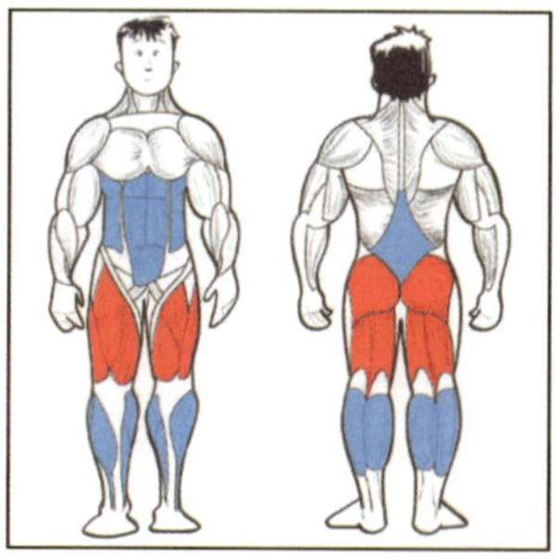

Why?

Treadmill ramp training increases physical conditioning and is a step up in cardio intensity from your previous cardio treadmill training. This method of training requires more balance and stability than walking on a flat terrain.

How?

Step 1 - Step onto the treadmill and press **QUICK START** or select a **MANUAL PROGRAM**.

Step 2 - Increase the speed to a comfortable walking pace, somewhere between 2.5 to 4.0 mph. Your speed will vary depending on your physical condition.

Step 3 - Next, walk at zero percent incline for one minute.

Step 4 - At the one minute mark, increase your incline by one, two, or three percent. Decrease your speed if necessary.

Step 5 - At the two minute mark, increase your incline again by one, two, or three percent.

Step 6 - Continue to increase your incline in one minute intervals until you have reached your peak incline. Your peak incline can be one or up to fifteen percent. It can vary depending on the brand of your treadmill and level of your conditioning.

Step 7 - If you lose control or experience extreme muscle fatigue in your stabilizers, you have reached your peak.

Step 8 - Once you have reached your peak, the point at which you are losing form and technique, decrease your incline back to zero percent and start all over again.

Step 9 - Walk on the treadmill for up to 15 minutes in addition to the 15 minutes on the EFX. Remember to work out at medium intensity, a breathing rate at which it's a little hard to hold a conversation.

Range of Motion Techniques

Dos

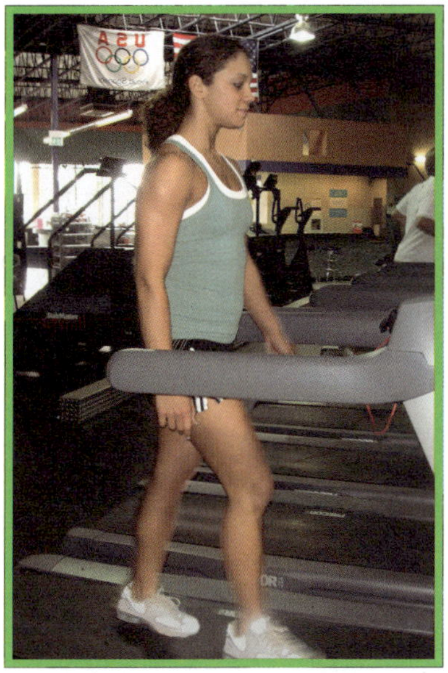

Maintain Long Strides

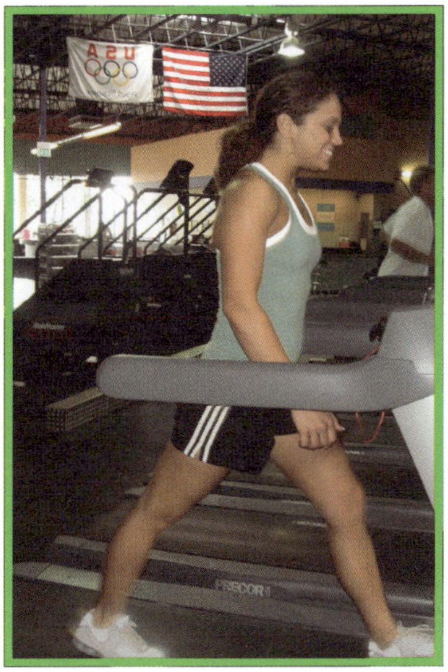

Allow Arms to Swing Naturally

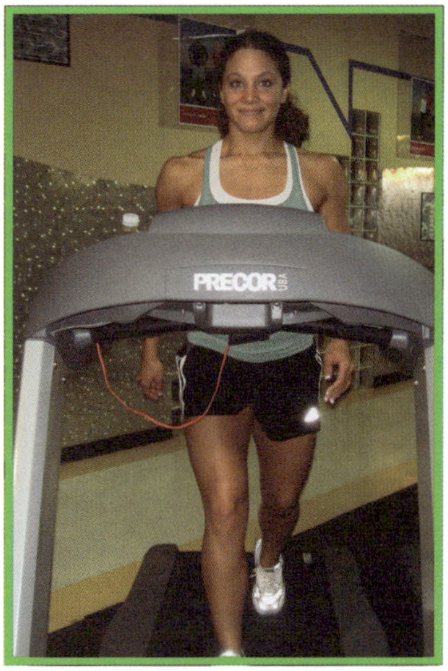

Shoulders Should be Even and in Proper Alignment

Visualize

"Cloud Effect"

By now you should be working out consistently. The consistency in your workouts should be increasing your physical and cardiovascular conditioning as well as making your visualizations more successful.

You already know how to visualize walking on water and walking quietly. In addition to these visualizations, imagine yourself walking on clouds.

The cloud visualization provides you with another tool to assist you in walking softly. It allows you to walk with the least amount of impact by bending your knees to the correct degree. As you walk, your strides will lengthen, which allows you to walk with the least amount of impact and reduce the risk of injury.

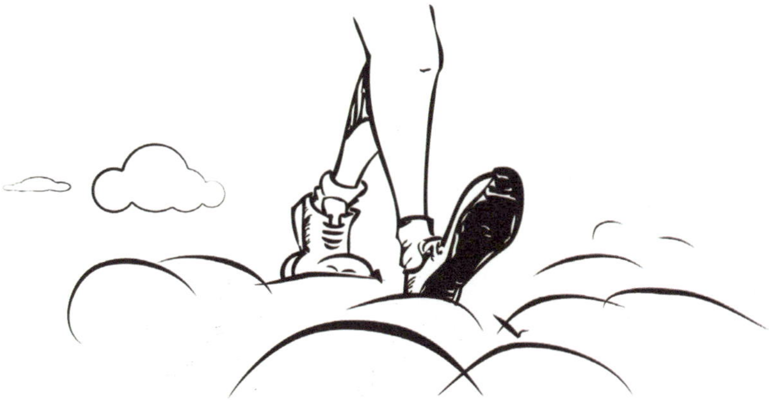

Questions and Answers

Can I hold on?

If you feel the need to hold on, you're probably walking too fast. Holding on doesn't allow your natural walking form and gait to take place. Decrease your speed enough to continue to increase your incline without holding on. You need to maintain proper technique and stay in control as you increase the incline as high as possible.

This is difficult! Do I have to complete ramp training?

Yes, ramp training challenges your body. If you continue to walk on the treadmill, eventually your body will adapt to the exercise and you will stop seeing results. Anytime you perform the same repetitive motion, without challenging your mind or body, you will increase your risk of mental and physical plateaus. You have to challenge your body to get results. If ramp training seems too challenging for you, try decreasing your speed a little so that you can complete the exercise.

I feel pain in my shins! Should I stop?

Well, that depends on what you are feeling. If you are experiencing tension or a slight burning sensation in your shins, then it is OK to continue. However, if you are feeling any sort of pain you'll need to decrease speed and/or incline to the point of avoiding the pain. Pushing through the pain in your shins is a bad idea. It increases your risk of shin splints, an injury that takes time to heal. If you are feeling pain, your body is trying to warn you that you could be in danger of seriously injuring yourself. Injuries slow your progress and make it difficult to achieve your goals. It is best to listen to your body and avoid pushing through your pain.

Do I need to continue stretching?

Yes! Stretch your hamstrings and calves for two sets of 15 seconds. Remember, stretching reduces your risk of injury and injuries prevent you from reaching your goals. Stretching should be relaxing and not too intense. Now, we will add another stretch, which will be for your quads. Complete one of the three following quad stretches for two sets of fifteen seconds:

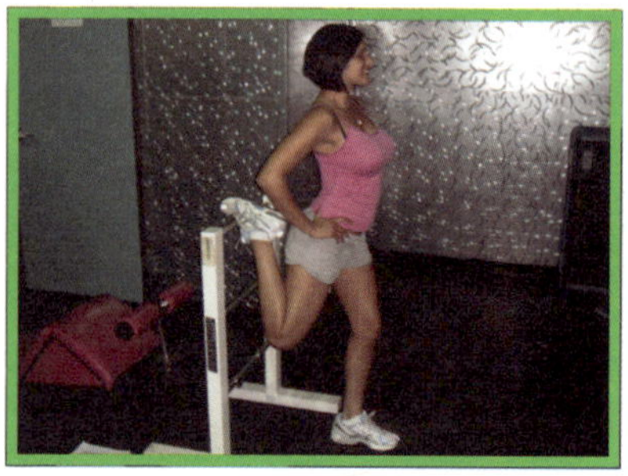

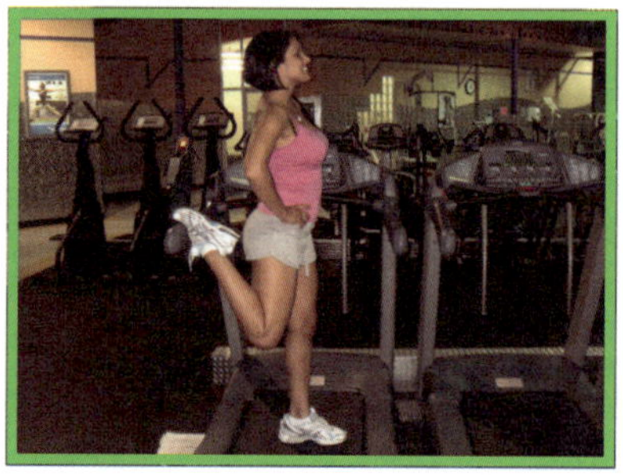

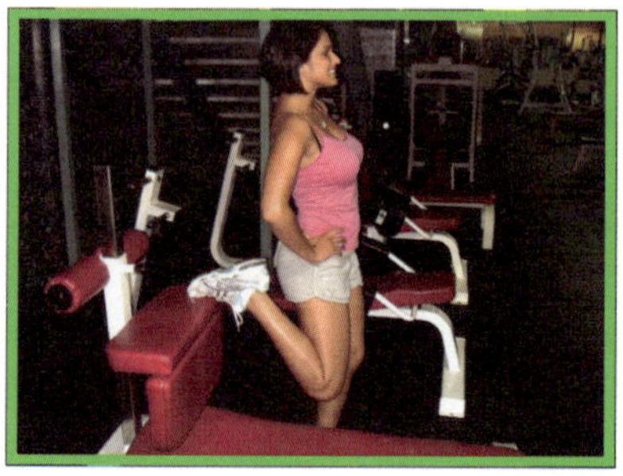

1. Stand or kneel with heels lifted up and toes secure.
2. Pull your hip flexors forward.
3. Lean back without arching and lower yourself slightly by bending your front knee.
4. Stretch and hold lightly for two sets of 15 seconds.

The Secrets to Success!

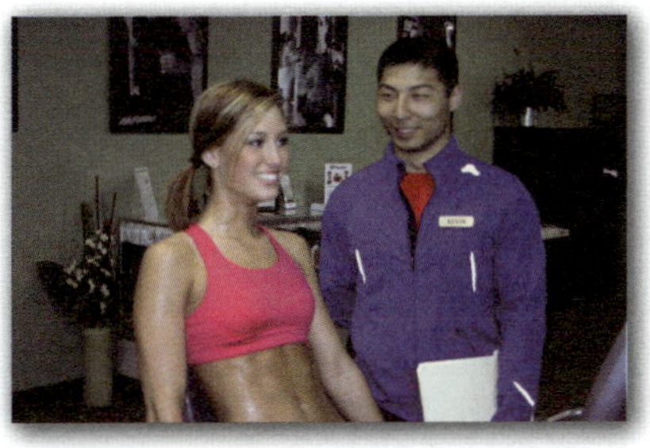

From Your Personal Trainer, Kevin Orr

I hope you have enjoyed your weight training workouts. You may feel burning and fatigue after each set. That's good! It is what you really want to feel. Your goal is to be a little sore for a few days after you work out. If you're not sore after at least every other workout, you may not be working out hard enough. The number of sets, the number of reps, the amount of weight, or the intensity might not be enough to really work your muscles. Soreness is a sign that you have damaged your muscles and now they need time to recover to get stronger. Go for the burn! This is a positive sign that you are training your muscles effectively at the right intensity. Feeling the burn is the secret! If you are too sore–painful to sit, stand up, comb your hair, hold a pencil–ease up. A little sore is good. Really sore is not good!)

Example Weight & Cardio Routine

Continue to choose a workout routine based on your level of fitness and your schedule before progressing to Week Four. Write it down in your schedule, on page 249. If none of the example routines work for you, configure a routine that fits your needs, and write it down. Planning ahead will help you set yourself up for success.

Weight Routine 1

Sunday	Monday	Tuesday	Wednesday	Thursday	Friday	Saturday
	Arms/Abs 2x15		Chest/Back/ Shoulders 4x15		Arms/Abs 3x15	

Weight Routine 2

Sunday	Monday	Tuesday	Wednesday	Thursday	Friday	Saturday
		Arms/Abs 2x15		Chest/Back/ Shoulders 4x15		Arms/Abs 3x15

Weight Routine 3

Sunday	Monday	Tuesday	Wednesday	Thursday	Friday	Saturday
	Arms/Abs 2x15		Chest/Back/ Shoulders 4x15	Arms/Abs 3x15		

Continue to choose routine 1, 2, or 3 to begin your weekly cardio routine, or rearrange your cardio training to best fit you. **Note**: Tread: R means ramp training on the treadmill.

Cardio Routine 1

Sunday	Monday	Tuesday	Wednesday	Thursday	Friday	Saturday
	EFX: 15 Tread:R 15		EFX: 15 Tread:R 15		EFX: 15 Tread:R 15	

Cardio Routine 2

Sunday	Monday	Tuesday	Wednesday	Thursday	Friday	Saturday
		EFX: 15 Tread:R 15	EFX: 15 Tread:R 15	EFX: 15 Tread:R 15		EFX: 15 Tread:R 15

Cardio Routine 3

Sunday	Monday	Tuesday	Wednesday	Thursday	Friday	Saturday
	EFX: 15 Tread:R 15	EFX: 15 Tread:R 15	EFX: 15 Tread:R 15	EFX: 15 Tread:R 15	EFX: 15 Tread:R 15	

Example Schedule

On your schedule, page 249, continue to write down which cardio machines along with the duration you plan to complete this week.

	Sunday	Monday	Tuesday	Wednesday	Thursday	Friday	Saturday	
Week 1 Weight: Body fat: Cardio: Duration:		226 31% EFX: 5	EFX: 10	EFX: 15	EFX: 20	EFX: 20		Why Too Tired Solution Pace Yourself
Week 2 Weight: Body fat: Weights: Sets: Cardio: Duration:		224 Chest/Back Shoulders: 2x15 EFX: 15 Tread: 15	EFX: 15 Tread: 15	Chest/Back Shoulders: 2x15 EFX: 15 Tread: 15	EFX: 15 Tread: 15	Chest/Back Shoulders: 3x15 EFX: 15 Tread: 15		Why Still too sore from Monday Solution Weight train when recovered
Week 3 Weight: Body fat: Weights: Sets: Cardio: Duration:		222 30% Arms: 2x15 Abs: 2x20 EFX: 15 Tread:R 15	EFX: 15 Tread:R 15	Chest/Back Shoulders: 4x15 EFX: 15 Tread:R 15	Arms: 3x15 Abs: 3x20 EFX: 15 Tread:R 15	EFX: 15 Tread:R 15		

Before moving on...

Did you follow through with your plan? If not, cross out what you did not complete on your schedule and write in what you did complete before moving on to the next week.

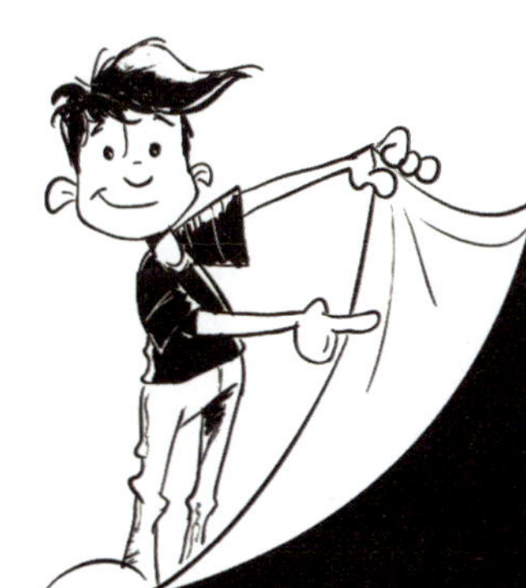

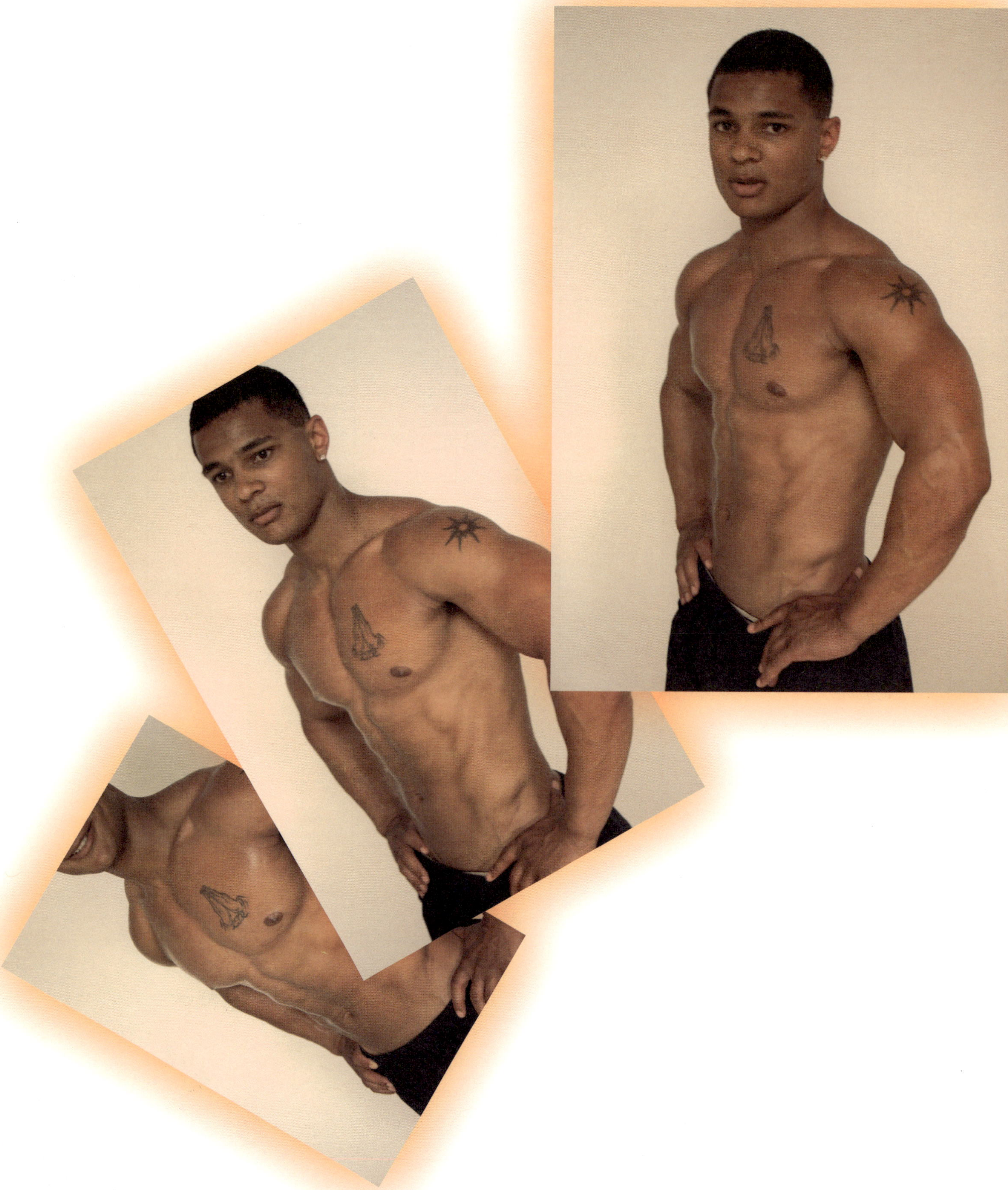

Week 4

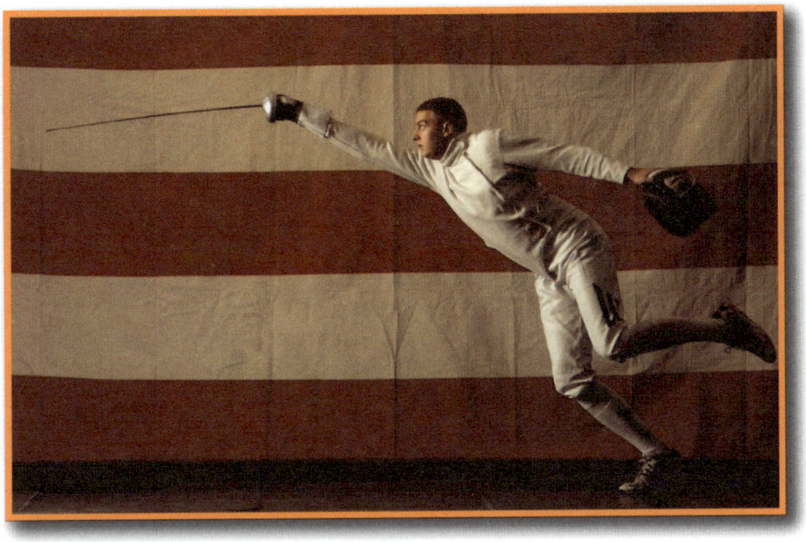

Learning the fundamentals of Kevin Orr's training helped me to leap into competitive fencing. I was once uncoordinated but became one of the finest athletes with the help of his rigorous training and nutrition programs.

-Seth Kelsey, 2004 and 2008 Olympian and Air Force Olympic Fencing Team

Goal:

Avoid processed foods.

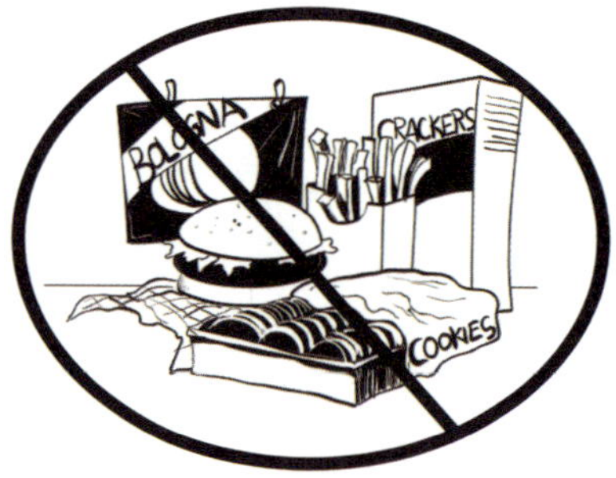

Why?

Processed foods are another form of empty calories that provide few, if any, nutrients. They are calorie-dense and digest very quickly. They do not replenish the nutrients lost in the digestion process. It is OK to eat processed foods occasionally in moderation, but you should avoid them as much as possible. Do not eat processed foods on a daily basis!

Processed foods can digest as fast as sugar and white flour due to their lower nutrient density. They also play a similar role in fuel utilization and body fat storage. If you are not using this "fuel" through some form of activity, the excess calories in the processed foods will be stored as body fat!

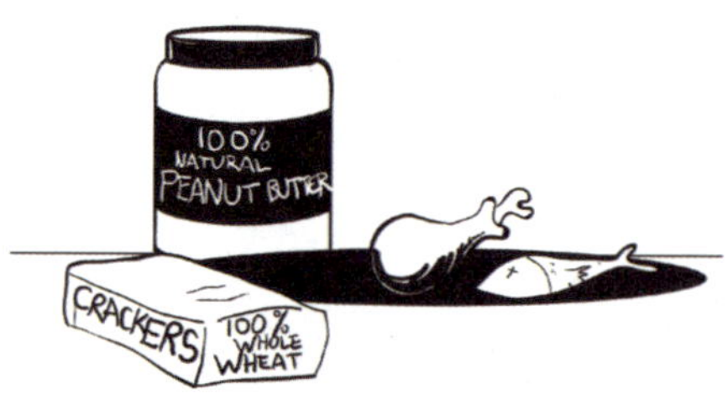

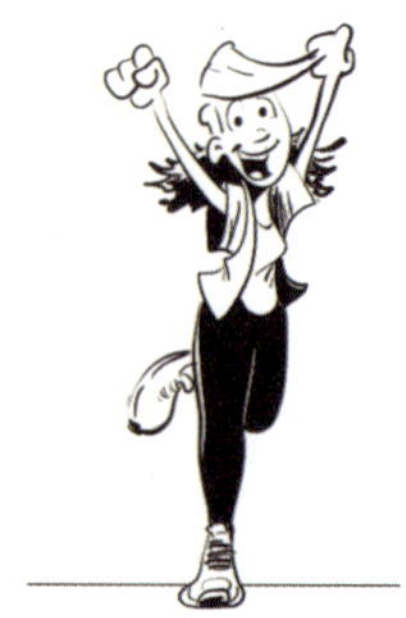

Balanced Blood Sugar = Optimal Metabolism and Energy

How?

Replace processed foods with 100% natural food products. These healthy substitutions will help to balance your blood sugar levels, optimize your metabolism and boost your energy. Try some of the following healthy substitutions:

100% Natural Peanut Butter contains protein, vitamins, minerals, fiber, and most importantly, mono- and polyunsaturated oils (good fats!). Jif® and Skippy® are processed and contain trans-fats and hydrogenated oils (bad fats). They have fewer nutrients and do not provide the health benefits of 100% natural peanut butter. **Recommendation:** Eat one serving (2 Tbsp) of 100% natural peanut butter a day. Pour out the oil that rises to the top of the jar to reduce more fat.

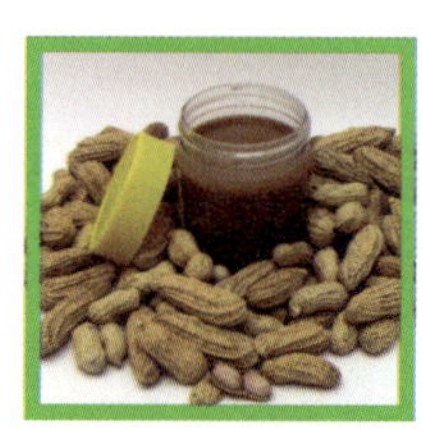

VS

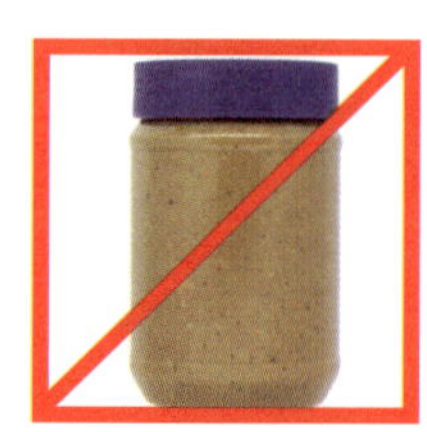

Lean Meats such as chicken and fish are good sources of quality protein. They contain essential amino acids, B-complex vitamins, and minerals. Processed meats like most packaged meats, hot dogs, bacon, pepperoni, on the other hand, are typically lower in nutrients and are known to be linked to various forms of cancers.
Recommendation: Eat one to three servings (4 oz. per serving) of lean meat a day.

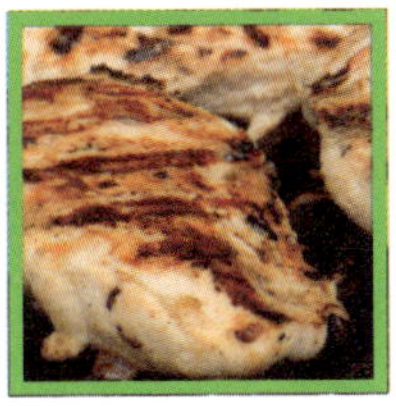
VS
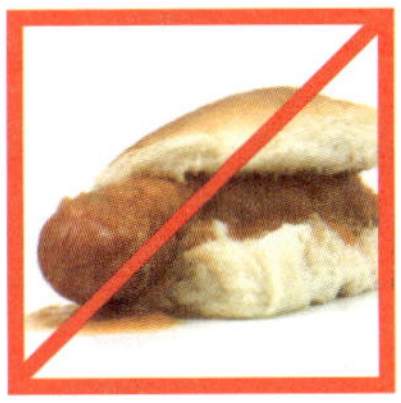

Whole wheat crackers are nutrient dense. Most other types of packaged cookies and crackers are processed and contain excess fats, sugars, and carbohydrates and fewer nutrients.
Recommendation: Replace all processed snack foods with whole wheat and 100% natural snacks.

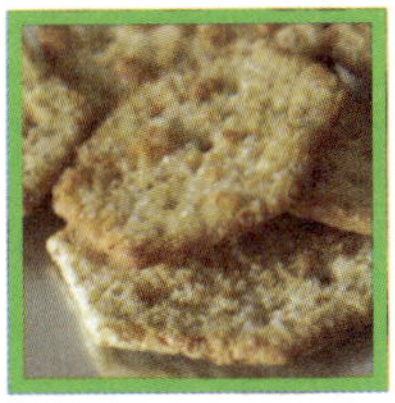
VS
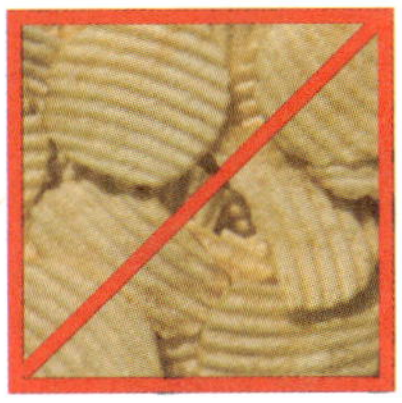

Making healthy choices is not always easy. Packaging can be very deceptive and you may think you are making a healthy choice, when in fact, you are not. For example, color is not necessarily an indicator of whole grains. Just because bread is brown doesn't mean it is healthy or made with whole grains. You have to read the food labels.

Time to review your nutrition log.

1. Cross out all processed foods.

2. Next to the foods you crossed out, write down your healthy alternative.

3. Keep your "better choice" food selections simple. Don't forget, too many food decisions can lead to indecisive eating habits that can lead to overeating.

4. Continue to record everything you eat and drink in your nutrition log daily.

For Example:

Time	Food and Amount	Substitute
7:00 AM	Pancake, sausage	**WW toast, Adam's® PB**
10:00 AM	Chips, snack dips	**WW crackers, Hummus**
12:30 PM	Canned soup	**Home-made Soup**
3:00 PM	Macaroni and cheese, hot dogs	**WW pasta, lean hamburger**
6:00 PM	Workout	Workout
8:00 PM	Lunch meat, salad, salad dressing, boxed rice	**4 oz. Chicken**, salad, salsa, brown rice

WW = 100% whole wheat

Questions and Answers

I see processed foods on every grocery aisle. Are they really that bad?

Yes! Foods are processed to lengthen their shelf life. Most packaged foods, such as ready-made snacks, low fat dressings, dips, and chips are made with chemical ingredients used to color, stabilize, emulsify, bleach, texturize, soften, preserve, sweeten, add or cover smells, add flavor, help maintain the taste, appearance, and increase the shelf-life. Yuck! These chemicals are used in the growing as well as the processing of the products.

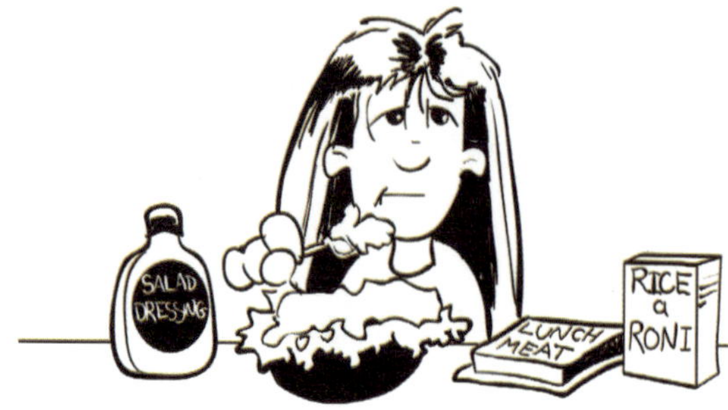

Processed foods deplete you of your own nutrients because they don't replace many of the nutrients that have been utilized by your body. And, as if all that wasn't bad enough, most processed foods contain trans-fats and partially hydrogenated fats. Trans-fats are a by-product of the hydrogenation of plant oils that happens during processing. The link between trans-fats and cancer, heart disease, and obesity is undeniable. No scientific studies have shown that processed foods provide **any** health benefits. Besides, they are full of empty calories that digest very quickly, causing fluctuations in your blood sugar, and leading to lower energy! So yes, they really are *that bad*!

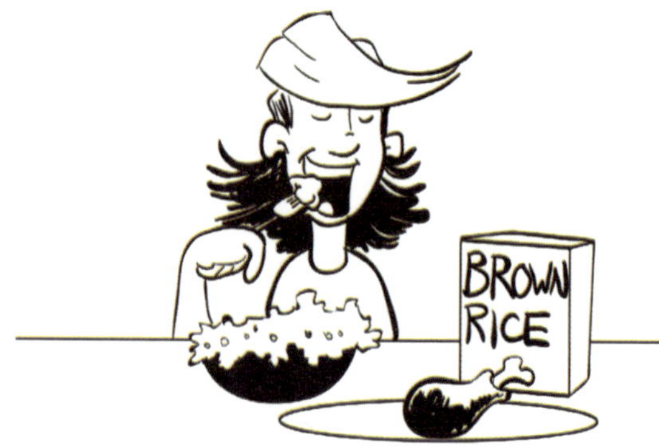

Which foods contain trans-fats and hydrogenated fats?

Some of the most popular fast food items, including french fries, as well as many other fried foods, cookies and crackers, donuts, scones, and muffins, ready-made meals, pastries, canned soups, juice drinks, breakfast cereals, boxed desserts, salad dressings, bread, cakes, pasta, mayonnaise, ice cream, candy, and processed meats contain trans fats and should be avoided. Whew! The good news is that most of these foods, when prepared at home, do not contain all the bad chemicals and fats, and can be part of a healthy diet when eaten in moderation.

Kevin gave me the skills to move forward with my fitness training for life. He 'walks the walk' and 'talks the talk'. He lives what he teaches and his goal is to give everyone the skills and knowledge to keep fit for life. He gave me the knowledge of what to eat and how to eat for balance and energy, while at the same time he taught me the principles of fat loss and maintenance. Sometimes, everyday life makes it hard to stay on track, but the skills that Kevin has taught me lingers forever and I know I will never return to the unhealthy lifestyle I lived before. He is truly amazing. Without his guidance, I would not have been able to go forward with the discipline, the understanding, the courage, or the self-esteem I now have. When I walk into the gym (four to five times a week), I walk in knowing that living a healthy lifestyle, keeping fit, and eating right is a part of everything I do and everything I think.

- Kathaleen Crawford

He has taught and inspired me in areas such as proper nutrition, injury prevention and rehabilitation, proper weight training, self visualization, lifestyle management, and much more.

- Ken Taylor

Nutrition Log

Date:____________	Sun Mon Tues Wed Thurs Fri Sat	
	Plan	**Actual**
Meal 1	*Food & Amount*	*Food & Amount*
Time:______		
Meal 2		
Time:______		
Meal 3		
Time:______		
Meal 4		
Time:______		
Meal 5		
Time:______		
Meal 6		
Time:______		

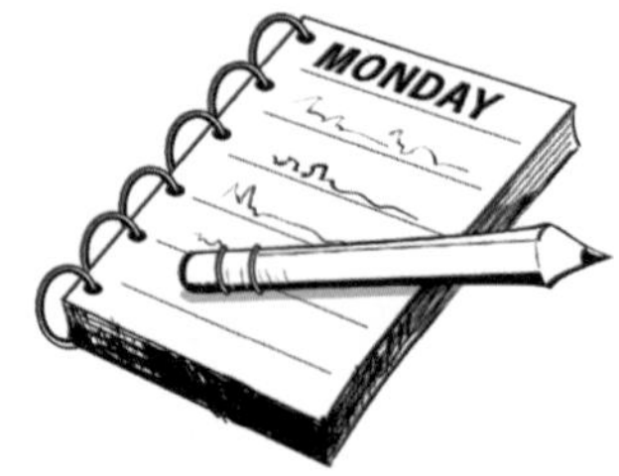

Checklist

Achieved:

✓ Consume meal or snack every 3 hours

✓ Water every 3 hours

✓ Sleep optimal hours

✓ Intake multivitamin

✓ Weights and cardio

Avoided:

✓ Sugars

✓ White flour

✓ **Processed foods**

Key Points

Week 1

- Eat a small meal or snack once every three hours – five to six meals per day.
- Drink at least 1 cup (8 ounces) of water per meal and at least one cup before, during, and after your workouts.
- Keep a nutrition log.
- Sleep is vital!
- Take a daily multivitamin.

Week 2

- Avoid bad sugars.

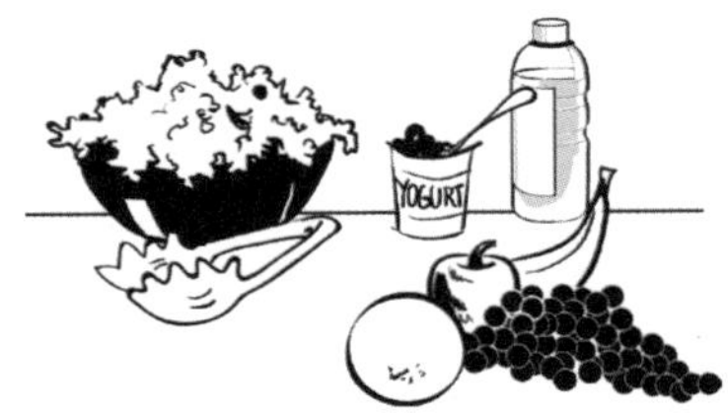

Week 3

- Avoid white flour and white rice.

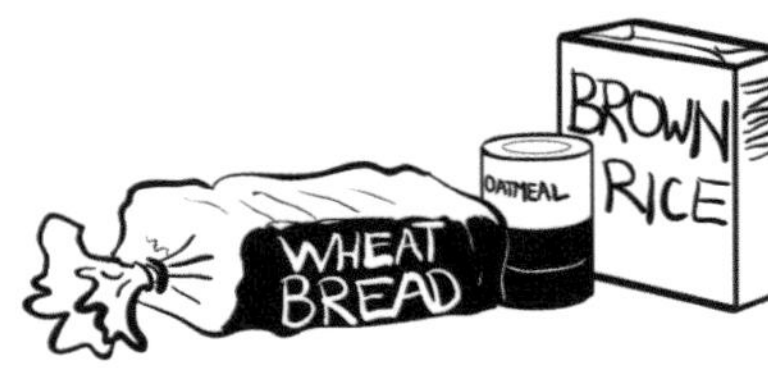

Week 4

- **Avoid processed foods.** They are unnecessary calories that do not provide nutrients lost in the digestion process. They contain bad fats and chemicals that lead to many health risks. Replace all processed foods with 100% natural food products.

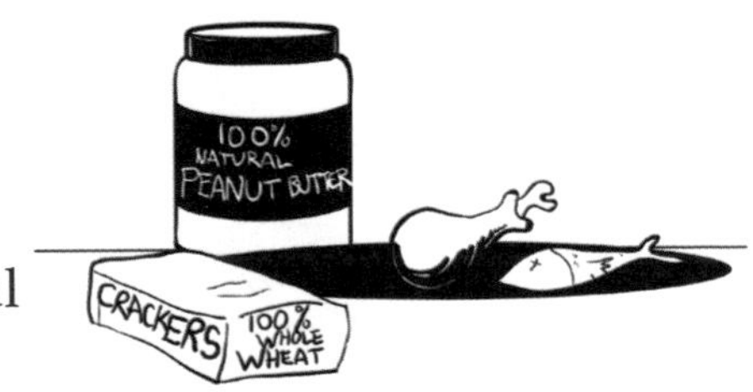

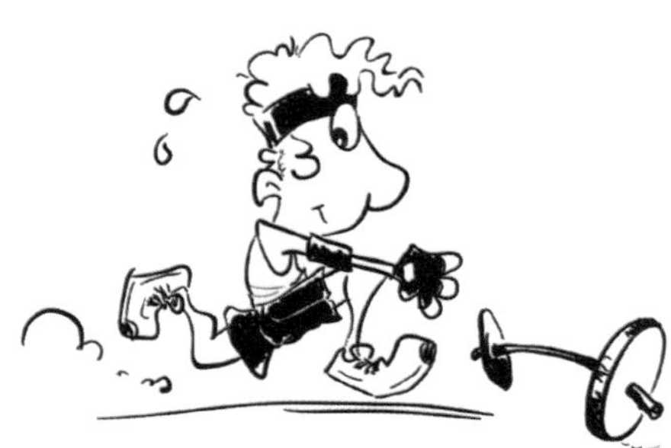

Legs

Goal:

Complete two sets of 20 reps of **squats**.

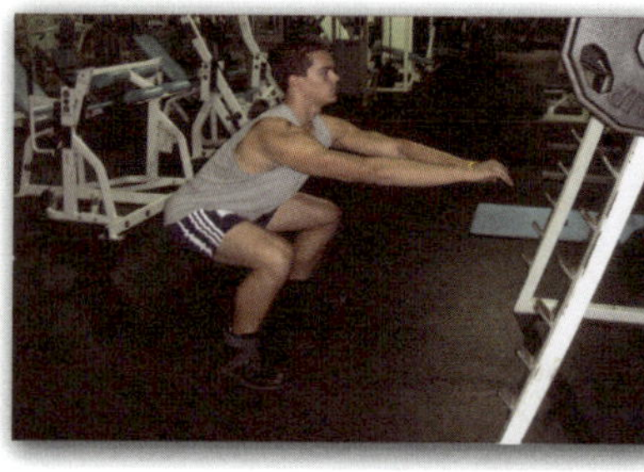

Primary
Quads
Glutes
Hamstrings

Stabilizers
Lower back
Core
Calves
Shins

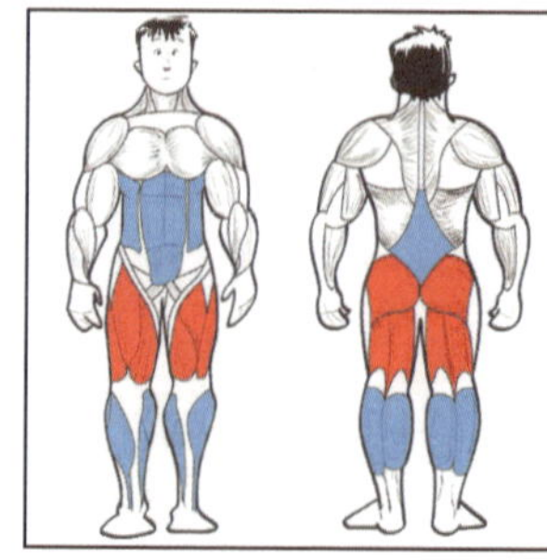

Why?

Squats are a free weight, compound exercise targeting the major muscle groups of your legs: glutes, quads, and hamstrings. The muscle stabilizers include your lower back, calves and shins. Squats are a demanding exercise. In order to maintain and stabilize the squat motion, your body has to utilize stabilizers throughout the entire body. Squats are, by far, one of the best leg exercises to improve strength conditioning and lung capacity.

How?

Step 1 - Begin by standing with your feet slightly wider than shoulder-width. You may want to stand in front of a mirror to provide you feedback.

Step 2 - Squeeze your abs to protect your lower back.

Step 3 - Lift your arms up, palms down, and hold with your elbows slightly bent.

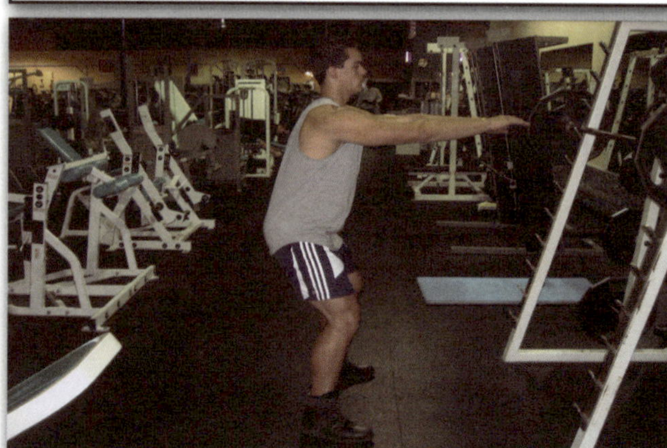

Step 4 - Bend your knees, stick your glutes out, and lean your upper body slightly forward.

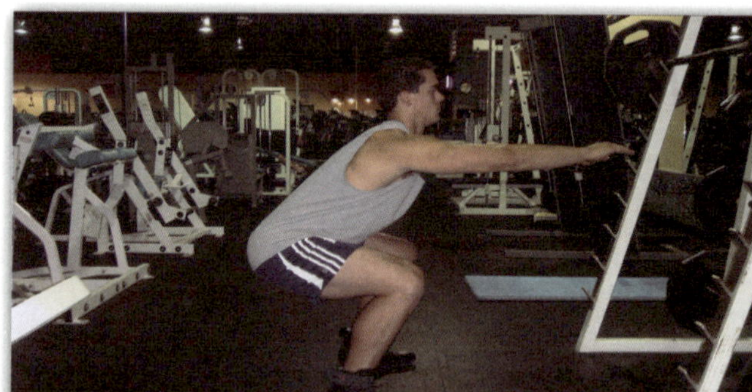

Step 5 - Slowly lower yourself to a 90-degree angle and keep your weight on your heels.

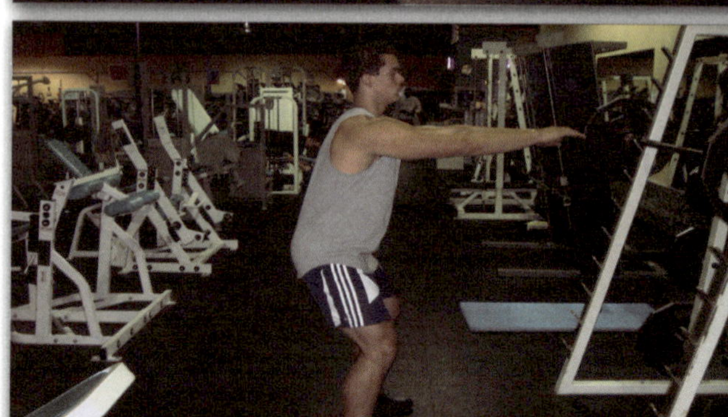

Step 6 - Push up to your starting position and repeat.

Your goal is to complete two sets of 20 (2 x 20).

Range of Motion Techniques

To Maximize Muscle Tension and Minimize Overcompensation

Dos

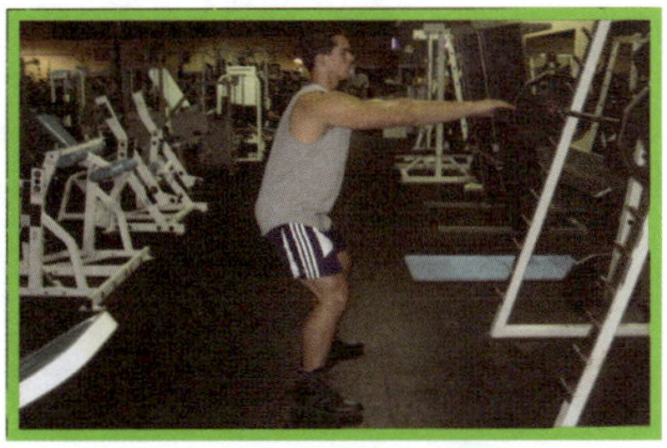

Begin With Knees Bent

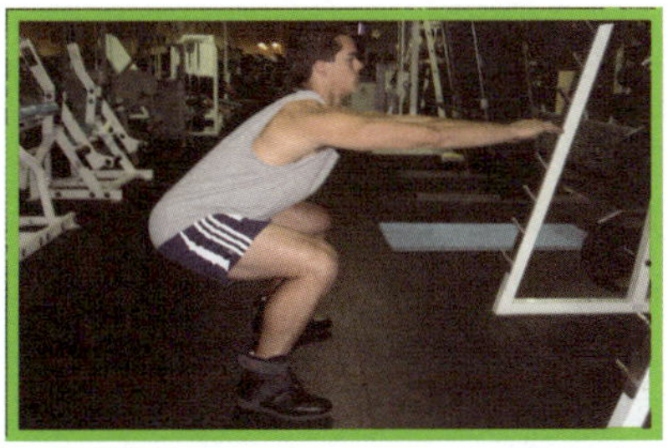

Upper Thighs Should Almost be Parallel With Floor

Don'ts

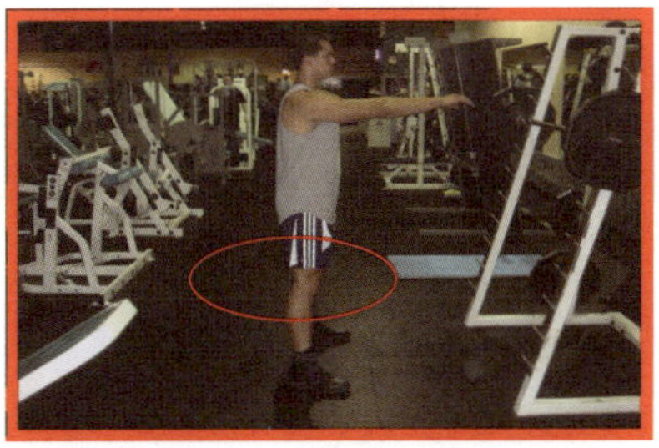

Avoid Locking Out Knees and Coming Up Too High

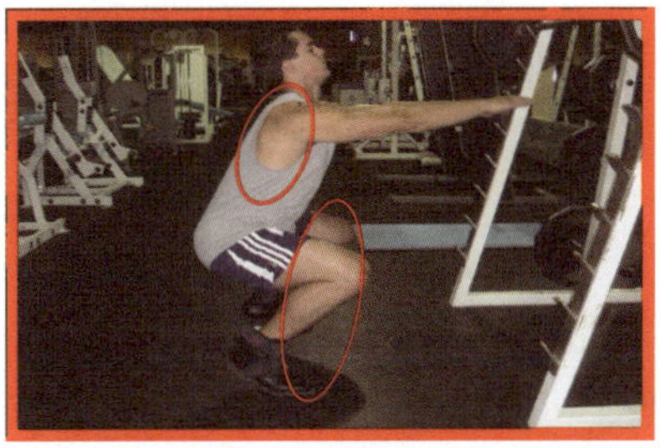

Avoid Allowing Knees to Go Beyond Toes and a Vertical Lower Back Posture

Visualize

"Cable Effect"

Stand in a squat stance. Visualize a cable attached to your hips, pulling your hips back. Another cable is attached to your arms, pulling your arms forward as you squat down and stand up.

Visualizing while staying within the proper range of motion will maximize muscle tension in your glutes, quads, and hamstrings. It also minimizes overcompensation in your lower back and knees. Due to the strength requirements of squats, you may need to develop more strength in your legs to visualize correctly.

If you have trouble keeping your weight in your heels while squatting, try raising your toes up inside your shoes. You can also imagine a rope pulling your toes up to the ceiling. This helps to keep your heels on the floor as you move through the squat motion. By shifting the pressure from the balls of your feet to your heels, you will naturally reduce joint tension in your knees and increase the effectiveness of the exercise.

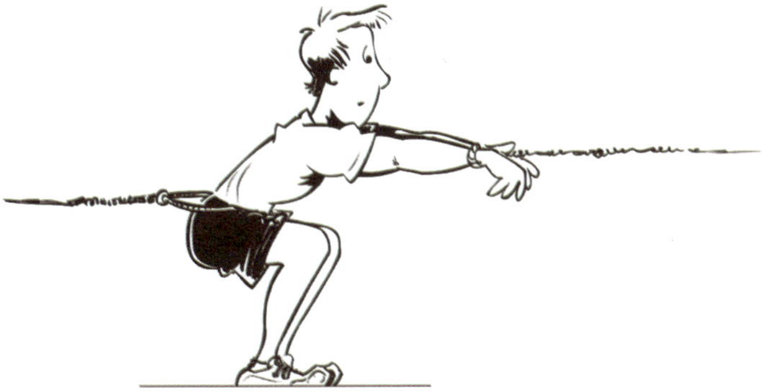

Questions and Answers

I lose balance! What should I do?

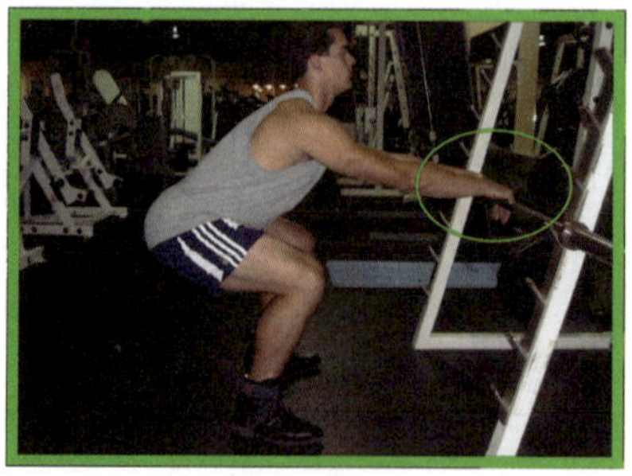

If you are having a hard time squatting, you can hold onto a post or bar. This will help to increase your stability and balance until you get a little stronger. As your muscles develop and your stabilizers strengthen, you will be able to do squats without holding on.

Why do I need to lean so far forward?

Leaning forward, arching your lower back, and keeping your knees bent are all necessary to reduce joint tension. By decreasing tension in your joints, you increase the tension in your muscles and you will get a much more effective leg workout.

Why do I need to keep my weight on my heels?

Keeping your weight on your heels saves your knees! When your weight is on your heels, the pressure is placed on your leg muscles. If you allow your weight to shift forward, your heels will lift off the floor and the pressure will be in your knees. In order to keep the pressure off of your knees, you have to keep your weight on your heels. Keeping your weight on your heels decreases joint tension, forcing your legs to do the work, which increases the effectiveness of the exercise. Lastly, make sure your knees stay above or behind your toes to further minimize knee tension.

I can't squat down low enough. What can I do to improve my form?

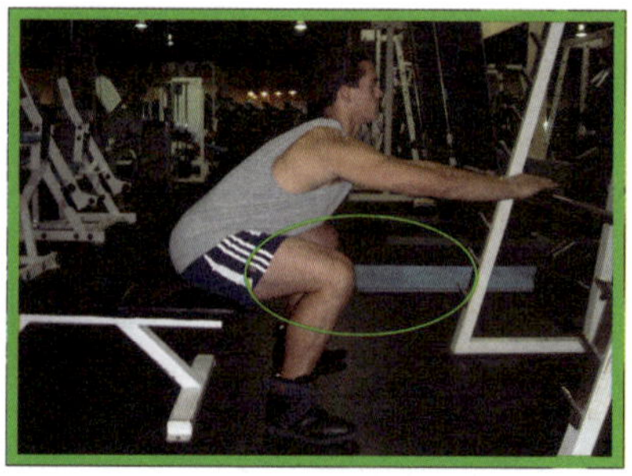

Try replacing squats with bench squats. Lower yourself down lightly, as if you were going to sit down. When your glutes touch the bench, stand back up. This will help you to build the foundation of strength needed to perform squats.

Can I perform more than two sets of 20 reps?

Yes. If you're ready, you can perform up to six sets of twenty reps. Just beware, if you do too much too fast, you may find yourself in a world of hurt! Sitting and then standing can be uncomfortable.

What should I feel after performing squats?

You should feel a burning sensation in your legs by the end of each set. You should also feel a slight pump and/or a "wobble" effect in your legs. This is very positive feedback from your muscles. It is your body's way of telling you that you are training at your optimal intensity.

I feel pain in my lower back and knees! What should I do?

If you are feeling pain in your lower back or knees, you are probably allowing them to overcompensate for your legs. Allow your leg muscles to provide balance and stability rather than your lower back and knees.

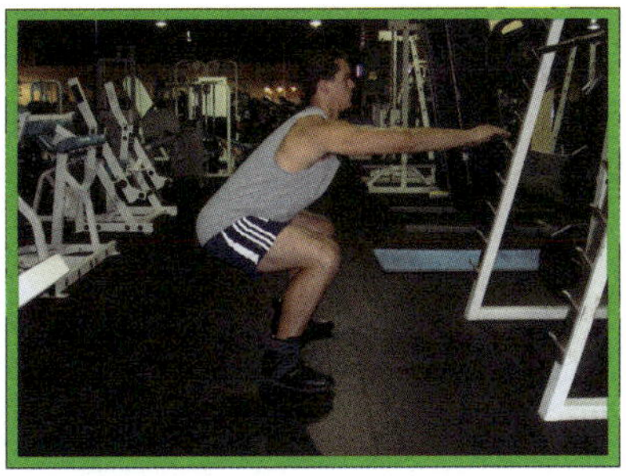

Be sure to use proper form and technique. Stick your glutes out, pull your knees back, and lean forward. Pushing your glutes out enables your leg muscles to do the work. Pulling your knees back forces your leg muscles to provide stability and balance. Leaning forward allows you to push your glutes out. By allowing your leg muscles to do the work, you can avoid the use of your knees and lower back to stabilize. Remember, your goal is to let your leg muscles do the work, not your joints, tendons, or ligaments. However, if you continue to feel tension or a dull pain, make sure it's decreasing throughout your workout.

I don't feel comfortable performing squats.

If you're not used to physical activity, you may not feel comfortable performing squats. Squats can be a very difficult exercise to perform. However, squats are one of the most effective leg exercises. Not only do they work all the major and minor muscle groups of your legs, they also utilize all of the stabilizers that assist the body in movement and motion. Squats provide both a strength and cardio workout. If you're not comfortable performing squats at your current fitness level, it is OK to build up to them. Practice the bench squats until you build up enough strength to perform squats. As soon as you strengthen, you will notice the results.

When should I breathe?

You should always inhale at your starting position and exhale as you complete the range of motion. In squats, inhale as you lower yourself down and exhale as you lift yourself up. As an analogy, would you exhale before lifting a heavy box off the floor? Probably not, otherwise, you will lose much of your strength very quickly.

Calves

Goal:

Complete two sets of 20 reps of **calf raises**.

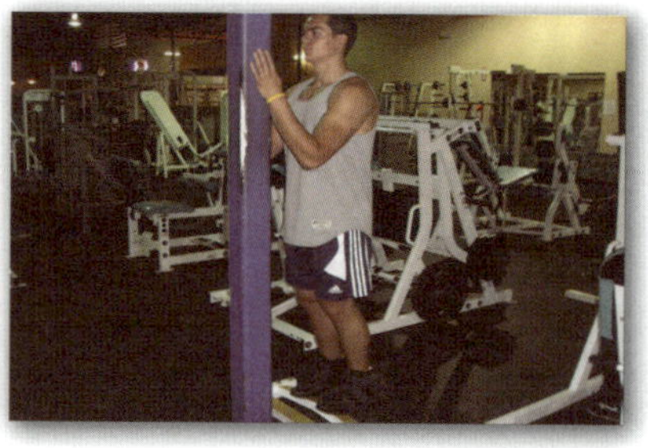

Primary
Calves

Stabilizers
Quads
Hamstrings
Core

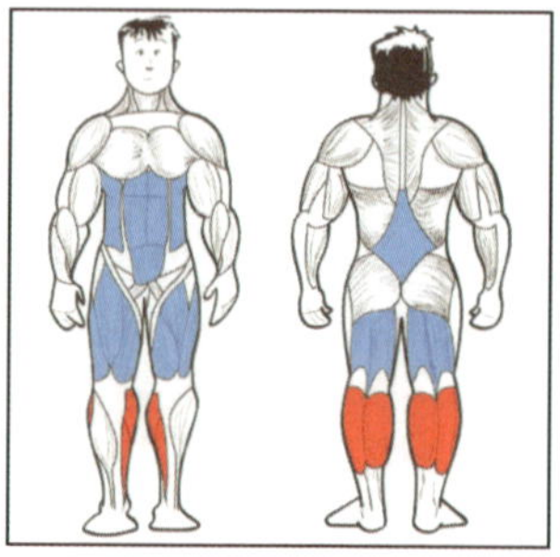

Why?

Calf raises are a free weight exercise targeting your calves. Your calves serve as a stabilizer for walking, running, and performing leg exercises. The muscle stabilizers for calf raises include your quads and hamstrings, as well as the rest of your core.

How?

Step 1 - Stand on the balls of your feet on the edge of a calf stand.

Step 2 - Squeeze your abs to push your lower back into a neutral position.

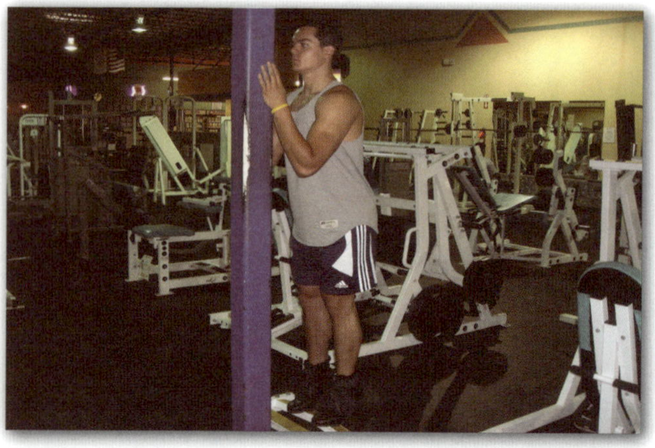

Step 3 - Pull your hips slightly back and lean slightly forward.

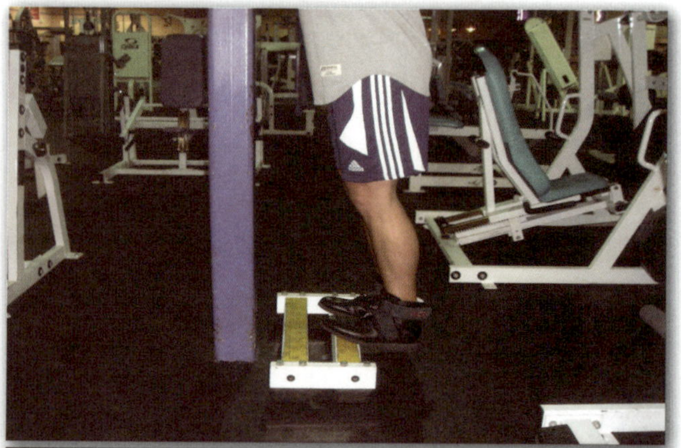

Step 4 - Lower your heels to the point of feeling a slight stretch in your calves.

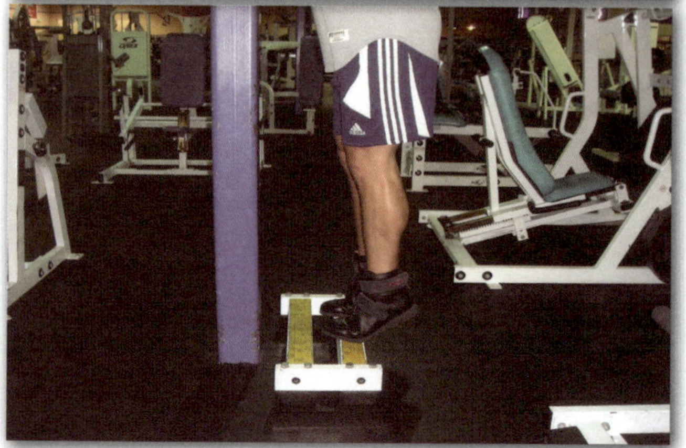

Step 5 - Lift and squeeze up to the peak contraction of your calf and repeat.

Your goal is to complete two sets of 20 (2 x 20).

Range of Motion Techniques

To Maximize Muscle Tension and Minimize Overcompensation

Dos

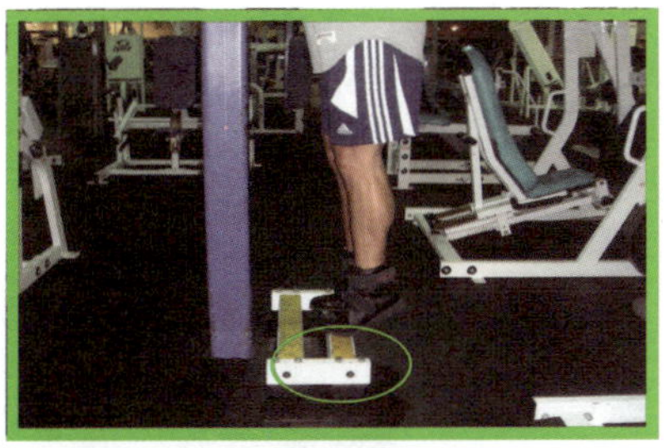

Begin With Squeezing Calves at Top

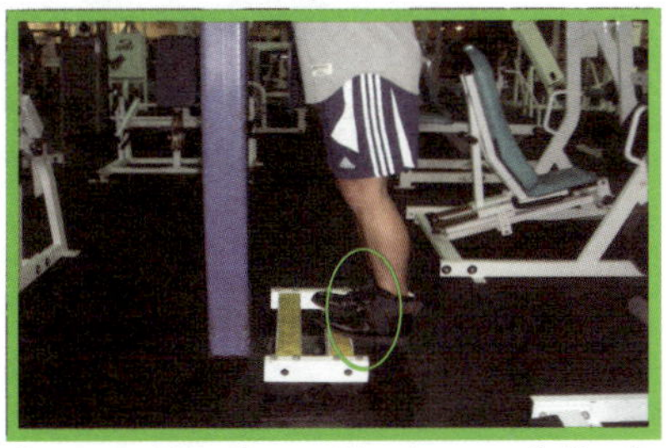

Lower Heels to Resist and Feel Calves Stretching

Don'ts

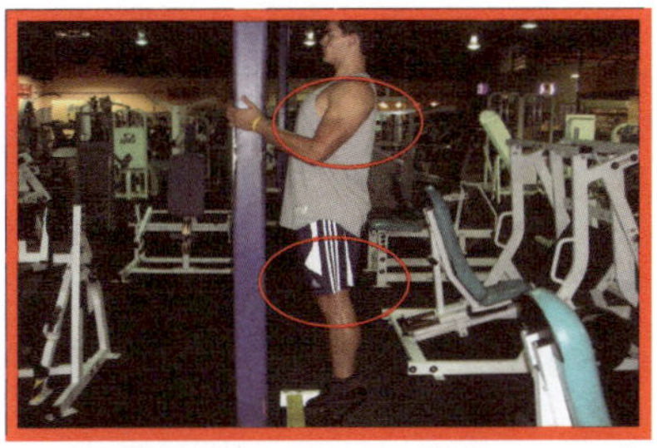

Avoid Locking Out Knees and Arching Lower Back

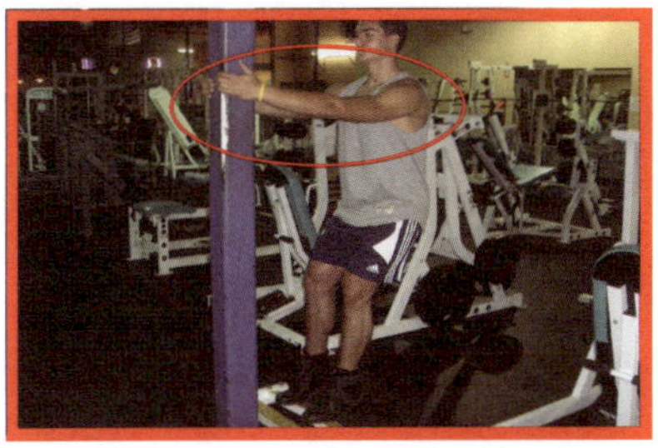

Avoid Leaning Too Far Back or Using Arms for Help

Visualize

"Balloon Effect"

Imagine yourself standing on a balloon that cannot be popped as you are performing calf raises. You are resisting and stretching your calves as you lower yourself down. When you feel the stretch in your calves, you contract them, pushing yourself up. Your goal is to move softly from a stretch to a contraction without popping the balloons beneath your feet.

The balloon visualization helps to create a smooth and controlled motion. The smooth motion allows for greater calf muscle utilization and a more effective workout. Explosive or jerky motions allow the entire body to overcompensate by creating momentum.

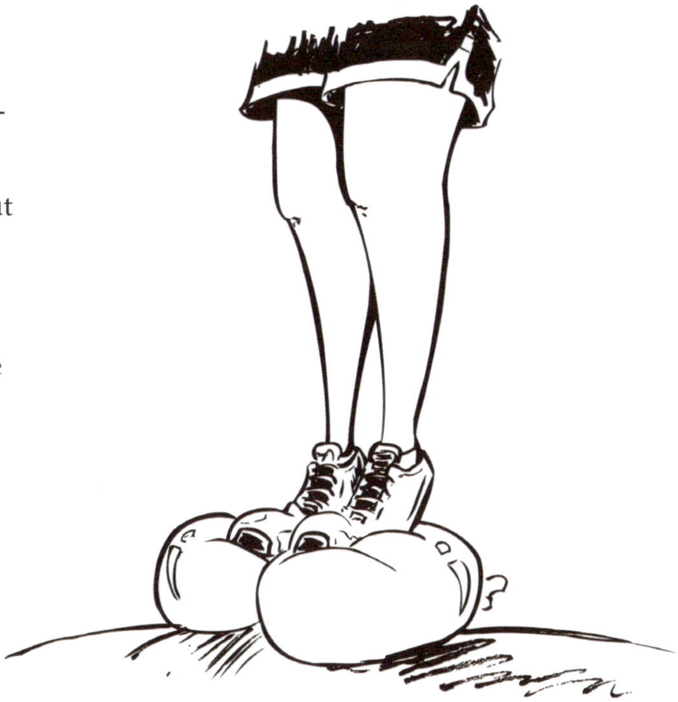

Questions and Answers

How do I position my feet for calf raises?

Place the balls of your feet on the edge of the calf stand with your heels hanging off the edge of the stand. This forces the calves to do the work and keeps your toes from overcompensating.

Why do I need to maintain a neutral lower back position when I'm training my calves?

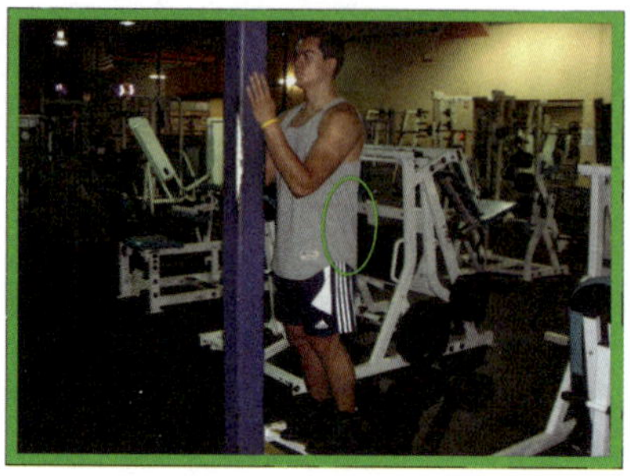

The neutral lower back position is proper posture. It relieves the pressure in your lower back, helps to prevent overcompensation, and forces your calves to do most of the work. For that reason, pull your hips back, lean slightly forward, and squeeze your abs to push your lower back into a neutral position.

When should I breathe?

You should always inhale at your starting position and exhale as you complete the range of motion. In calf raises, inhale as you lower yourself down and exhale as you lift yourself up.

Staying on a routine that focuses on good nutrition and exercises that fit into my lifestyle is definitely what got me over my plateau. Under Kevin's guidance, I was able to successfully train and run the Portland Marathon three times in the past four years. Without routine and discipline, no program that you set yourself up for will be successful. You are the only one who can make that decision for yourself and once you have committed yourself, you will begin to see 'the new you.'

- Marcie Mueller

Kevin was inspirational, always positive and motivating. He lived what he preached. Everything I worked on was set at levels I could achieve and felt successful at. There was also enough change-over/variety to the routines and nutrition that I stayed motivated. I wanted to complete a half marathon before I got pregnant and that was why I joined the club initially; though I had to postpone that goal until now, I know I completed it because Kevin helped boost my confidence in my ability to achieve it. I had three back-to-back auto accidents and shoulder issues in 2000. I was told to give up my first sport swimming, etc. I'm going back to swimming soon as a result of my success with the half marathon. While I'm not looking for competitive success, I consider it a milestone already that I can get back in and try regardless of the doc's pessimism. While I don't think he specifically said as much, I know I left our workout sessions feeling it wasn't about everyone else out there what "they" looked like, how fast, how strong, how accomplished–but about me- my goals, my own personal bar I set for myself–and that was okay. That confidence to set my own bar and be proud has stayed with me and I owe Kevin thanks!

- Mary Unruh

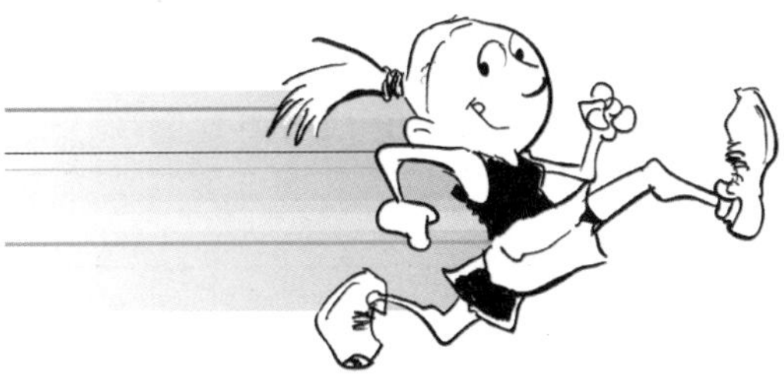

Cardio

Goal:

Complete 15 minutes on the **stair stepper** and 15 minutes of treadmill: ramp training.

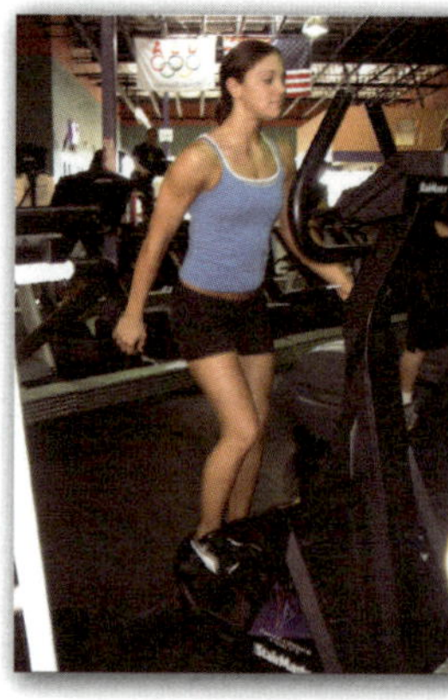

Primary
Quads
Glutes
Hamstrings

Stabilizers
Calves
Shins
Core

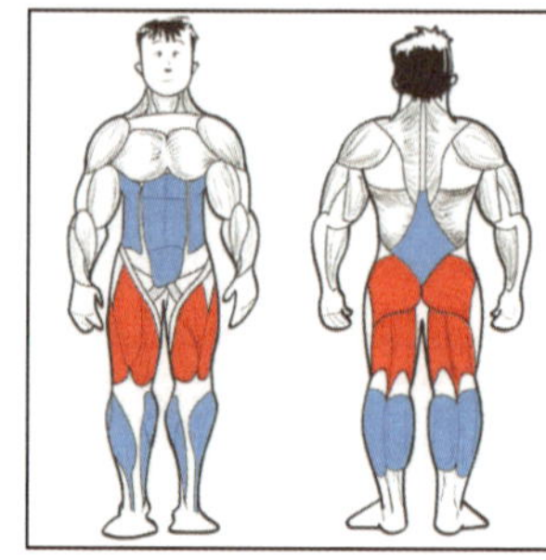

Why?

The stair stepper is a cardio machine that utilizes the major muscle groups of the legs. This stepping machine can be very challenging. It is a higher intensity exercise than walking on the treadmill. It increases your lung capacity, and strengthens and conditions your legs.

How?

Step 1 - Step onto the stair stepper and press a program showing gradual up and down hills.

Step 2 - Choose an intensity level from 1 up to 10, based on your physical condition.

Step 3 - Enter 15 minutes and begin stepping up and down.

Step 4 - Hand position should be nearly shoulder level.

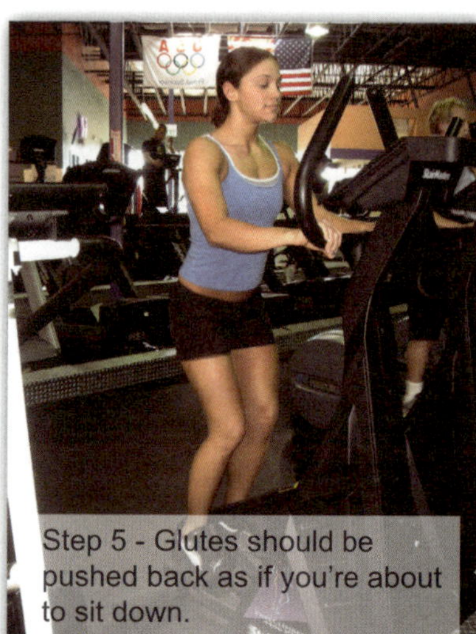

Step 5 - Glutes should be pushed back as if you're about to sit down.

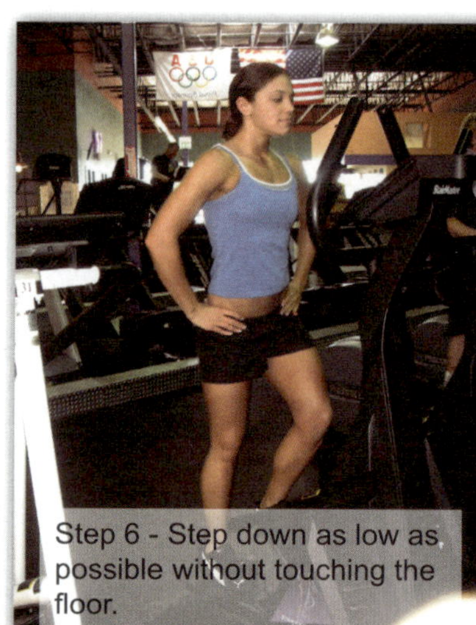

Step 6 - Step down as low as possible without touching the floor.

Step 7 - Step up as high as possible without touching the top.

Your goal is to pace yourself for 15 minutes at medium intensity in addition to completing 15 minutes on the treadmill.

Range of Motion Techniques

To Maximize Muscle Tension and Minimize Overcompensation

Dos

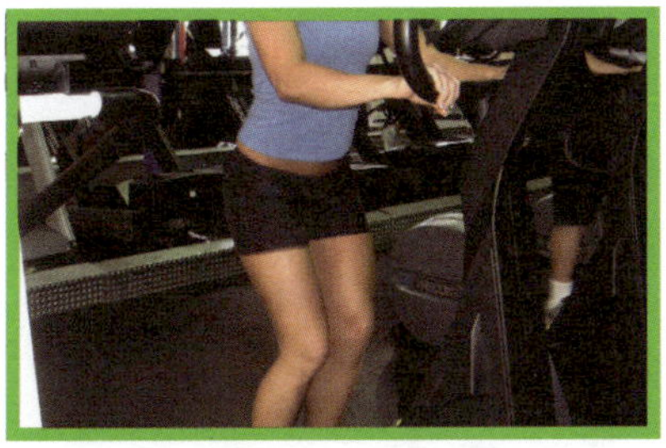

Begin with Proper Posture: Glutes Back, Knees Bent, Lean Slightly Forward

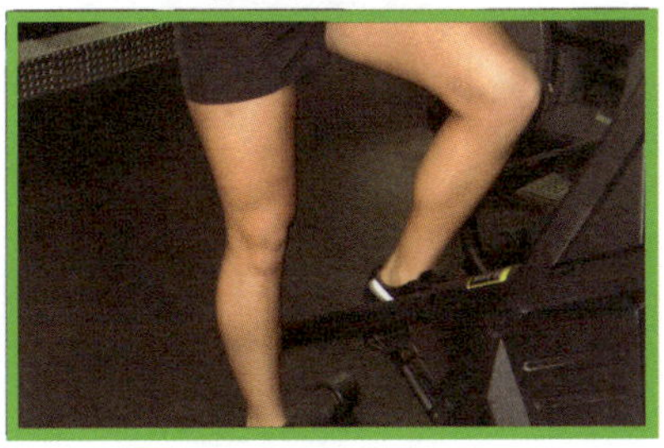

Take Large Steps

Don'ts

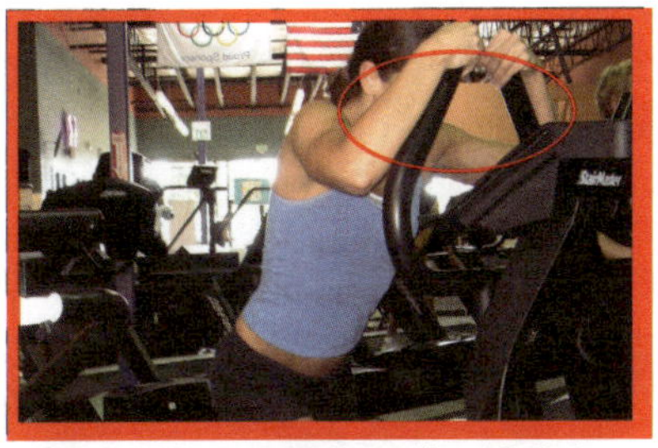

Avoid "hanging on" to Maintain Proper Posture

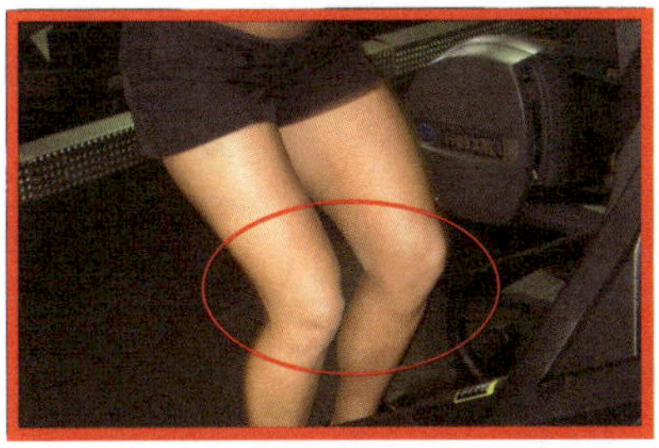

Avoid Knee and Joint Tension When Taking Small Steps

Visualize

"Hill and Balloon Effect"

As you step up and down on the stair stepper, imagine yourself walking up a steep hill. You have a balloon beneath each of your feet and your steps are large and soft. As you climb the hill, your goal is to take the biggest steps possible without "popping" the balloons.

This visualization technique corrects your posture. It places you in the position to maximize the use of your glutes, quads, hamstrings, and calves. It also reduces joint overcompensation in the knees and lower back.

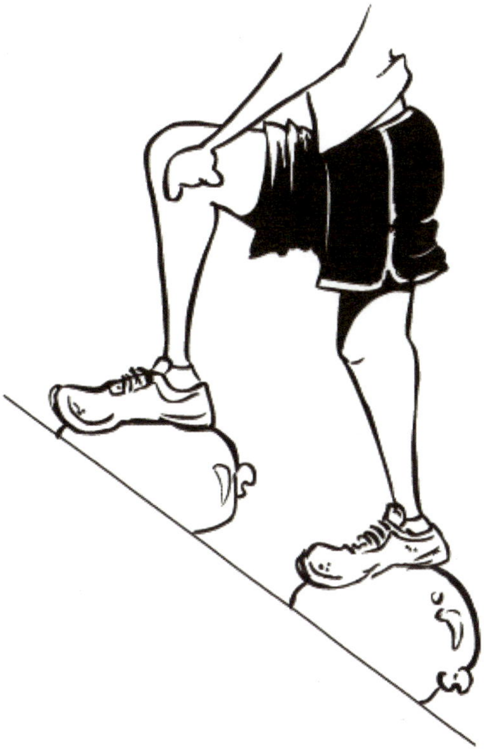

Week 4

Questions and Answers

Is it OK to hold on?

This is one of the most common questions in the gym. Eventually, you'll be able to place your hands on your hips or let them hang naturally in motion with your strides. But, until then, you can lightly hold the handles at shoulder height. If you feel the need to grip tightly or to hang on to the bar, you are probably stepping too fast. Decrease your speed enough to step up and down with a light grip.

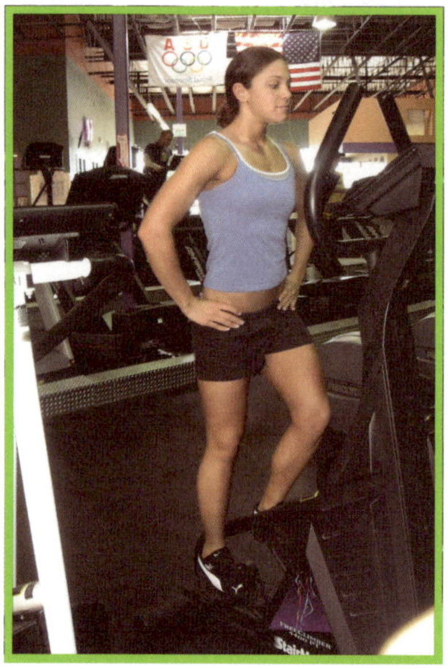

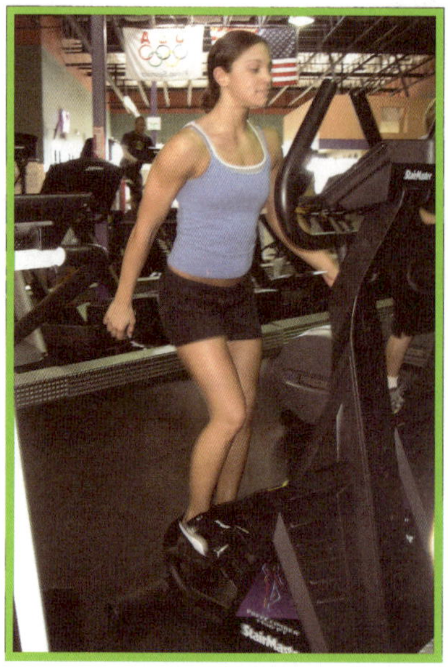

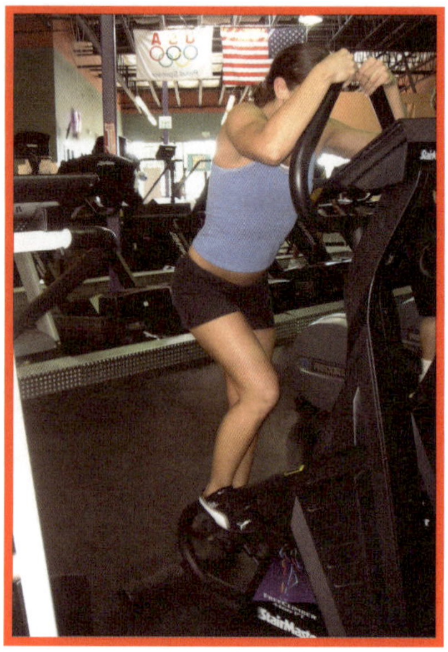

My knees hurt! Should I keep going?

That depends on your definition of hurt. Some people view a burning sensation or slight tension as painful, while others view it as a positive burn. If you feel actual knee pain, you need to reduce your intensity. Most knee pain is a result of improper form and technique. In this case, your glutes may not be far back enough. If your hips are back and your glutes are out, shift your weight to your heels and point your toes up. This relieves the pressure in your knees and allows your quads and glutes to do the work. If you continue to experience pain, you will need to stop and go back to the treadmill.

My lower back hurts! Should I keep going?

It's OK to feel a light burning sensation or tightness in your lower back muscles, but feeling pain is a different story. Slow down and make sure you are using proper form. Your glutes should be pushed back and your weight should be in your heels. Never allow your knees to travel beyond your toes. Proper technique minimizes joint and ligament pressure in your knees and lower back, which ultimately decreases the risk of injury. Most muscle and joint pains are due to a lack of activity, cardio, and strength training. If you continue to feel pain in your lower back, then you may need to stop to avoid aggravating your pain. In this case, go back to the treadmill or EFX until you strengthen a little more.

It's difficult to take large steps. Can I take smaller steps?

Your goal is to take the largest steps possible. Taking large steps is the most effective way of using the stair stepper. The bigger your steps, the better the workout. As you step up, your pedal should nearly touch the top and as you step down, your pedal should almost touch the bottom of the step. Maintaining proper form and technique is your number one priority. Therefore, you may need to decrease your intensity in order to maintain form and control.

Do I need to continue stretching?

Yes! Stretch your hamstrings, quads, and calves after your cardio training for two sets of 15 seconds!

Hamstrings

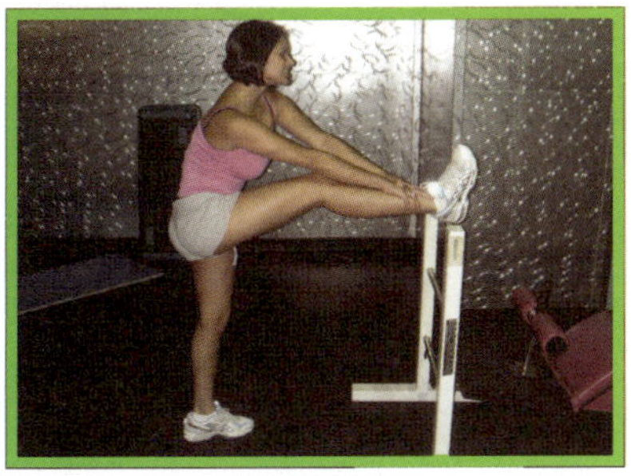

Quads

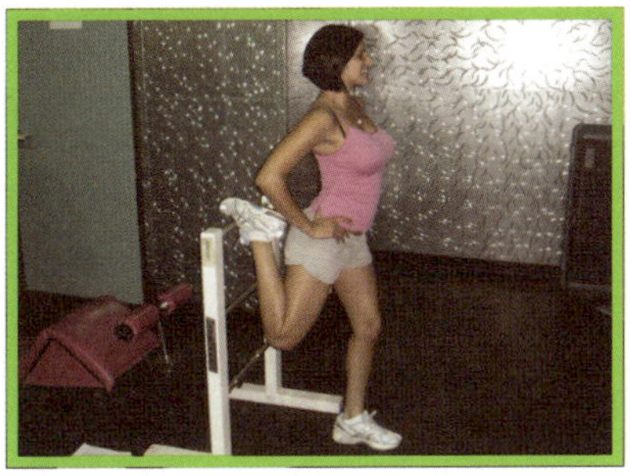

Calves

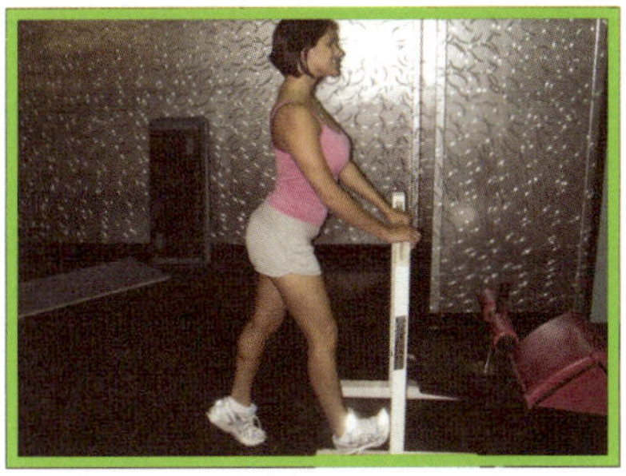

The Secrets to Success!

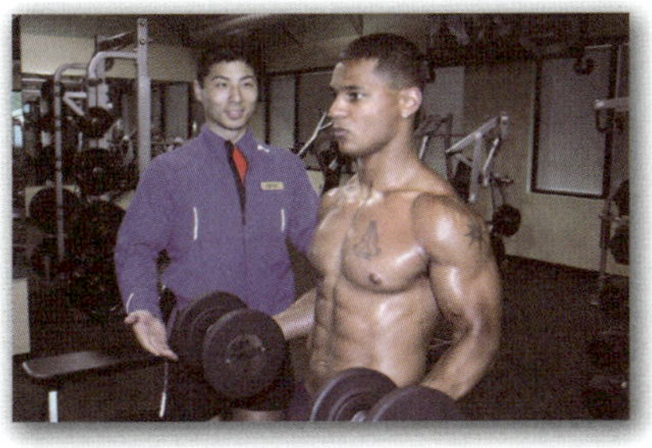

From Your Personal Trainer, Kevin Orr

Eating nutritionally correct meals frequently does not mean you can't live your life. It simply means that you have to be purposeful. Life itself will put obstacles in your way every day. If you find yourself in situations where there is absolutely nothing healthy to eat, then choose the healthier food out of all of your options and eat it in moderation. Bringing a sack lunch to a restaurant for a business meeting or going to a social event and eating nothing may be frowned upon by colleagues and friends. In this case, have fun and learn to go with the flow. Enjoy the situation. Make the best food choices you can make. Simply stick with the basics: not too full; not too hungry; simply satisfied and ready to eat your next meal in about three hours. Moderation really is the secret!

Example Weight & Cardio Routine

Continue to choose a workout routine based on your level of fitness and your schedule before progressing to Week Five. Write it down in your schedule, on page 249. If none of the example routines work for you, configure a routine that fits your needs, and write it down. Planning ahead will help you set yourself up for success.

Weight Routine 1

Sunday	Monday	Tuesday	Wednesday	Thursday	Friday	Saturday
	Legs 2x20		Chest/Back/ Shoulders 4x15		Legs: 3x20 Arms: 4x15 Abs: 4x20	

Weight Routine 2

Sunday	Monday	Tuesday	Wednesday	Thursday	Friday	Saturday
		Legs 2x20	Chest/Back/ Shoulders 4x15	Arms: 4x15 Abs: 4x20		Legs 3x20

Weight Routine 3

Sunday	Monday	Tuesday	Wednesday	Thursday	Friday	Saturday
	Legs 2x20	Chest/Back/ Shoulders 4x15	Arms: 4x15 Abs: 4x20	Legs 3x20		

Continue to choose routine 1, 2, or 3 to begin your weekly cardio routine, or rearrange your cardio training to best fit you.

Cardio Routine 1

Sunday	Monday	Tuesday	Wednesday	Thursday	Friday	Saturday
	Stepper: 15 Tread:R 15		Stepper: 15 Tread:R 15		Stepper: 15 Tread:R 15	

Cardio Routine 2

Sunday	Monday	Tuesday	Wednesday	Thursday	Friday	Saturday
		Stepper: 15 Tread:R 15	Stepper: 15 Tread:R 15	Stepper: 15 Tread:R 15		Stepper: 15 Tread:R 15

Cardio Routine 3

Sunday	Monday	Tuesday	Wednesday	Thursday	Friday	Saturday
	Stepper: 15 Tread:R 15	Stepper: 15 Tread:R 15	Stepper: 15 Tread:R 15	Stepper: 15 Tread:R 15	Stepper: 15 Tread:R 15	

Example Schedule

On your schedule, page 249, continue to write down which cardio machines along with the duration you plan to complete this week.

	Sunday	Monday	Tuesday	Wednesday	Thursday	Friday	Saturday	
Week 1 Weight: Body fat: Cardio: Duration:		226 31% EFX: 5	EFX: 10	EFX: 15	EFX: 20	EFX: 20		Why Too Tired Solution Pace Yourself
Week 2 Weight: Body fat: Weights: Sets: Cardio: Duration:		224 Chest/Back Shoulders: 2x15 EFX: 15 Tread: 15	EFX: 15 Tread: 15	Chest/Back Shoulders: 2x15 EFX: 15 Tread: 15	EFX: 15 Tread: 15	Chest/Back Shoulders: 3x15 EFX: 15 Tread: 15		Why Still too sore from Monday Solution Weight train when recovered
Week 3 Weight: Body fat: Weights: Sets: Cardio: Duration:		222 30% Arms: 2x15 Abs: 2x20 EFX: 15 Tread:R 15	EFX: 15 Tread:R 15	Chest/Back Shoulders: 4x15 EFX: 15 Tread:R 15	Arms: 3x15 Abs: 3x20 EFX: 15 Tread:R 15	EFX: 15 Tread:R 15	EFX: 15 Tread:R 15	Why Worked Over-time Solution Can you make it up another day?
Week 4 Weight: Body fat: Weights: Sets: Cardio: Duration:		220 Legs: 2x20 Stepper: 15 Tread:R 15	Chest/Back Shoulders: 4x15 Stepper: 15 Tread:R 15	Arms: 4x15 Abs: 4x20 Stepper: 15 Tread:R 15	Legs: 3x20 Stepper: 15 Tread:R 15	Stepper: 15 Tread:R 15		

Before moving on...

Did you follow through with your plan? If not, cross out what you did not complete on your schedule and write in what you did complete before moving on to the next week.

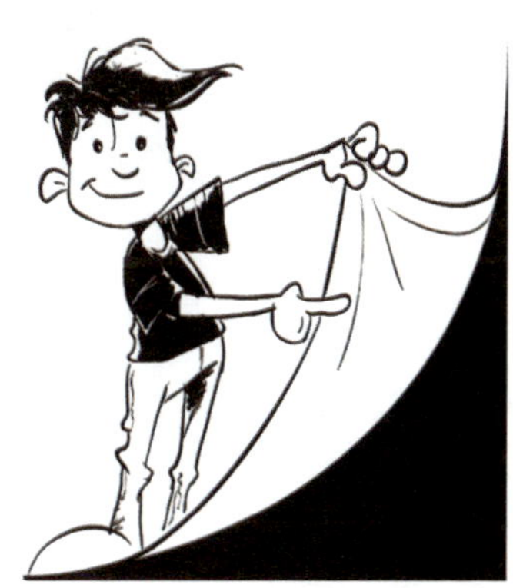

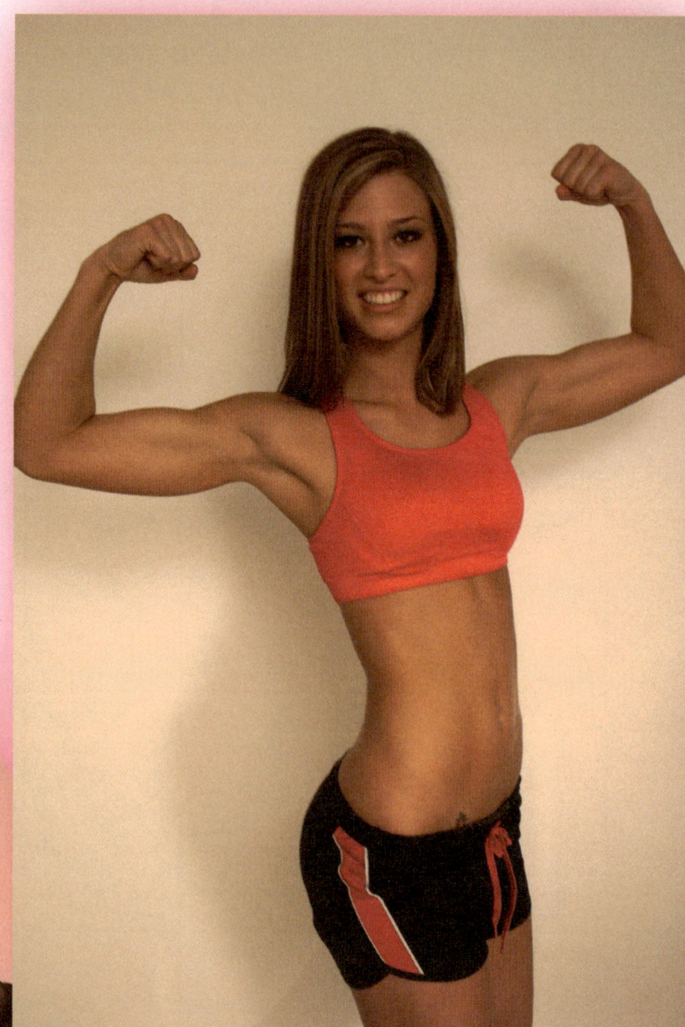

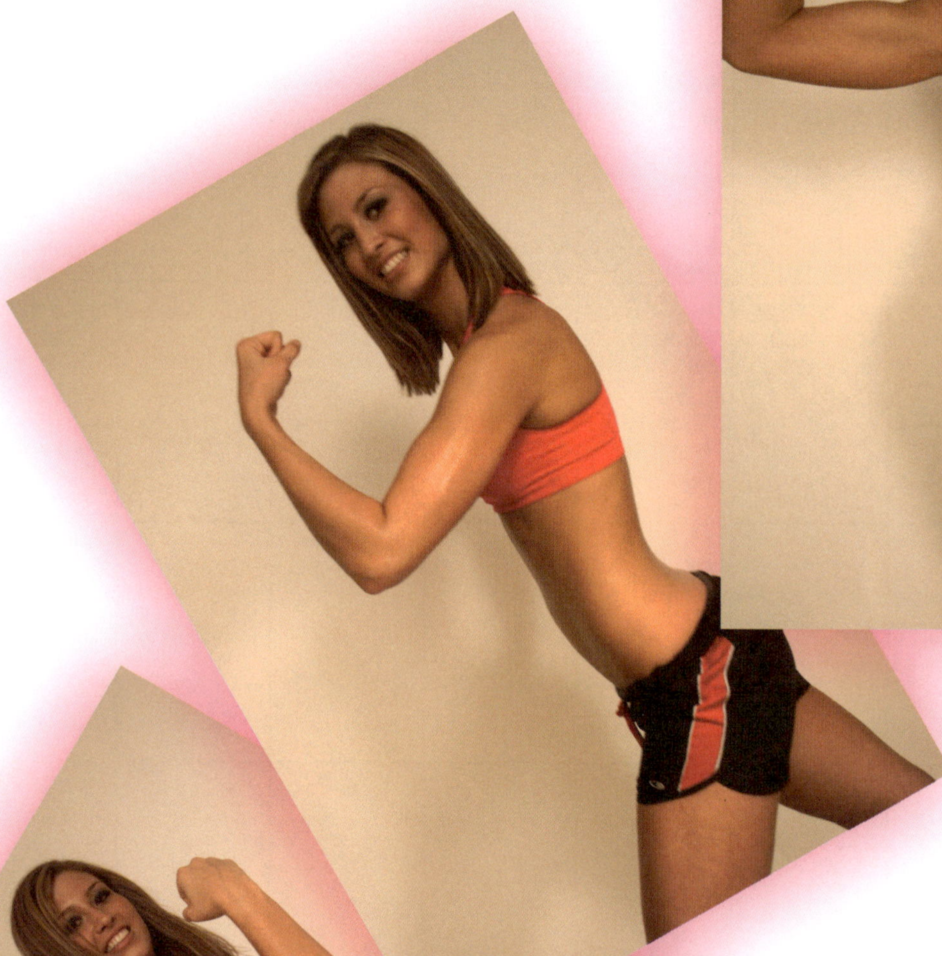

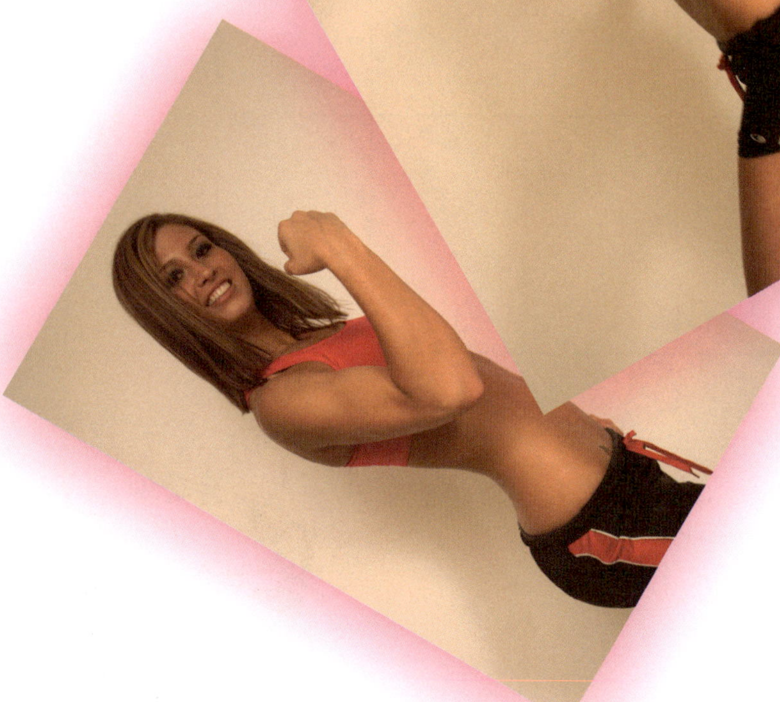

Week 5

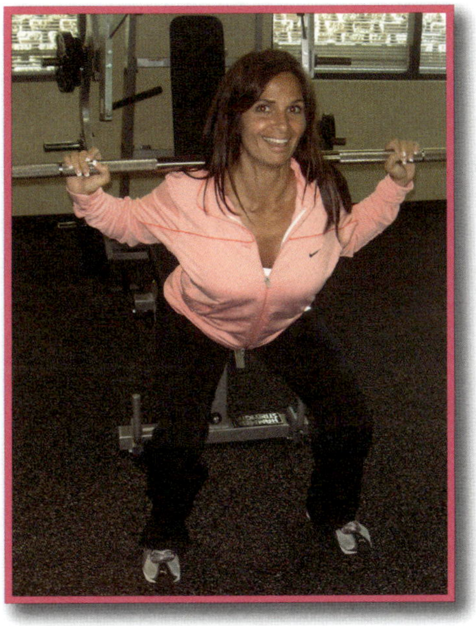

The lifestyle change with the weight training and nutrition program that Kevin provided my husband and I was a wonderful experience. The knowledge that he equips you with to continue training on your own is priceless. Whether your goal is to lose body fat, weight loss, enhance endurance, strengthen muscles, or tone up your body, Kevin provides the most natural way possible to do so. To see results in this manner and continue to maintain them is quite different than the yo-yo effect that a multitude of programs saturate our society with today.

-Hallie Kofstad

Goal:

Include a combination of proteins, fats, and carbohydrates in all of your meals and snacks.

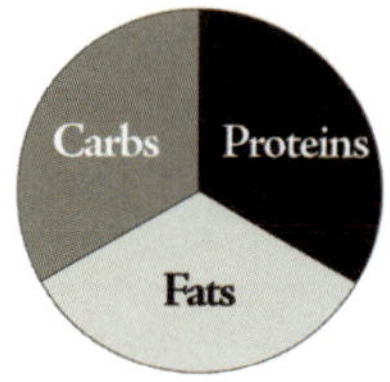

Why?

Eating the three macronutrients–proteins, fats, and carbohydrates–will further stabilize your blood sugar. As you already know, a stable blood sugar level promotes optimal energy and high metabolic rate. Eating a combination of proteins, fats, and carbohydrates balances the nutrition in your meals and snacks. Proteins and fats affect the blood sugar the least while carbohydrates cause greater fluctuations in the blood sugar, which is why it is important to include all three in each of your meals and snacks. The macronutrients balance each other out and their cumulative effect is more stabilizing than their individual effect.

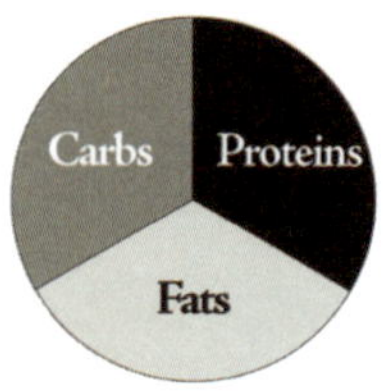

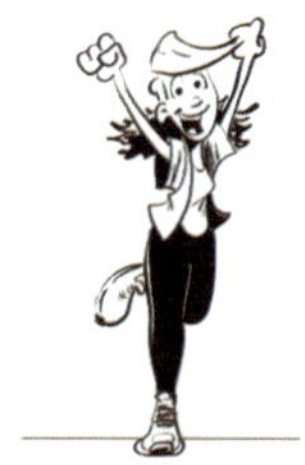

Balanced Blood Sugar = **Optimal Metabolism and Energy**

How?

Try some of the folowing healthy changes*:

Protein found in chicken, turkey, ham, fish, and lean red meat contain complete essential amino acids, B-complex vitamins, and minerals. Protein plays a key role in the repair of muscle tissue and cells. Other good protein sources are eggs, low-fat dairy products such as cottage cheese, low-fat white cheese, yogurt, and for those vegetarians: tofu. Avoid eating processed meats and cheeses as your protein source.
Recommendation: Eat protein with each meal and snack.

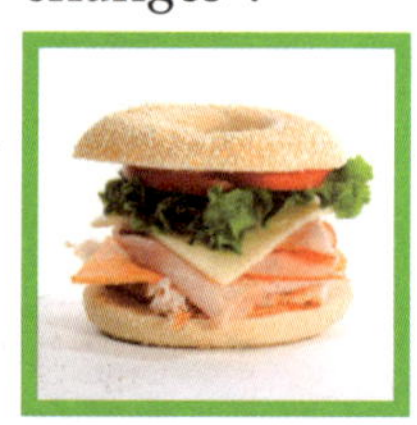 VS 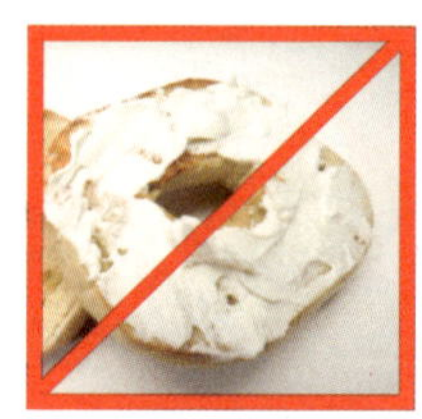

Fat, the type found in 100% natural peanut butter, most nuts, avocados, olives, and olive oil, are good fats with heart-healthy benefits.
Recommendation: Include a good fat with at least every other meal and snack.

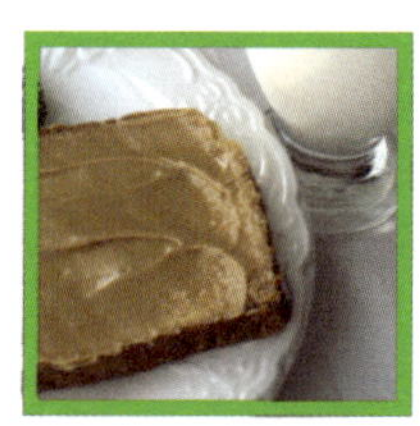 VS 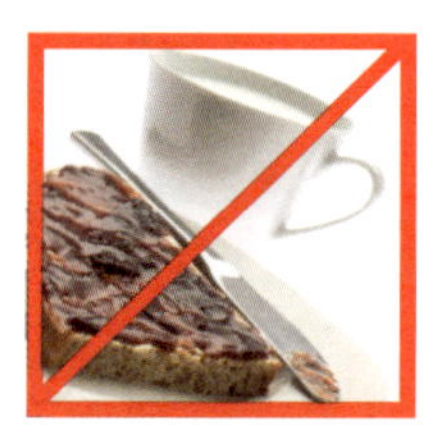

Carbohydrates, such as 100% whole wheat bread, fruits, and vegetables, are nutrient dense and provide many health benefits. These foods provide fuel for your brain and body and help your muscles recover from activities such as cottage cheese and strawberries instead of only yogurt.
Recommendation: Include carbohydrates with each meal and snack.

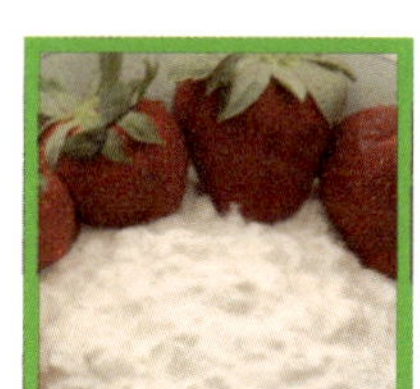 VS 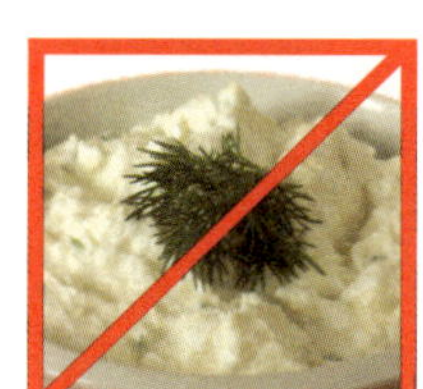

*Substitutions are based on calories per serving

Time to review your nutrition log.

1. Next to the foods you wrote down, add proteins, fats, and carbohydrates, so you include all three macronutrients in each meal and snack.

2. Keep your "better choice" food selections simple.

3. Continue to record everything you eat and drink in your nutrition log daily.

For Example:

Time	Food and Amount	Substitute
7:00 AM	WW Toast, Adam's® PB	WW toast, Adam's PB, ½ **cup cottage cheese**
10:00 AM	WW crackers, Hummus	WW crackers, swiss cheese, **lean meats e.g. turkey, chicken, tuna**
12:30 PM	Home made soup	Home-made soup with **chicken**
3:00 PM	Apple	Apple, **string cheese**
6:00 PM	Workout	Workout
8:00 PM	Salad, almonds, mixed vegetables, vinaigrette	Salad, almonds, mixed vegetables, vinaigrette, **lean meats, eggs, or cottage cheese**

WW = 100% whole wheat

Week 5

Questions and Answers

I'm not a big fan of protein-based foods. Do I have to eat protein?

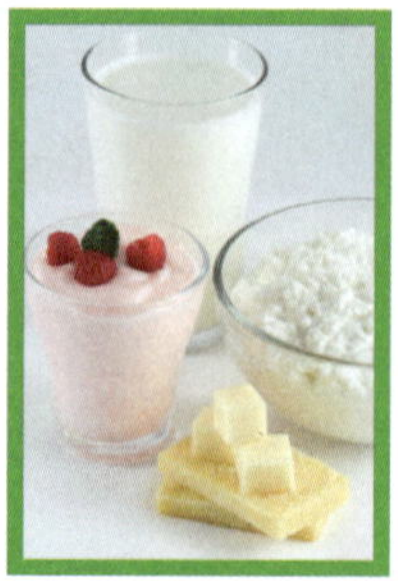

Of course! Protein is a crucial component in your nutrition plan. Your body utilizes the essential amino acids found in complete proteins for the repair, recovery, and maintenance of your muscles. Proteins are the building blocks of muscle. Each and every muscle fiber in your body consists of protein. They enable your muscles to contract and support the movement of joints, ligaments, and tendons. They are also one of the building blocks of hormones, enzymes, and your immune system. Without proteins, your body would be lacking the essential amino acids needed to build and repair your muscles. If you're not a fan of meat, try tofu and other soy-based food products.

What are good proteins?

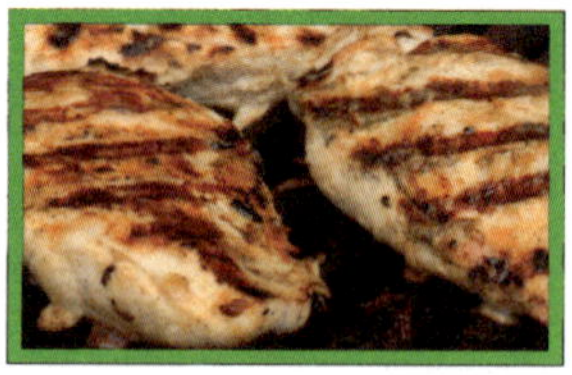

Good proteins are complete proteins such as the protein found in lean meats, eggs, and dairy products. Complete proteins contain all of the essential and non-essential amino acids required for your body to utilize for muscle recovery and repair. There is also protein in breads, nuts, and beans; however, the protein is incomplete, which means it doesn't contain all of the essential and non-essential amino acids. You can combine an incomplete protein with another incomplete protein, such as peanut butter on whole wheat bread, rice and beans, and peanuts and sunflower seeds, to make a complete protein source.

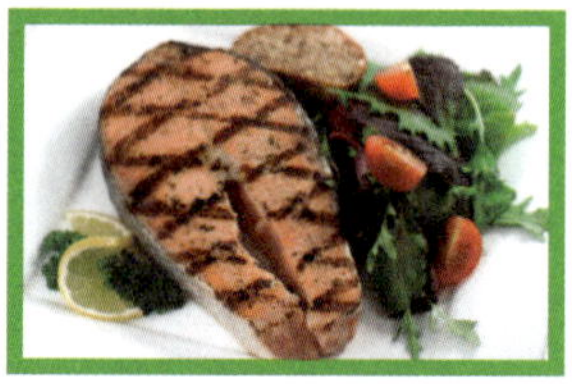

Is it possible to eat too much protein?

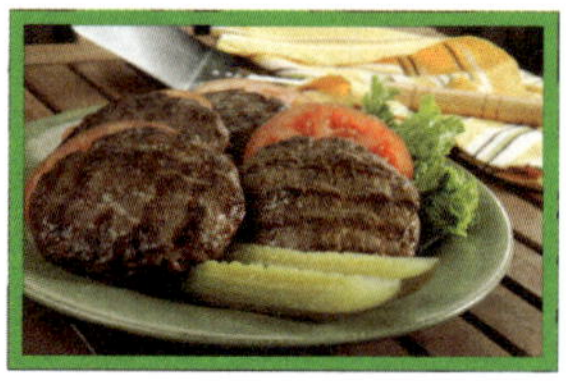

Yes, you can eat too much protein! Your body can only utilize so much protein (up to 30 grams) per meal. When you eat, your body sucks up as many proteins as it can into your muscle cells, but when they are full, they are full. Any excess protein will eventually be converted to fats and sugars. Unlike carbohydrates and fats that can be stored for later utilization as an energy source, protein is not stored for repair, recovery, and maintenance. When your primary source of calories is coming from protein, your body can use it as energy. However, it is a very inefficient energy source! Nevertheless, there is a specific time when it is OK to consume more protein, up to 45 grams of protein. This is in your post-workout meal. Your muscles are screaming for protein to optimize recovery. Keep in mind though, proteins digest at a much slower rate than carbohydrates, resulting in healthy, balanced blood sugar levels.

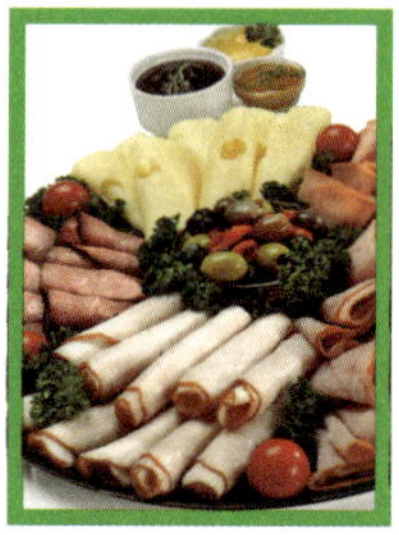

I thought all fat was bad for you.

Some fat is important for balanced nutrition. Everybody needs some fat in their diet. Fat plays a vital role in nutrient absorption, nerve transmission, and maintaining cell membrane integrity. It helps you maintain a balanced blood sugar due to its slower digestibility. Fats leave you feeling satisfied. They take much longer to digest than proteins and carbohydrates and as a result, they provide you with a sense of fullness to get you from one meal to the next. They are the main source of fuel for endurance exercise. However, there are good fats and bad fats.

What are good fats?

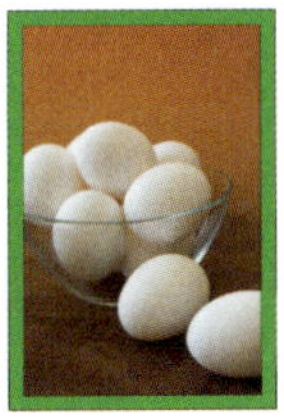

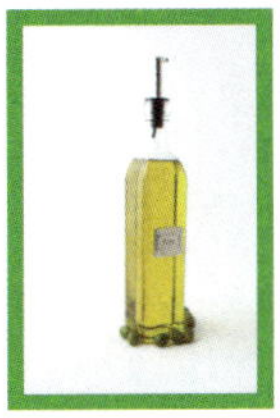

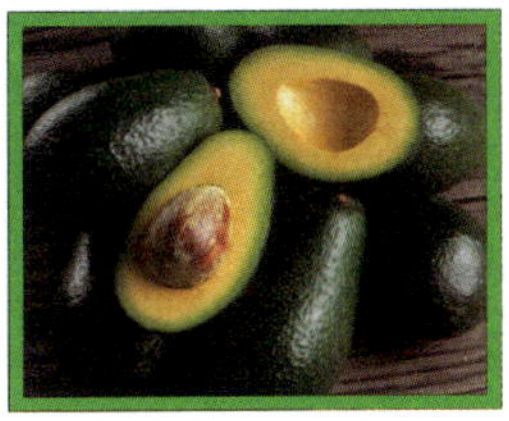

The two most common good fats are mono- and polyunsaturated fats. These fats are considered good fats because they provide a number of health benefits, like lowering cholesterol and minimizing the risk of heart disease.

Which foods contain good fats?

Monounsaturated fats are found in olive and peanut oils, peanut butter, and avocados. Polyunsaturated fats are found in sunflower, safflower, soy, sesame oils, and nuts. Some polyunsaturated fats are also known as essential fatty acids (EFAs) - omega 3 and omega 6. Like vitamins and minerals, EFAs are essential because your body does not produce them. They are vital to decreasing the risk of diabetes, high blood pressure, rheumatoid arthritis, skin conditions such as eczema and psoriasis, PMS, depression, Alzheimer's, and many other common health conditions. High amounts of omega 3 fatty acids can be found in fatty fish like salmon, mackerel, herring, sardines, and albacore tuna, fish oils, and flaxseeds and oils. High amounts of omega 6 fatty acids can be found in plant-based foods such as cereals, whole-grain breads, corn, soy, and most vegetable oils. It is also found in eggs.

Since good fats are good for you, is it possible to eat too much good fat?

You bet! Fats have more than double the number of calories per gram as proteins and carbohydrates. Regardless of where it came from, if you eat more than you need, your body is forced to store the excess calories as fat. Eat too much fat and you'll gain fat. Everybody needs fat in their diet. Fat plays a vital role in nutrient-absorption, nerve transmission, maintaining cell membrane integrity, and providing satiety. It helps you maintain a balanced blood sugar due to its slower digestibility.

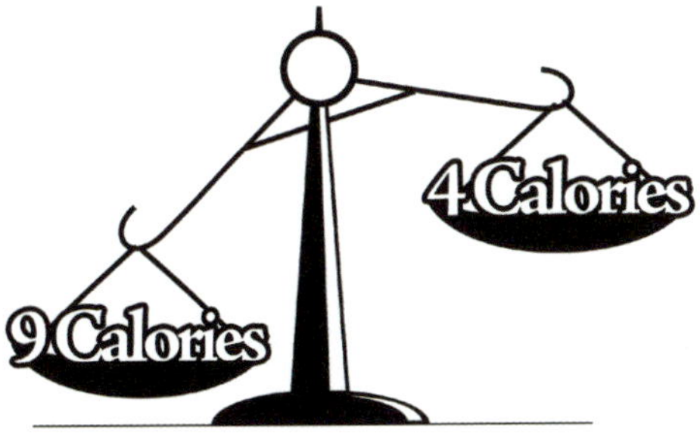

Do I have to eat carbohydrates?

Yes, carbohydrates are your body's preferred energy source. There are two types of carbohydrates: simple and complex. Proteins, fats, and carbohydrates supply your body with energy, but carbohydrates are the most efficient energy source, especially for quick bursts of activity. They provide fuel for movement, as well as mental and physical performance. Of the three macronutrients, carbohydrates affect your blood sugar the most. By fine tuning your nutrition you can keep your blood sugar balanced and under control.

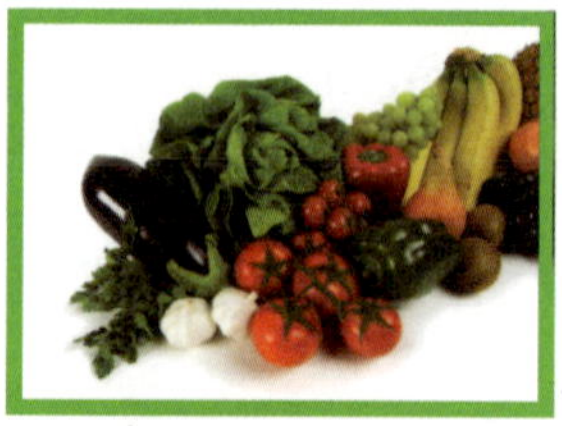

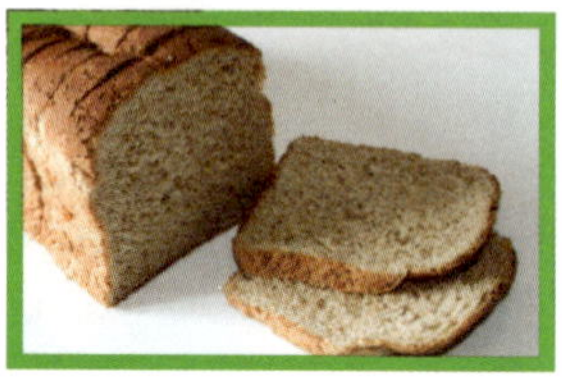

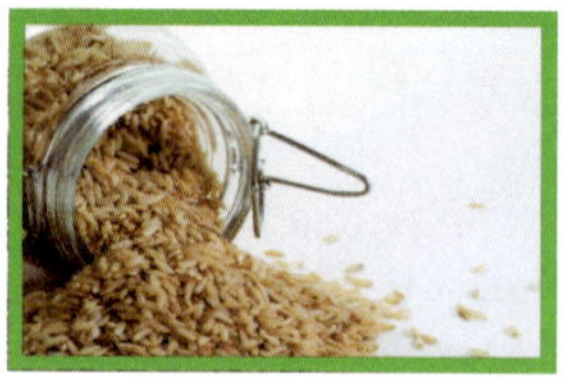

Can I eat extra carbohydrates for more energy and faster recovery?

It is possible, but be cautious when consuming extra carbohydrates. In order to successfully master your nutrition, you must be in tune with your body. If you eat too many carbohydrates, your body will not utilize the carbohydrates for energy and recovery. Instead it will store them as body fat!! However, if you eat extra carbohydrates and you are hungry at your next meal, it was the correct amount and your body will utilize the extra carbohydrates to refuel your muscles. Remember, carbohydrates have a significantly higher digestibility rate and cause the most fluctuations in your blood sugar. Your blood sugar can be stabilized if you eat a moderate amount of proteins and fats with your carbohydrates.

I came to Kevin injured, out of shape, and lost. He educated me in proper nutrition, weight and cardio training, and goal-setting, along with many other things. Without the training help from Kevin, I would be a drunken, fat couch potato. I would do anything to help repay Kevin for every thing he has done to help change my life forever.

- Jim Hicks

Kevin makes a constant effort to educate, support, and drive each of his clients to achieve goals both in the short- and long-term. The friendly smile and unassuming presence welcomes all those Kevin comes in contact with. His drive is truly inspiring! Patient, yet forceful; quiet, yet well-heard. Each and every workout session with Kevin is sure to cover all the bases: nutrition, mental attitude, fitness, and overall personal improvement. The best part of working with Kevin is knowing that he is honestly interested in helping improve lives.

- Dave Williams

Nutrition Log

Date:___________ Sun Mon Tues Wed Thurs Fri Sat		
	Plan	**Actual**
Meal 1	*Food & Amount*	*Food & Amount*
Time:______		
Meal 2		
Time:______		
Meal 3		
Time:______		
Meal 4		
Time:______		
Meal 5		
Time:______		
Meal 6		
Time:______		

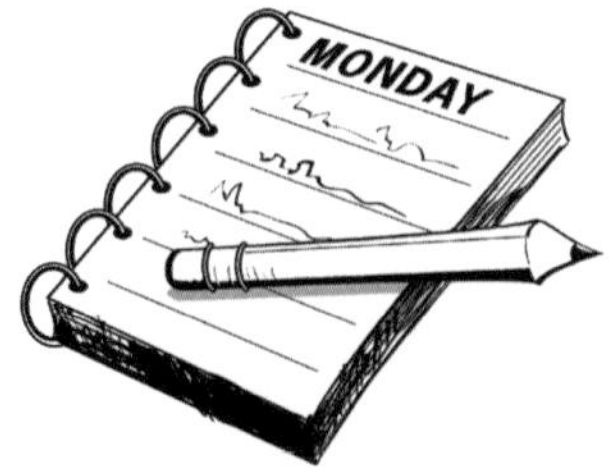

Checklist

Achieved:

- ✓ Consume meal or snack every 3 hours
- ✓ Water every 3 hours
- ✓ Sleep optimal hours
- ✓ Intake multivitamin
- ✓ Weights and cardio
- ✓ **Consume PFCs every meal or snack**

Avoided:

- ✓ Sugars
- ✓ White flour
- ✓ Processed foods

Key Points

Week 1

- Eat a small meal or snack once every three hours – five to six meals per day.
- Drink at least 1 cup (8 ounces) of water per meal and at least one cup before, during, and after your workouts.
- Keep a nutrition log.
- Sleep is vital!
- Take a multivitamin daily.

Week 2

- Avoid bad sugars.

Week 3

- Avoid white flour and white rice.

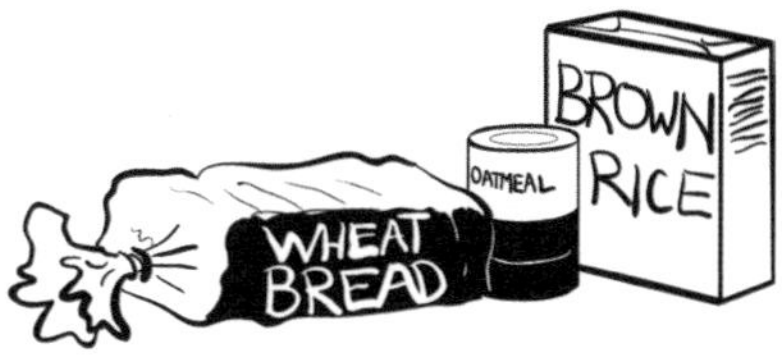

Week 4

- Avoid processed foods.

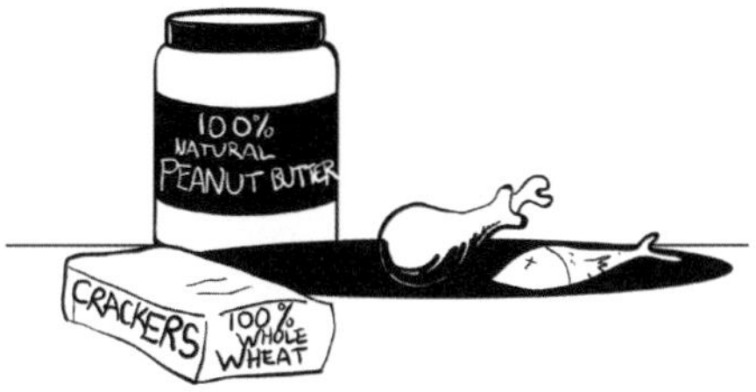

Week 5

- **Balance your meals and snacks with a combination of proteins, fats, and carbohydrates** to stabilize blood sugar levels to promote optimal energy and high metabolic rate.

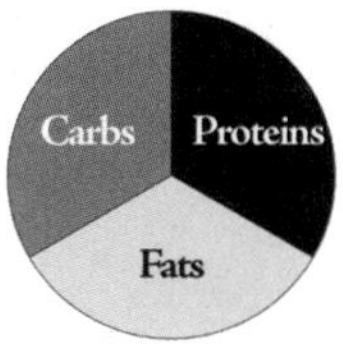

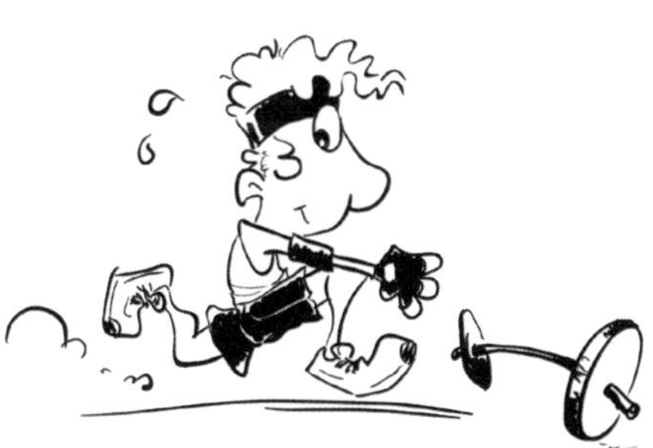

Chest

Goal:

Complete four sets of 15 reps of the **dumbbell bench press**.

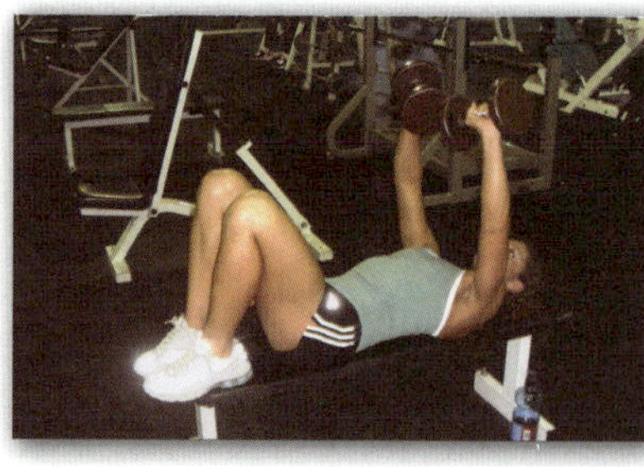

Primary
Chest

Stabilizers
Shoulders
Triceps
Forearms
Core

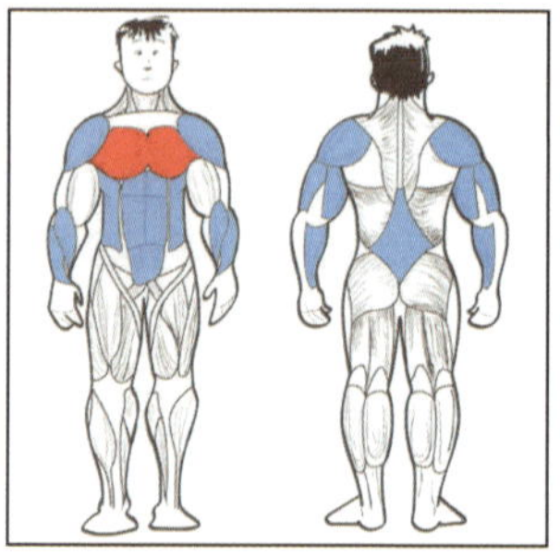

Why?

The dumbbell bench press is a free weight exercise targeting your chest. The muscle stabilizers include your shoulders, triceps, and forearms, as well as the rest of your core. Dumbbell exercises require both sides of your body to work independently in order to maintain the motion. Due to the independent movements, dumbbell motions require more stabilization than straight bar motions. In dumbbell bench press, all the stabilizers throughout your upper body are activated.

How?

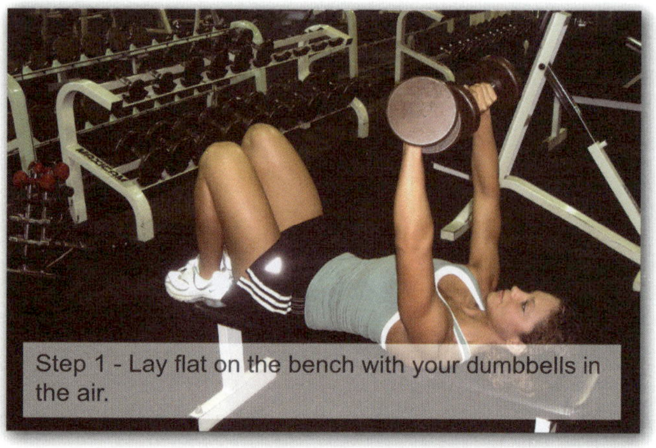

Step 1 - Lay flat on the bench with your dumbbells in the air.

Step 2 - Always squeeze your abs to assist the lower back's neutral position.

Step 3 - With a light grip, lower your dumbbells in a triangular motion.

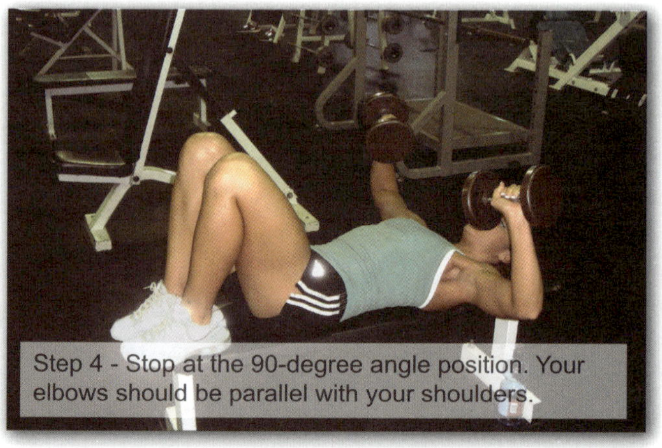

Step 4 - Stop at the 90-degree angle position. Your elbows should be parallel with your shoulders.

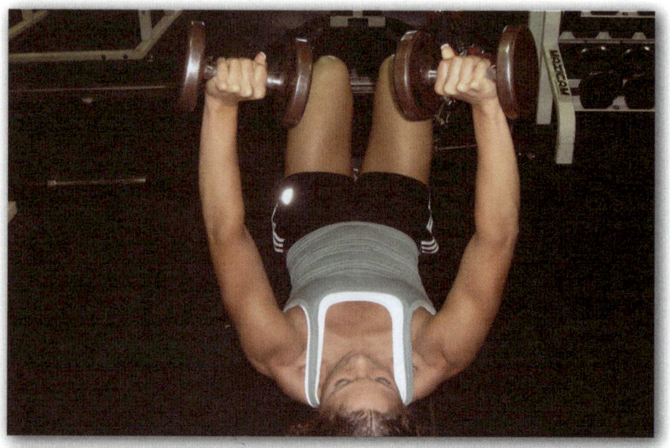

Step 5 - Push the dumbbells up in a smooth and controlled triangular motion.

Your goal is to complete four sets of 15 (4 x 15).

Range of Motion Techniques

To Maximize Muscle Tension and Minimize Overcompensation

Dos

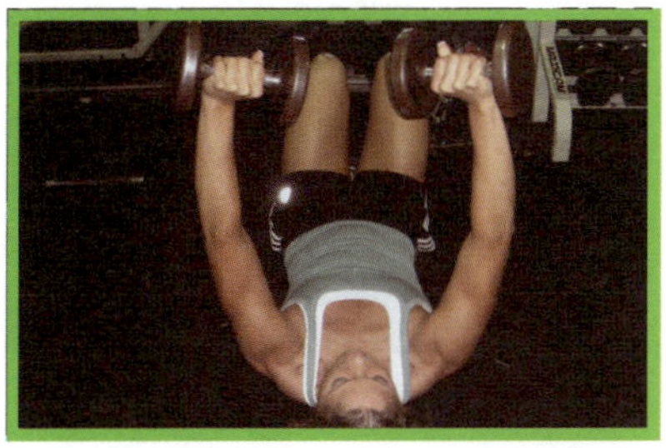

Squeeze Your Chest While Keeping Elbows Bent

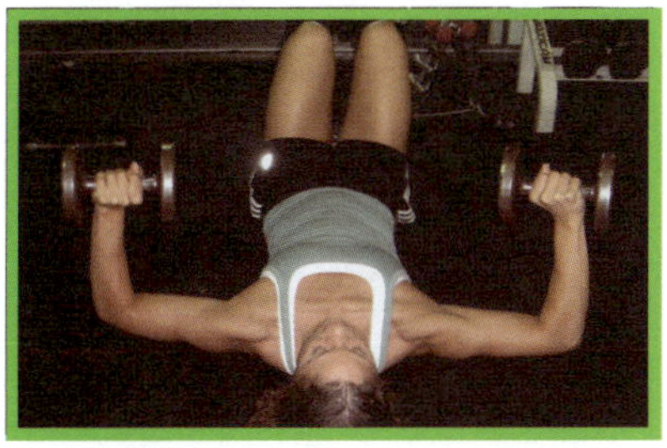

Feel Light Stretch in Chest While Elbows are Parallel with Shoulders

Don'ts

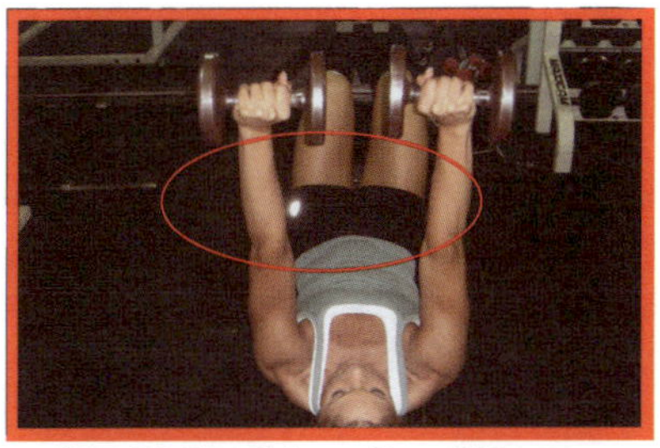

Avoid Locking Out Elbows

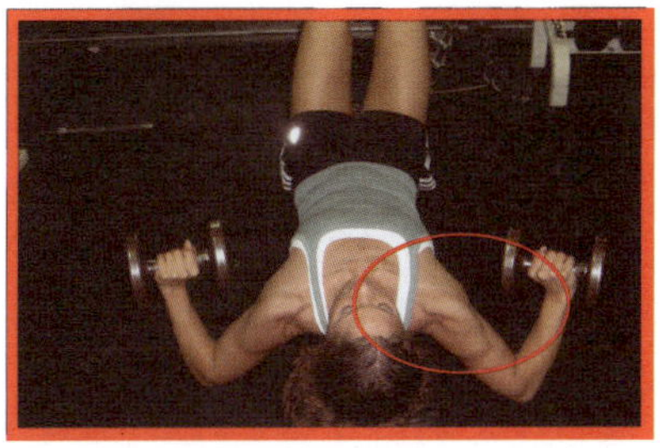

Avoid Dropping Elbows Below Shoulder Level

Visualize

"Semicircle and Cable Effect"

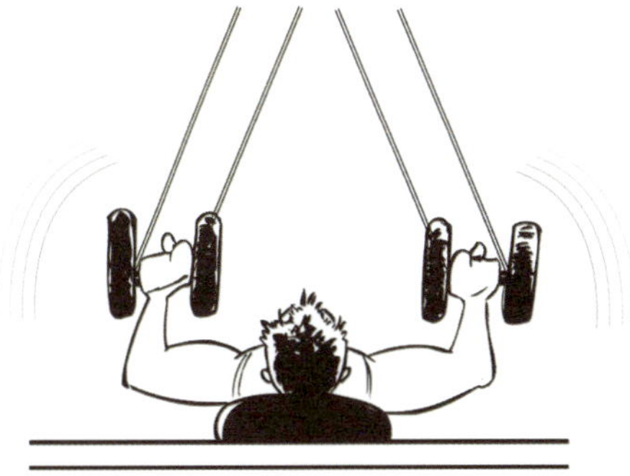

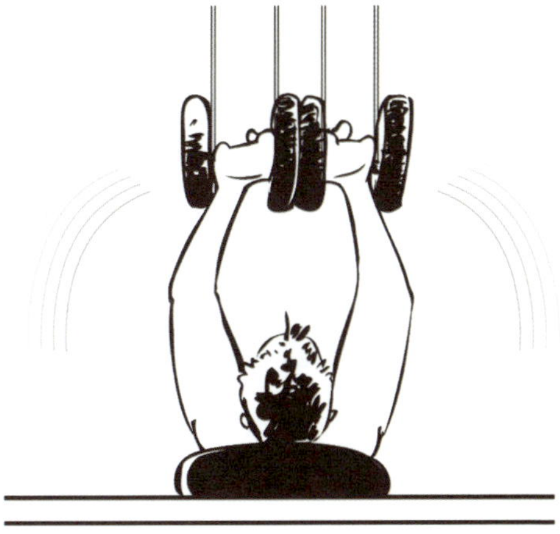

While you're lying on a bench, resist the dumbbells while lowering them down and while pushing them up. As you lower the dumbbells, focus on feeling the stretch in your chest. Squeeze and flex your chest muscles as you push the dumbbells up to your starting position.

Now, visualize a cable attached to each of your dumbbells. The cable pulls your dumbbells up and lowers your dumbbells down in a smooth semicircular motion. The semicircular motion utilizes your chest muscles more effectively, allowing you to get a better workout. Continue to visualize each rep throughout the entire range of motion.

At this stage of weight training, you may have a hard time feeling the targeted muscle group. As your muscles strengthen, it will be easier for you to feel them contract. Flexing and contracting your muscles takes practice, but the more you visualize, the easier it will become. As you discover your visualization techniques working, your goal is to stay within the proper range of motion. This will maximize the tension in your chest, minimize overcompensation, and decrease the risk of injury associated with poor technique.

Questions and Answers

Is it still important to keep my lower back flat?

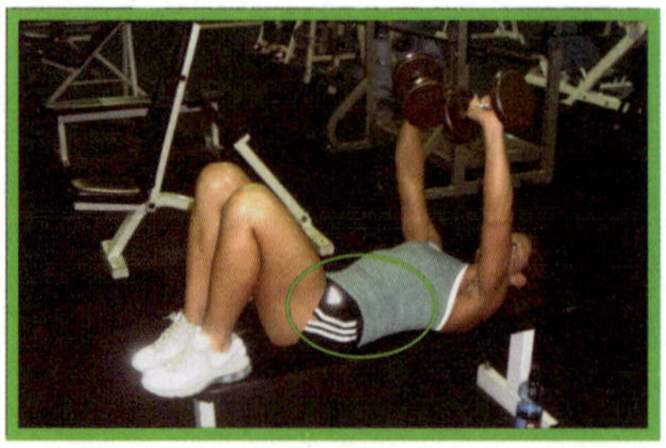

Yes. Keeping your lower back flat is very important because it relieves the pressure in your lower back, decreasing joint tension, and increasing the tension in the targeted muscle group. This means when you keep your back flat, you get a better workout. The best method for keeping your lower back flat is to squeeze your abs and place your feet on the bench.

Am I doing something wrong if I feel my shoulders burn?

Your shoulders are a stabilizer in this exercise. It is normal to feel your stabilizers burn if you are in need of more conditioning. As you get stronger, you will be able to work your chest without feeling your shoulders. Make sure to raise your dumbbells above your chest. Keeping your dumbbells aligned with your chest allows you to use more of your chest and less of your shoulders.

How fast should I perform my reps?

Again, your tempo should be two seconds down and two seconds up using a smooth and controlled motion. Since both sides of your body are having to work independently, you should expect to be more unbalanced and have less stability than you do when performing the bench press. As your stabilizers strengthen, it will be easier to stabilize yourself throughout the motion. In order to minimize your risk of injury, you need to maintain form and control. Your form is the most important, so you may have to start with a lighter weight until you get the form down. Once you have mastered the form, bump it up to a more challenging weight.

How do I practice visualization when I can't even maintain form?

Remember, visualization is the mental focus and concentration that allows you to strengthen your targeted muscles. Visualization requires practice and you may not feel your chest contract and reach the "pump" effect, yet. Of course, building some muscle does help to physically contract your targeted muscle group, so you may have to wait until you've strengthened a little more. For now, visualize maintaining control and it will come together as you maintain consistency in working out.

When can I pause on this exercise?

If you need to pause, you should pause at your starting position. Pausing is an effective way to gain control of your motion. If you are tired and beginning to lose form, pausing can also serve as a short one to two second break before ultimately fatiguing.

How do I get into my starting position without feeling awkward?

To decrease the risk of injuring your lower back and shoulders, you should always use proper technique. When lying down into your starting position, use the following steps:

1

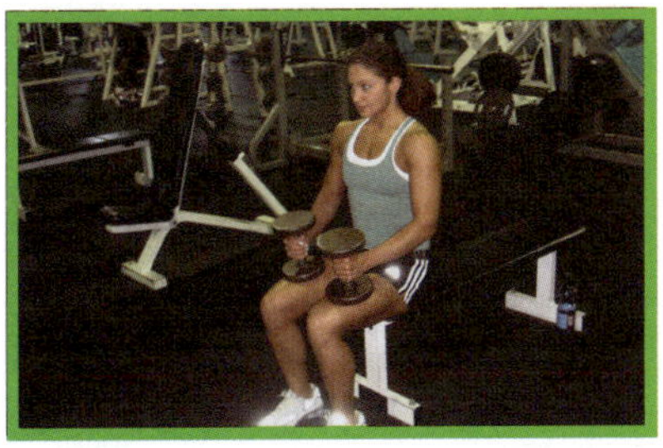

Place your dumbbells on your thighs.

2

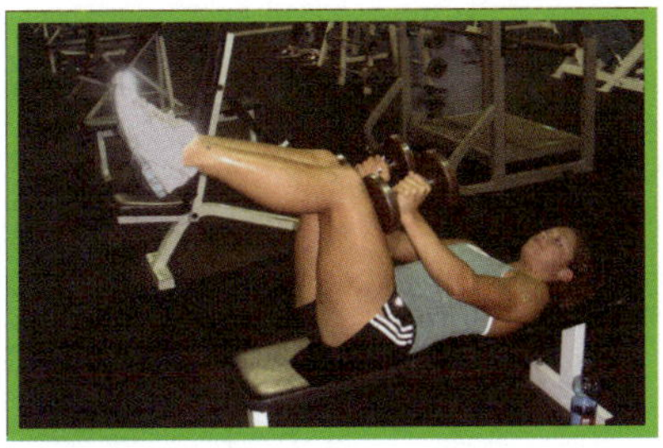

Roll onto your back, knees up, and dumbbells on your thighs.

3

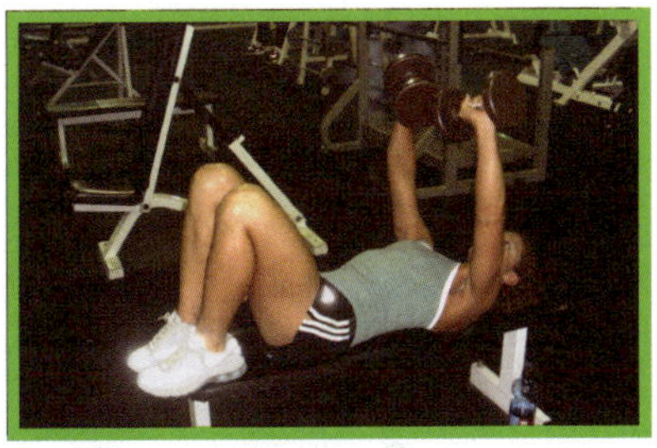

Lift the dumbbells up and position them into your starting position.

When completed with your set, place the dumbells on your thighs, and slowly roll back to a stitting position.

Why do I need to perform a triangular motion?

A triangular motion allows you to maximize the tension in your chest and minimize overcompensation of your shoulder muscles and joints. Pushing the dumbbells straight up and down is easier. It allows your shoulder muscles and joints to assist your chest in moving the weight. You should avoid allowing your shoulder muscles and joints to overcompensate for your chest. If you want to get the most effective chest workout, you'll want your dumbbells to travel in the triangular motion.

Can I do more than four sets of 15 my first time?

If you have been consistent with your weight training, then yes. You can actually perform up to six sets of 15. If you feel the need to do more than four sets of 15, you may not be working out at a high enough intensity. Be sure you're fatiguing by the end of each set. You need to challenge yourself to get results. When you lift weights without challenging yourself, you are asking for mediocre results or no change in conditioning. So, do your best to train with intensity.

How much weight should I lift?

Again, weight varies from person to person when building a foundation of conditioning. Your goal is to complete four sets of fifteen reps. You should be fatigued by the end of each set. Use the following to determine the amount of weight you should be lifting:

• The first set should be a warm-up. It should be easy to achieve your first set of fifteen reps. Warming-up lubricates your joints, ligaments, and tendons in preparation for higher intensity exercise.

• The second, third, and fourth sets should be at a higher intensity. You can bump up your intensity by increasing the weight or performing more reps. Lift enough weight to fatigue by the fifteenth rep and do not forget to use proper form. If you're not fatigued by the fifteenth rep, you'll need to increase the weight for your next set or next workout. Remember, you will have to challenge yourself if you want to see results.

Back

Goal:

Complete four sets of 15 reps of **lat row**.

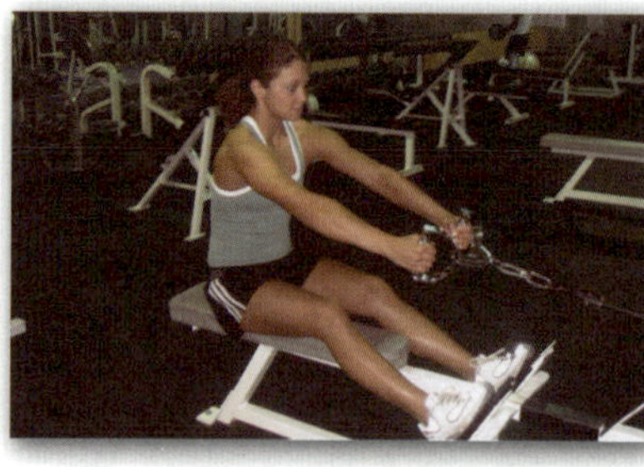

Primary
Lats

Stabilizers
Shoulders
Traps
Biceps
Forearms
Core

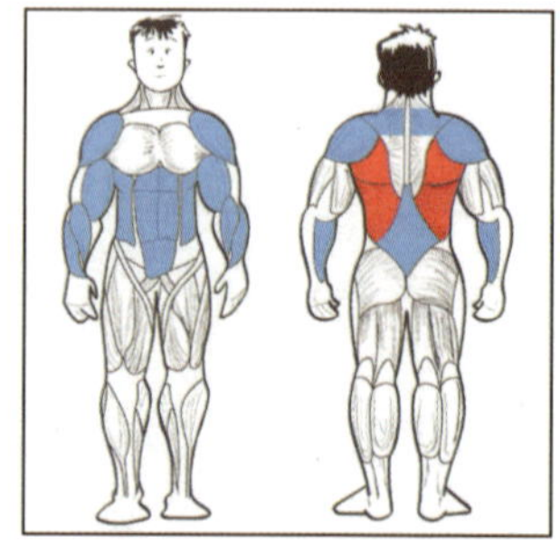

Why?

The lat row is an exercise machine that targets your lats. The muscle stabilizers include your shoulders, traps, biceps, and forearms, as well as the rest of your core. Lat row strengthens your back from a different angle than the lat pulldown. As you continue to work out, training variety will become very important. If you perform the same exercises at the same intensity, your body will adapt to the exercise and you will no longer get results. To continue to see great results, you will want to work the same muscles in a variety of different ways. The lat row is great for training variety.

How?

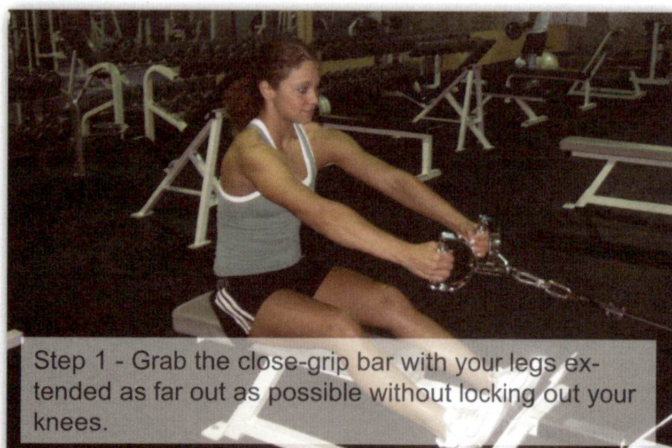

Step 1 - Grab the close-grip bar with your legs extended as far out as possible without locking out your knees.

Step 2 - Squeeze your abs to push your lower back into a neutral position.

Step 3 - Begin with a light grip and your elbows unlocked and slightly flared out.

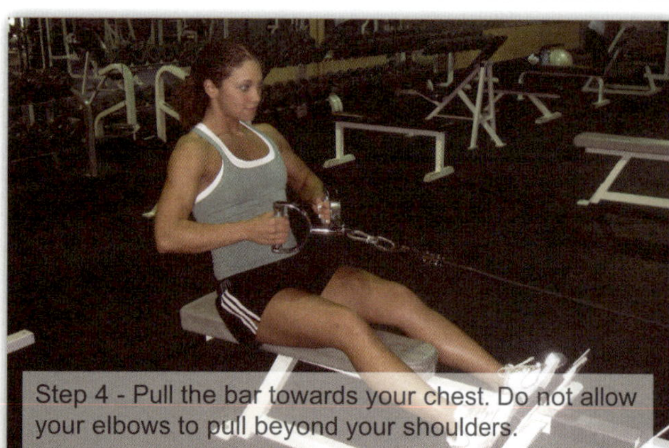

Step 4 - Pull the bar towards your chest. Do not allow your elbows to pull beyond your shoulders.

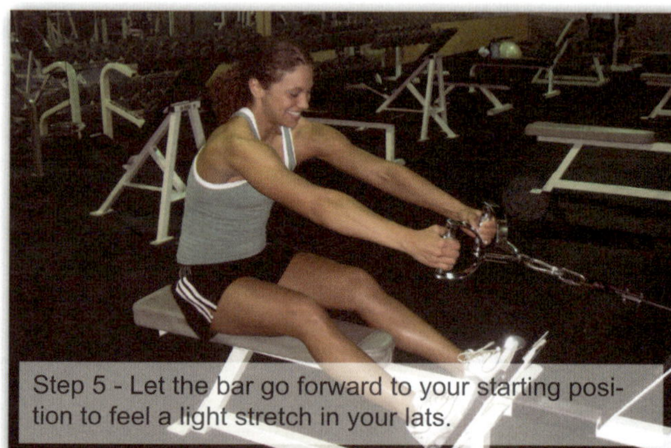

Step 5 - Let the bar go forward to your starting position to feel a light stretch in your lats.

Step 6 - Repeat using a smooth and controlled motion to maximize the tension in your lats.

Your goal is to complete four sets of 15 (4 x 15).

Range of Motion Techniques

To Maximize Muscle Tension and Minimize Overcompensation

Dos

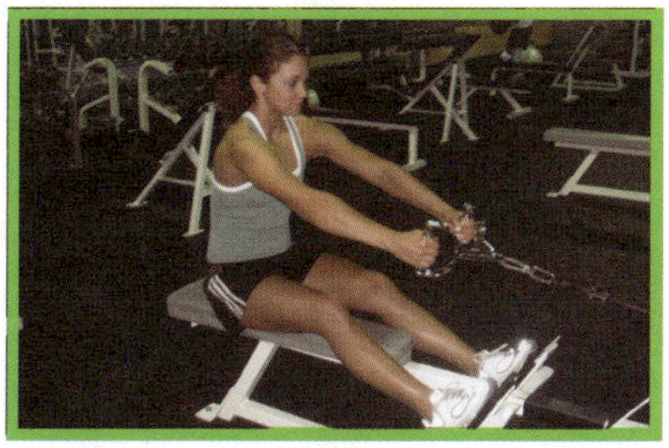

Stretch Lats While Keeping Elbows Bent

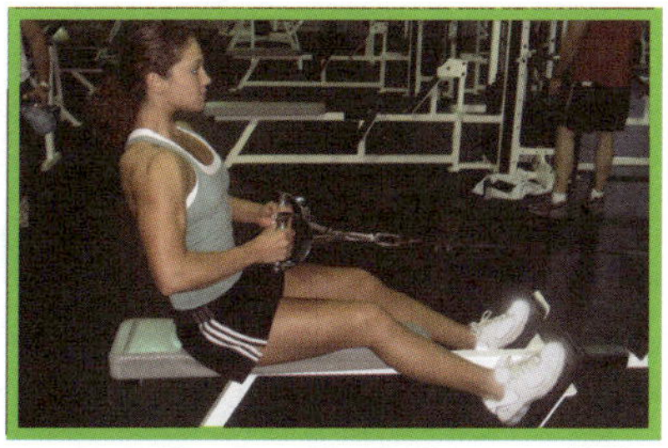

Keep Elbows Slightly Parallel with Shoulders

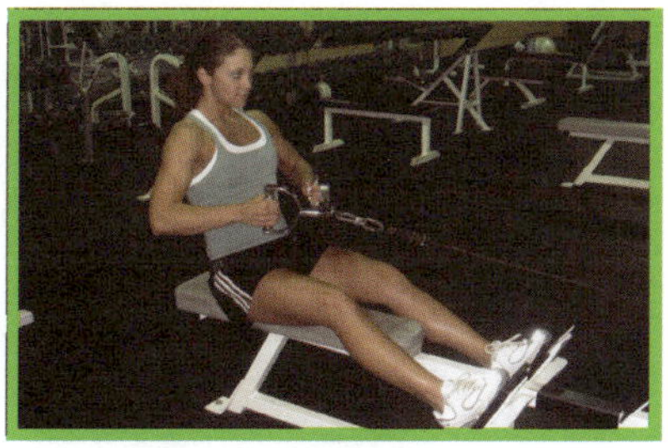

Maximize Lat Tension When Elbows Flared Out

Don'ts

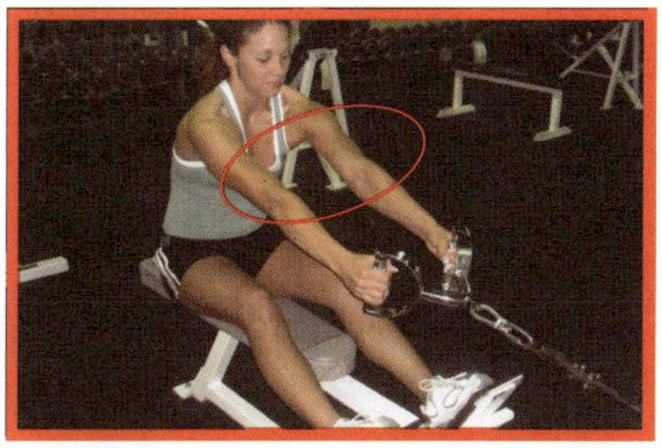

Avoid Locking Out Elbows

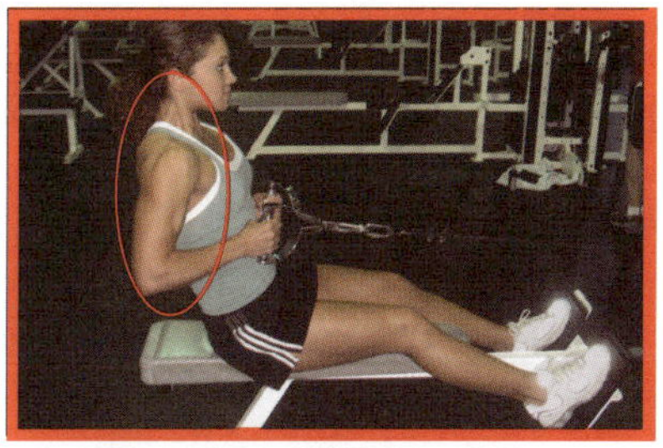

Avoid Pulling Elbows Beyond Shoulders

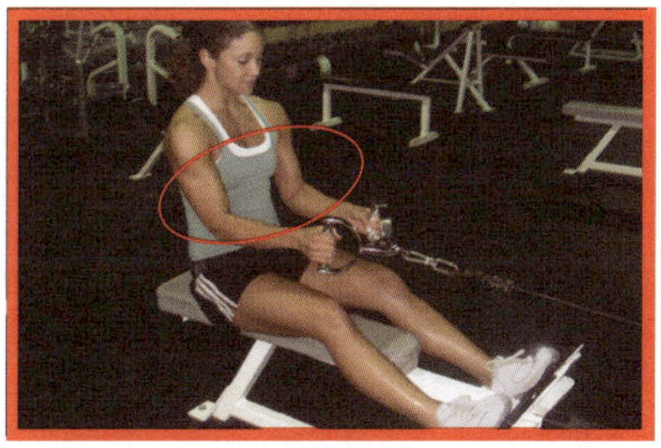

Avoid Pulling Elbows Together

Visualize

"Flare, Stretch, and Hook Effect"

Feeling the targeted muscle group stretch and contract is essential for an effective workout. The lat row is one of the most difficult exercises to feel your lats. That being said, you may be wondering why you should perform this exercise? Well, in short, the lat row provides variety for your lats and variety is the key to your training progression.

When seated in your starting position, imagine flaring out your lats, making your upper back look as wide as possible. Your elbows are pointed outward and your upper back is rounding out. Keeping your lats flared, pull the close-grip bar toward your chest to your peak contraction. Resist the weight as it pulls forward and focus on feeling the stretch in your lats. Also, imagine your hands are a hook, lightly holding the close-grip bar as you complete each rep.

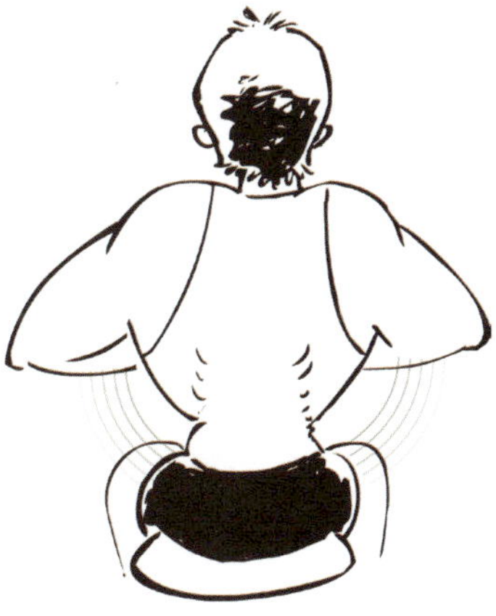

Continue to visualize your lats flaring outward and stay within the proper range of motion. This will maximize the tension in your lats and minimize the use of your biceps, wrists, and forearms.

Questions and Answers

I thought I was supposed to have an arch in my lower back! Isn't that correct form?

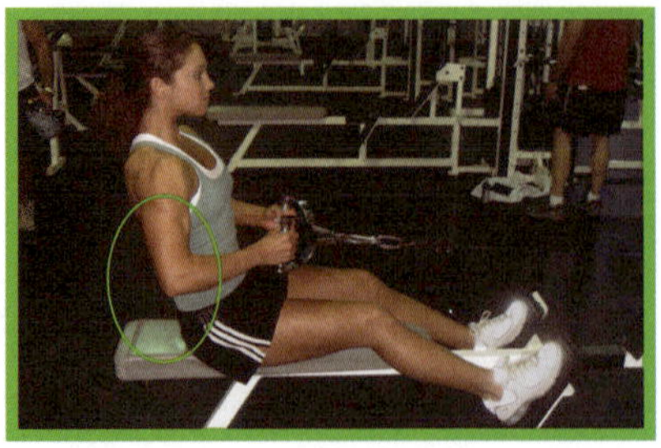

When your lower back is in an arched position, you are placing extra tension in your lower back joint. When your lower back is in a neutral position, it relieves the pressure in your lower back forcing your lats to do the work. Proper form decreases joint tension and increases muscle tension.

Can I pull the bar beyond my shoulders?

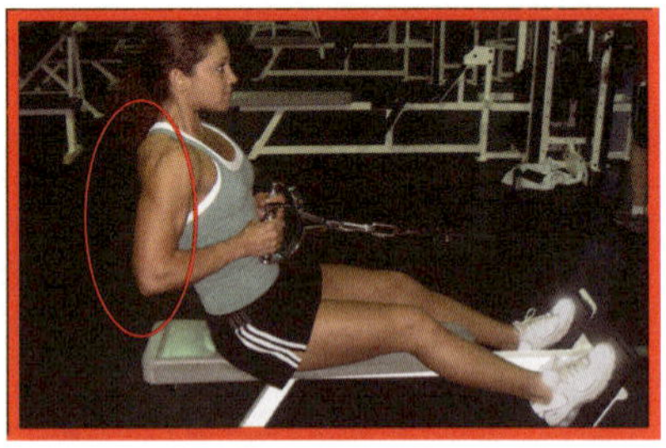

Your goal in performing this exercise is to work your lats. If you allow your elbows to pull past your shoulders, you are pulling beyond your peak contraction. This means that the tension and pressure will shift to other muscles and joints, allowing your lats to relax. When your lats are relaxed, it forces your shoulders, traps, biceps, and forearms to overcompensate. Overcompensation reduces the effectiveness of your workout. It allows you to work more of your stabilizers and less of your targeted muscle group.

Why do I need to feel a stretch in my lats?

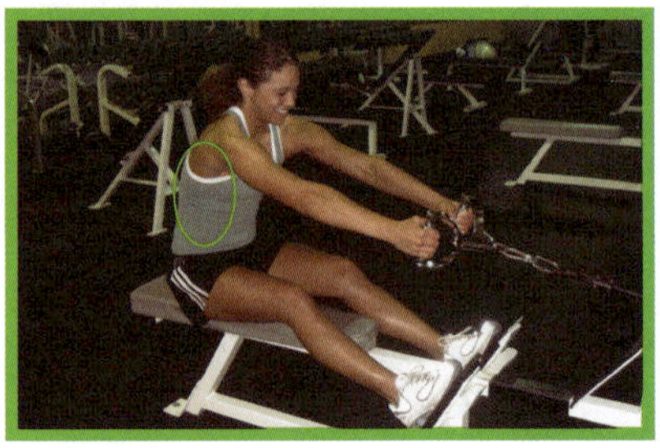

Feeling a stretch in your lats is the key in knowing whether your lat muscles are resisting. The lat row is the most difficult exercise to feel your lats. Feeling the stretch will take practice and some conditioning. As you get stronger and you become more aware of your body, it will be easier to feel the stretch and contraction of your muscles. If you can't feel the stretch in your lats, your lats are probably not resisting the weight. If your lats are not resisting, your shoulders and forearms are overcompensating.

How do I hold onto the close-grip bar?

Lightly hold the bar. Allow your thumbs to wrap around the bar to secure your wrists. Wrist stability helps to keep the wrists strong. Gripping too tightly increases wrist joint tension and allows your forearms and other stabilizers to overcompensate.

I still feel my biceps when my elbows are flared out. Why?

Your elbows should flare out for maximum lat contraction. If your elbows are flaring out too much, your biceps will overcompensate. As you already know, overcompensation leads to increased risk of injuries and reduces the effectiveness of your workout. Experiment with your elbow position to feel the most tension in your lats. The positioning is a little different for everyone.

Why is leaning back and swinging to pull the bar back incorrect?

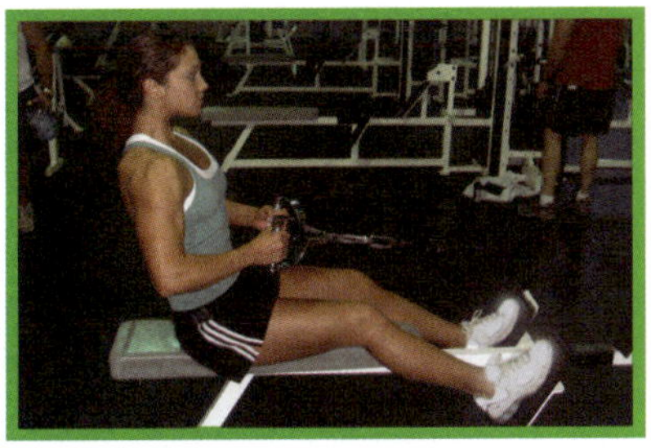

Leaning back and swinging emphasizes momentum and lower back tension. This allows your lower back to do the work of pulling the bar back instead of your lats. In order to get the most effective lat workout, you need to reduce lower back tension, momentum, and stabilizer utilization. Focus on keeping your lower back in a neutral position. This reduces overcompensation and forces your lats to do the work of pulling the bar back.

What If I don't feel my lats stretch?

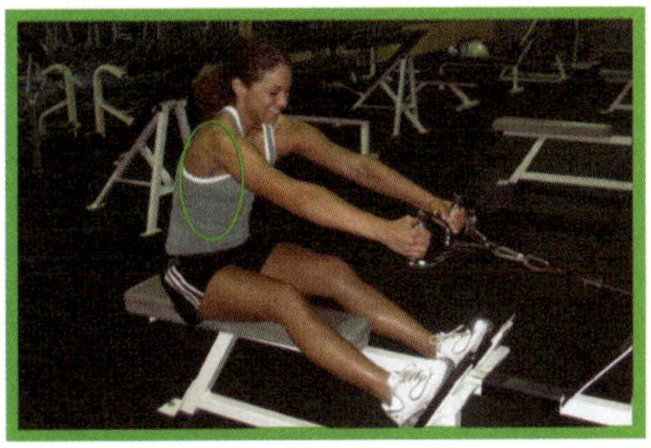

As you already know, feeling the stretch in your lats ensures that your lats are resisting the weight. This is very important. In order to feel your lats stretch, you need to lean forward enough to feel the weight pull on your lats. As you lean forward, you may also feel your lower back muscles. This means you are increasing your lower back strength. Remember, keep your grip light. Gripping too tightly will allow your forearms to overcompensate. If your forearms are resisting it will be even more difficult to feel the stretch in your lats.

Shoulders

Goal:

Complete four sets of 15 reps of the **dumbbell shoulder press**.

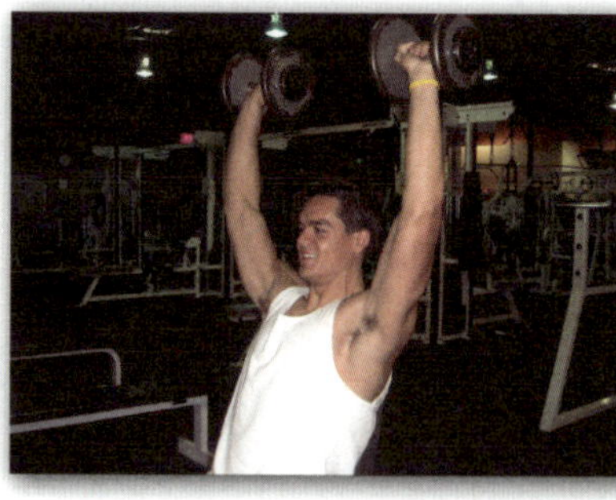

Primary
Shoulders

Stabilizers
Triceps
Forearms
Core

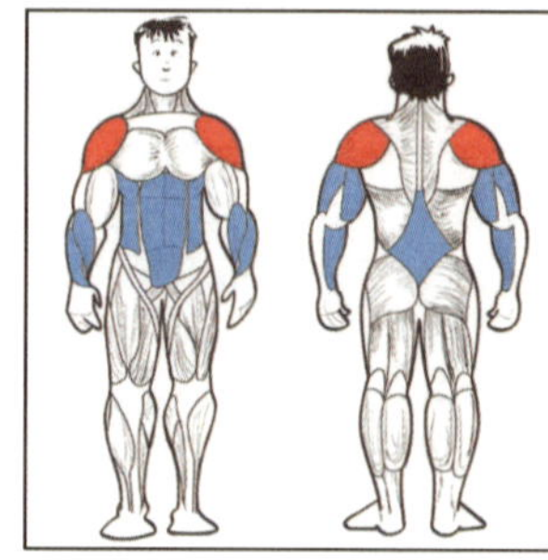

Why?

The dumbbell shoulder press is a free weight exercise targeting your shoulders. The muscle stabilizers involved include your triceps and forearms, as well as the rest of your core. This exercise improves your overall strength and conditioning by challenging your stability and balance. The dumbbell shoulder press is higher in intensity than the machine shoulder press because it requires more strength and stability to guide the press motion.

How?

Step 1 - Adjust the seat and lower back support, so your legs are parallel with the floor.

Step 2 - Squeeze your abs to push your lower back into a neutral position against the pad.

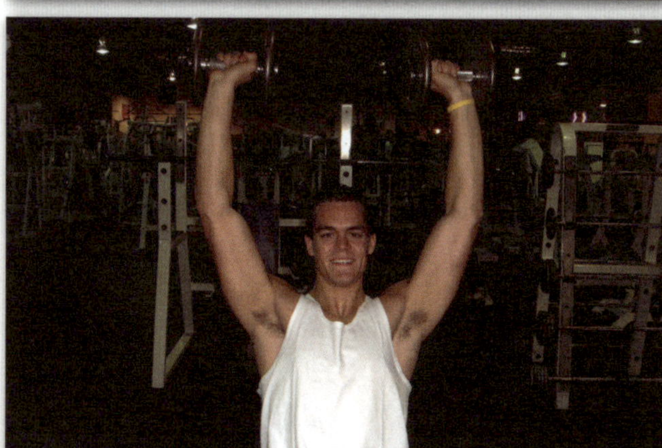

Step 3 - Push the dumbbells up as high as possible until your elbows nearly lock out. This is your starting position.

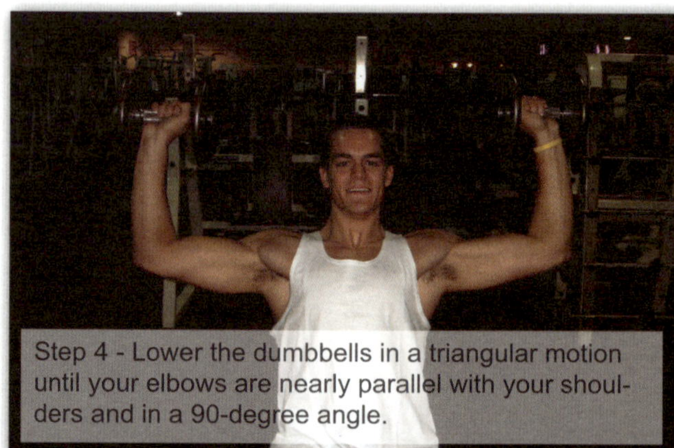

Step 4 - Lower the dumbbells in a triangular motion until your elbows are nearly parallel with your shoulders and in a 90-degree angle.

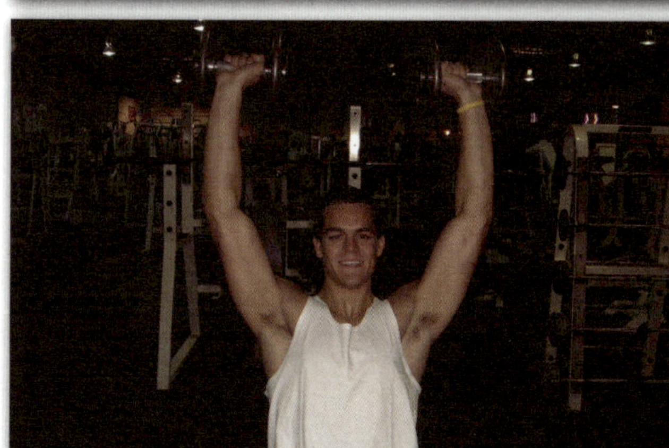

Step 5 - Push up in a controlled, smooth motion to complete one rep.

Your goal is to complete four sets of 15 (4 x 15).

Range of Motion Techniques

To Maximize Muscle Tension and Minimize Overcompensation

Dos	Don'ts
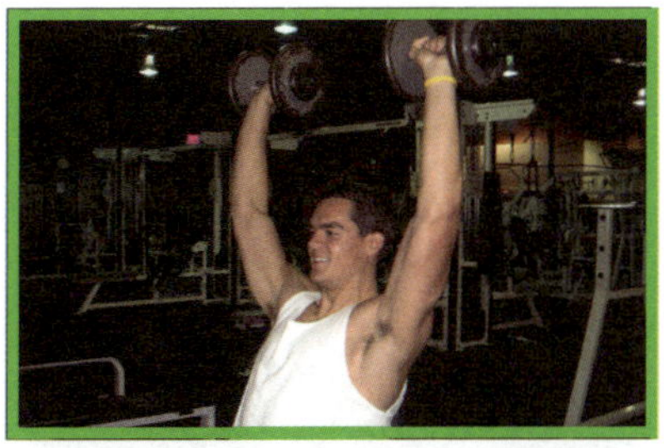 Begin with Elbows Bent	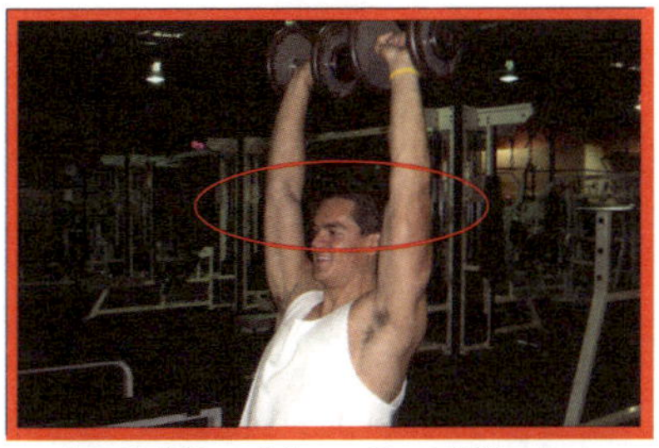 Avoid Locking Out Elbows
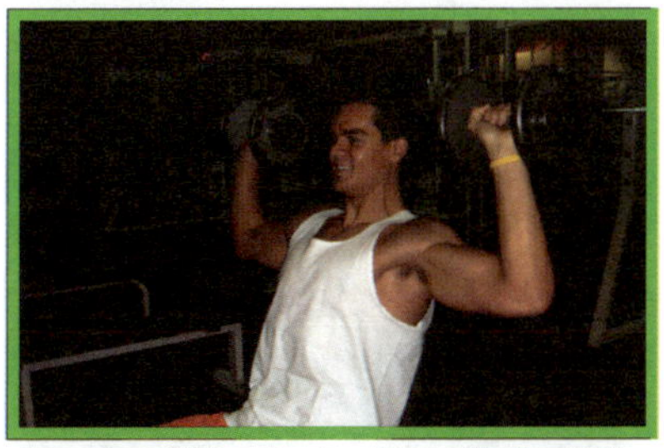 Lower Elbows to Parallel with Shoulders	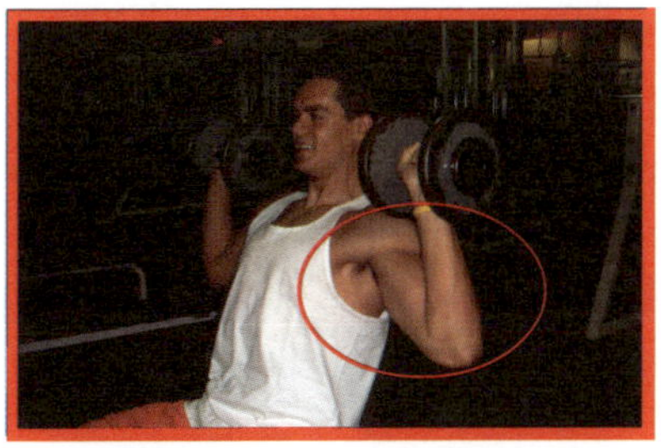 Avoid Dropping Elbows Below Shoulders
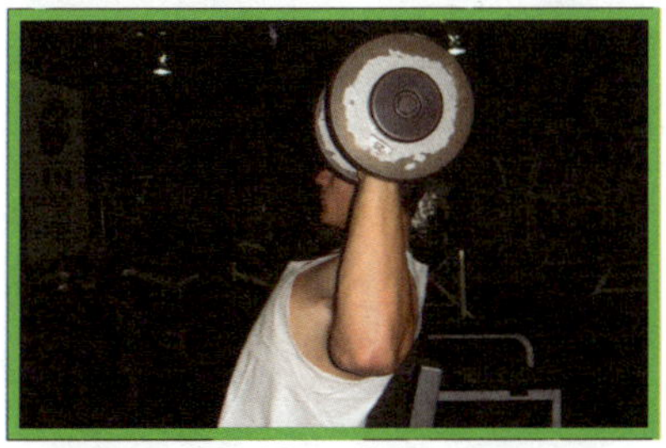 Maximize Shoulder Tension When Elbows are Vertical and Lower Back is Flat	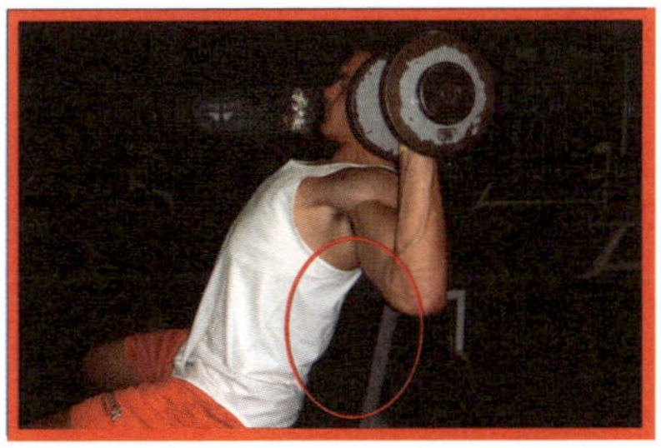 Avoid Arching Lower Back

Visualize

"Semicircle and Cable Effect"

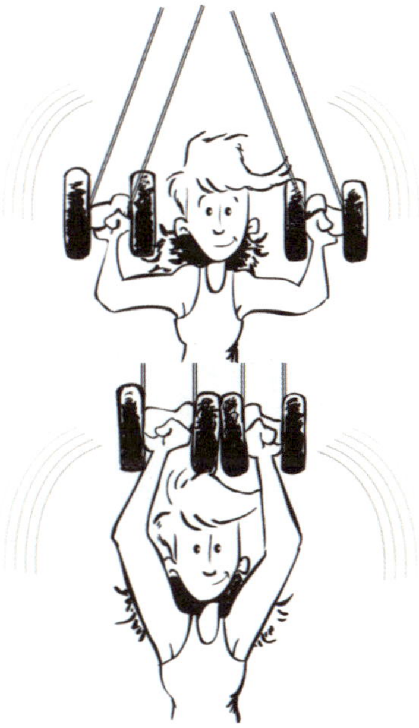

When performing the dumbbell shoulder press, resist the dumbbells as you lower them down and push them back up. Visualize completing a semicircular shape as you lower the dumbbells down. Focus on feeling the stretch in your shoulders by pulling your dumbbells apart before pushing them up.

Visualize a cable attached to each of your dumbbells. The cables are pulling them up in a semicircular shape. As you push the dumbbells up, imagine your hands touching together in your starting position.

Visualize every rep and stay within the proper range of motion. Practicing visualization will allow you to maximize the use of your shoulders and get the most effective workout. This reduces the use of your stabilizers and decreases your risk for injury.

Questions and Answers

I have a hard time keeping my back flat. Is this important?

Yes! Keeping your back flat relieves pressure in your joints, reduces overcompensation, and forces your shoulders to do the work.

Can I perform shoulder press with a full range of motion?

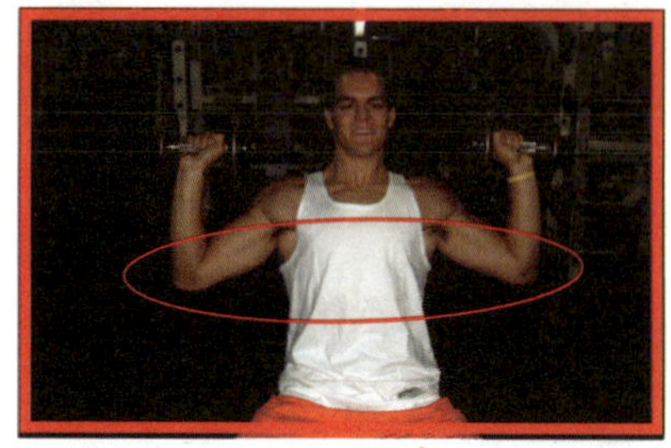

A full range of motion allows you to overcompensate with other muscles and joints. Lowering your elbows below your shoulders places unnecessary strain in your shoulder joints increasing your risk of injury and encouraging forearm overcompensation. Your goal is to maintain a safe range of motion while targeting your shoulder muscles.

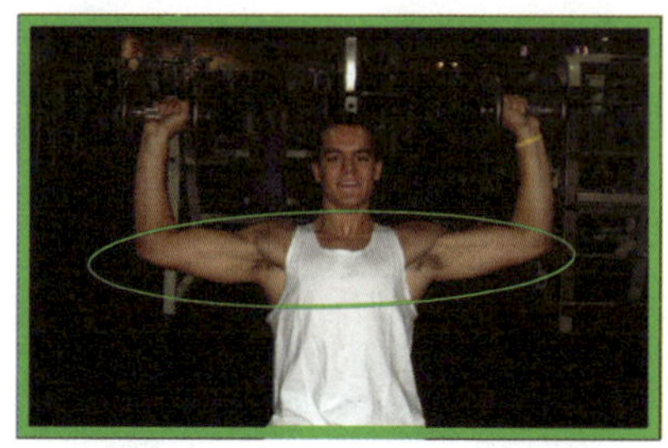

Where should my elbows be in this motion?

When performing the dumbbell shoulder press, your elbows should be in a vertical position throughout the motion. You may feel like your elbows are slightly forward when maintaining the correct position.

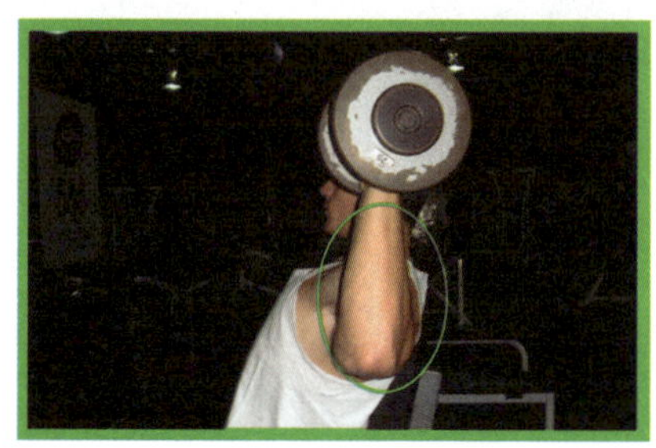

How do I get into my starting position without feeling awkward?

To reduce the risk of injuring your shoulders and lower back when lifting dumbbells into your starting position, use the following procedures:

1

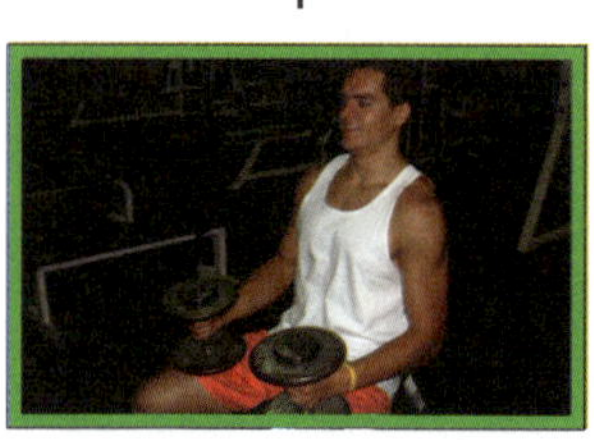

Place your dumbbells on your thighs

2

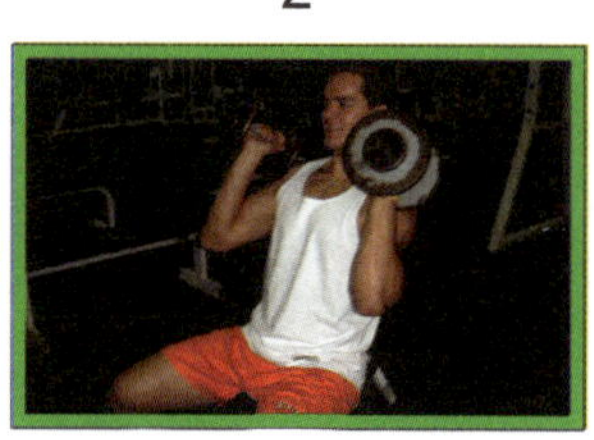

Lift the dumbbells on or close to your shoulders

3

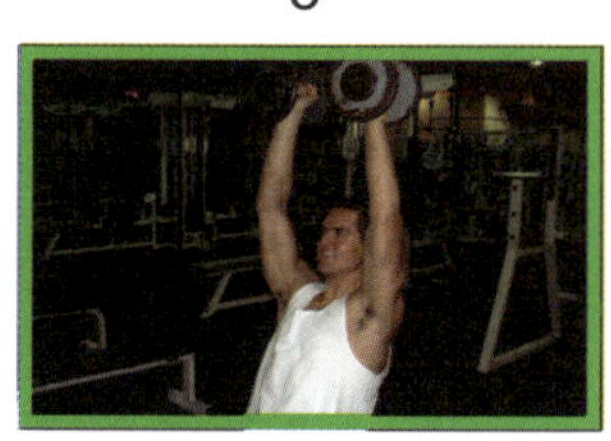

Lift the dumbbells up and place them into your starting position

4

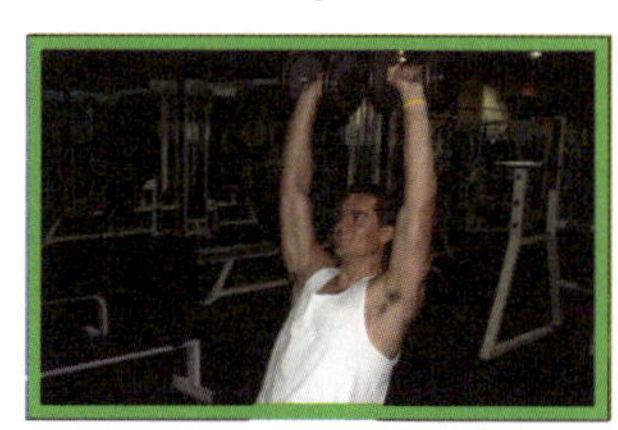

Turn your dumbbells, so your palms are facing forward

Why do I need to perform a triangular or a semicircular motion?

Dumbbell shoulder press is similar to dumbbell bench press. If you want to maximize the tension and contraction of your shoulders, you'll want your dumbbells to travel in the triangular or semi-circular motion. Pushing the dumbbells straight up and down is less effective in maintaining the tension in your shoulders and places unnecessary pressure in the shoulder joints.

Can I weight train with the two exercises I've learned and perform four sets each?

Weight training the same muscle groups with two different exercises and four sets each is not the most ideal weight training routine for foundation training. Foundation training prepares you to progress toward your next goal, whether that be body fat loss, strength, or endurance. Without a solid foundation, it would be difficult to achieve these goals.

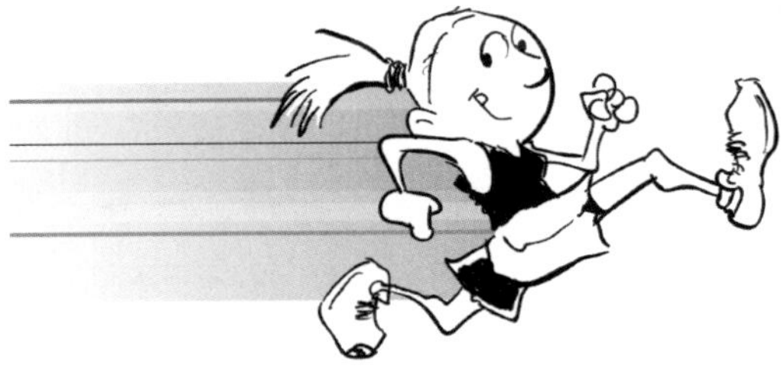

Cardio

Goal:

Complete up to 20 minutes on the **stationary bike** and 20 minutes on the stair stepper.

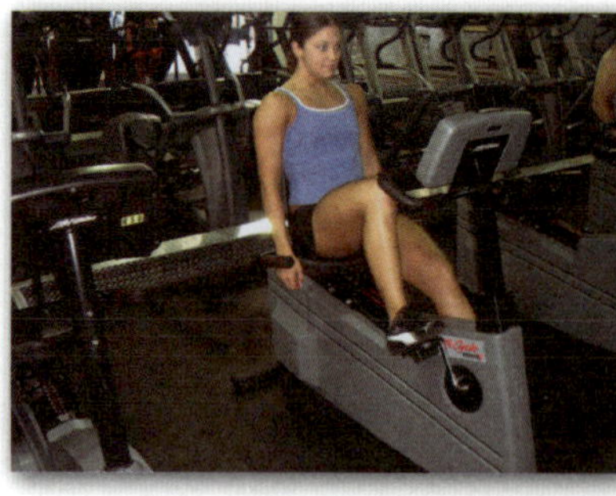

Primary
Quads
Glutes
Hamstrings

Stabilizers
Core
Calves
Shins

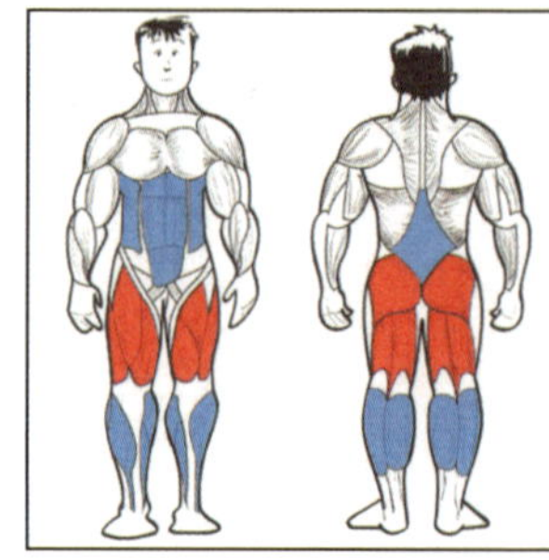

Why?

The stationary bike is a non-impact cycling machine that allows you to perform cardio without placing extra impact or tension in the joints of your ankles, knees, hips, or lower back. Ramp training on the bike provides you with another high intensity cardio workout to increase your physical conditioning.

How?

Sit down on the bike seat.

Step 1 - Adjust your seat according to your cycling motion. Your knees should be slightly bent throughout the entire cycling motion.

Step 2 - Press **START** and select **MANUAL**. This will allow you to have full control of your intensity level.

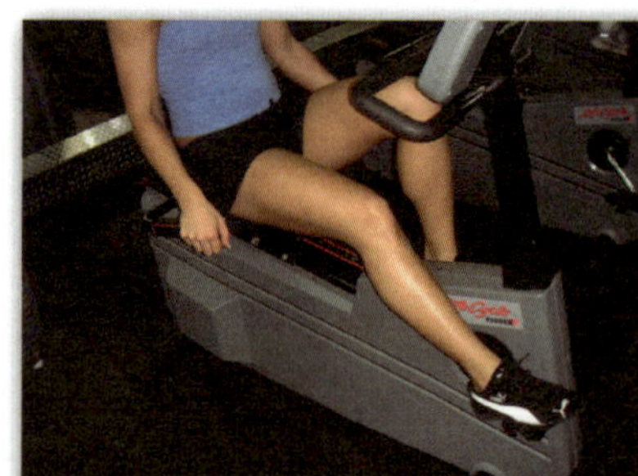

Step 3 - After selecting **MANUAL,** press intensity level one or higher for your warm-up.

Step 4 - Next, cycle above the minimum speed of 70 rpm for one minute and/or maintain an average speed of 80.

Step 5 - At the one minute mark, increase your intensity by one or two levels, depending on your conditioning.

Step 6 - At the two minute mark, increase your intensity by one or two levels again.

Step 7 - Continue to increase your intensity every minute until you reach your peak intensity, which may be resistance level four, six, or higher.

Step 8 - Once you reach your peak, you'll need to decrease your speed and start all over again at your base speed. Your base speed is your warm-up speed.

Step 9 - Your goal is to cycle for up to 20 minutes, in addition to the 20 minutes on the stair stepper. Maintain medium intensity, a breathing rate at which it's a little hard to hold a conversation, for both exercises.

Range of Motion Techniques

To Maximize Muscle Tension and Minimize Overcompensation

Dos

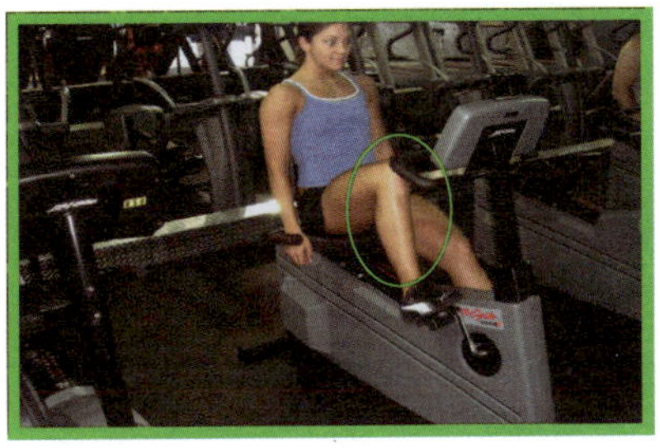

Maintain a Slight Bend in Your Knees

Don'ts

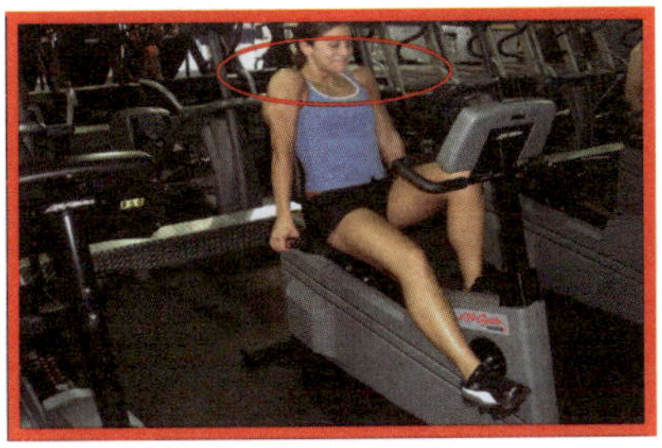

Avoid Shrugging Shoulders and Tight Grip

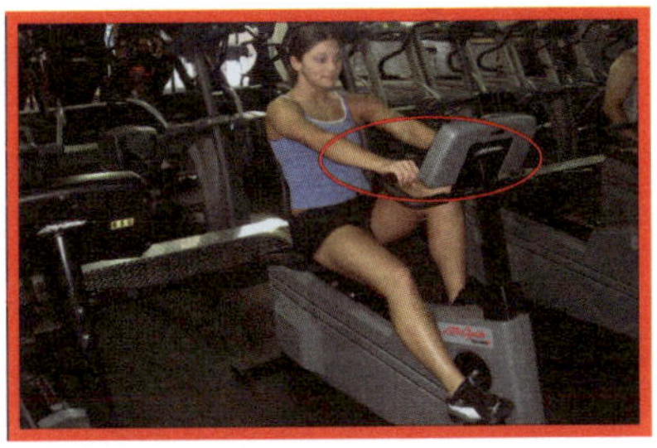

Avoid Holding Front Bar to Reduce Tense Shoulders

Visualize

"Balloon Effect"

When pedaling, you are pushing with your quads and pulling with your hamstrings as you complete the cycling motion. Imagine you have a balloon underneath each of your feet. As you pedal, place the least amount of pressure against the balloon to avoid popping it. This keeps you from pushing too hard and allows you to smoothly pull back with your hamstrings.

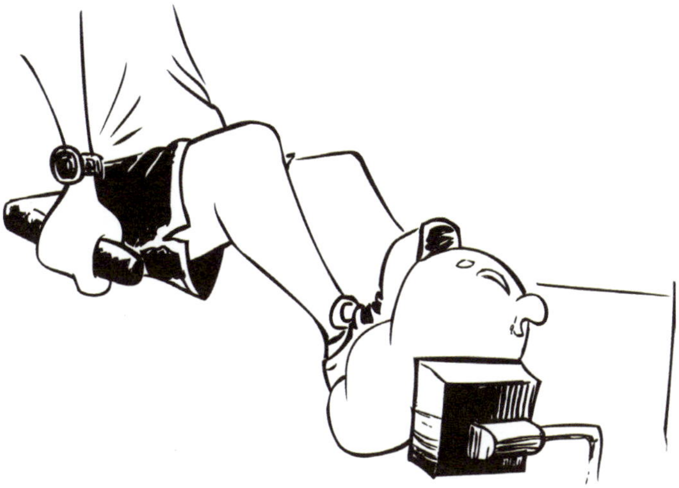

As you increase the intensity, it may become more difficult to visualize. If you lose your focus: POP! You've lost form and technique. If you can't maintain the visualization you'll need to back off. Drop the intensity level and start your ramp training over again to avoid overcompensating with your joints.

Questions and Answers

Why doesn't the seat stay still?

If your seat is jiggling back and forth, it is due to momentum in your cycling motion. Momentum is generally caused by a lack of resistance. Increase your resistance and visualize pushing with your quads and pulling with your hamstrings as you complete the cycling motion.

What is peak intensity when cycling?

Peak intensity is when you lose your cycling form after increasing your resistance level. There are a number of factors in losing form. You may feel more tension in your knees or you may notice your upper body swaying from side to side to assist your higher level of resistance. You may even find yourself gripping the handles tighter to assist stability or you just can't maintain the minimum speed of 70 RPM. Your goal is to maintain proper technique and to avoid going beyond peak intensity. This will minimize excessive joint and ligament pressure, decrease your risk of injury, and ultimately increase your muscle tension.

Can I work up to ramp training on the bike?

Ramp training may be too difficult to begin with. It just depends on your level of conditioning. If you are not quite ready for ramp training, cycle at a level of resistance high enough to maintain a cycling speed of 70 RPM or higher for the full duration. This can be a workout in itself.

Why perform ramp training on the bike?

Ramp training on the bike challenges your mind and body more than biking at a moderate speed. Biking at a low intensity does not challenge your mind or body. Performing repetitive motions at low intensity increases your risk of mental and physical plateaus. This means your body stops changing and you stop seeing results. Ramp training increases the intensity and pushes you toward achieving your desired results.

Do I have to maintain a slight bend in my knees while cycling?

Maintaining a slight bend in the knees throughout the entire cycling motion places more tension in the quads and hamstrings. This results in higher energy and calorie utilization and is the key for greater conditioning, body fat loss, and injury prevention.

What if maintaining a high speed of 70 RPM for instance, is too easy?

Your top speed may differ depending on the brand of the machine. If you find that 70 RPM is too easy, you'll need to increase your intensity. Your goal is to maintain a smooth and constant motion without feeling knee tension.

The sides of my knees are hurting. Should I keep going?

By now you should know the difference between good pain and bad pain. Typically, if the side of your knee is hurting, you're probably experiencing a bad pain.

Continued...

1. Take notice of your ankles, knees, and hips. Your goal is to align each joint by keeping it straight and aligned with the others.

2. Push with your quads and pull with your hamstrings while visualizing the balloon beneath your feet.

3. Reduce or increase your intensity enough to make your alignment and visualization correct. Otherwise, you'll continue to reinforce the incorrect form and technique.

Remember, you should feel an intense burning sensation and muscle tension. This is a positive feeling. However, if you feel actual knee pain, you will have to stop in order to avoid feeling the pain. Cycling on the bike may not be for you at this time. Use the treadmill until you establish a greater foundation of conditioning.

Do I need to stretch again?

Yes! Let's stretch again! Perform two sets of fifteen seconds each for your hamstrings, quads, and calves. Complete all of the following:

Hamstrings

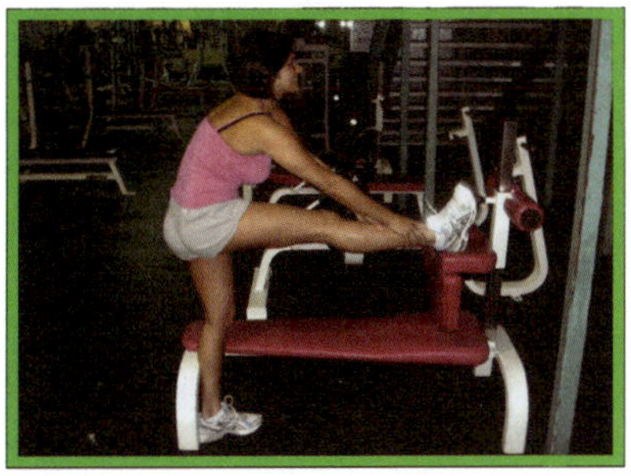

Quads

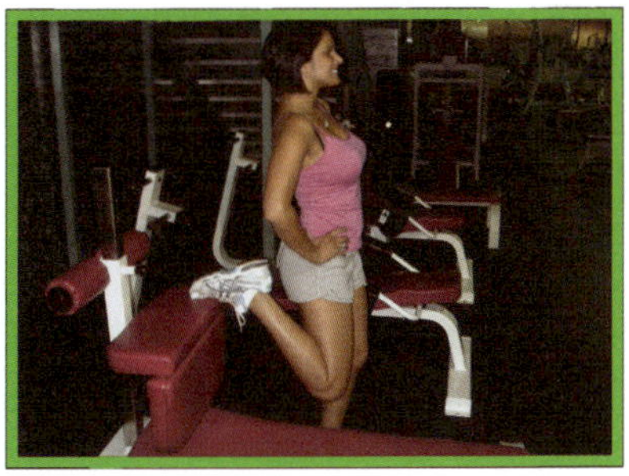

Calves

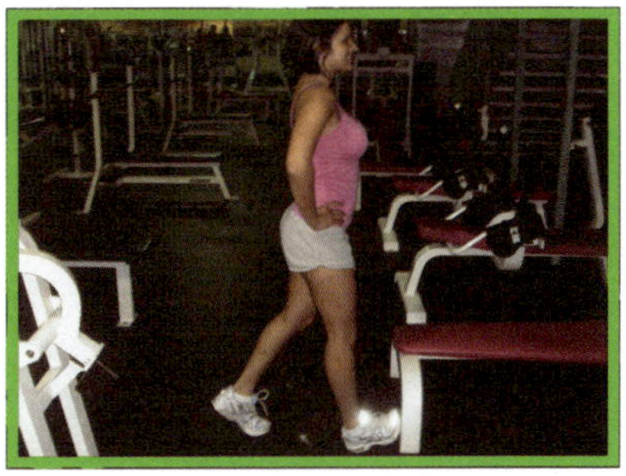

Can I stretch longer?

Fifteen seconds is optimal for injury prevention and recuperation. It doesn't hurt, however, to stretch more as long as you continue to feel the targeted muscle stretch without feeling extra tension in your joints and tendons. In fact, stretching longer increases flexibility and performance.

The Secrets to Success!
From Your Personal Trainer, Kevin Orr

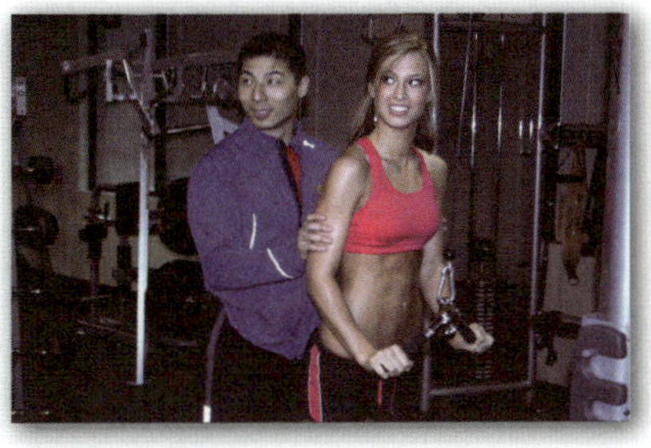

Achieving your fitness goals is not only about staying consistent with your workout schedule, but it's about getting back on course when you do miss a workout. There may be obstacles and challenges every day. That's life. Yes, it does help to stay perfectly consistent with your workouts. However, if you miss a workout due to work, family, or a social function, it is OK. You can simply make it up on another day during your week, so you can live your life. Missing one workout is not going to be the end of the world. Don't beat yourself up over one little mishap. Simply jump back onto your routine. Life happens! Staying the course is the secret!

Example Weight & Cardio Routine

Continue to choose a workout routine based on your level of fitness and your schedule before progressing to Week Six. Write it down in your schedule, on page 249. If none of the example routines work for you, configure a routine that fits your needs, and write it down. Planning ahead will help you set yourself up for success.

Weight Routine 1

Sunday	Monday	Tuesday	Wednesday	Thursday	Friday	Saturday
	Chest/Back/ Shoulders 4x15		Arms: 4x15 Abs: 4x20		Legs 4x20	

Weight Routine 2

Sunday	Monday	Tuesday	Wednesday	Thursday	Friday	Saturday
		Chest/Back/ Shoulders 4x15	Arms: 4x15 Abs: 4x20	Legs 4x20		Chest/Back/ Shoulders 4x15

Weight Routine 3

Sunday	Monday	Tuesday	Wednesday	Thursday	Friday	Saturday
	Chest/Back/ Shoulders 4x15	Arms: 4x15 Abs: 4x20	Legs 4x20	Chest/Back/ Shoulders 4x15		

Continue to choose routine 1, 2, or 3 to begin your weekly cardio routine, or rearrange your cardio training to best fit you.

Cardio Routine 1

Sunday	Monday	Tuesday	Wednesday	Thursday	Friday	Saturday
	Cycle: 15 Stepper: 15		Cycle: 15 Stepper: 15		Cycle: 15 Stepper: 15	

Cardio Routine 2

Sunday	Monday	Tuesday	Wednesday	Thursday	Friday	Saturday
		Cycle: 15 Stepper: 15	Cycle: 15 Stepper: 15	Cycle: 15 Stepper: 15		Cycle: 15 Stepper: 15

Cardio Routine 3

Sunday	Monday	Tuesday	Wednesday	Thursday	Friday	Saturday
	Cycle: 15 Stepper: 15	Cycle: 15 Stepper: 15	Cycle: 15 Stepper: 15	Cycle: 15 Stepper: 15	Cycle: 15 Stepper: 15	

Example Schedule

On your schedule, page 249, continue to write down which cardio machines along with the duration you plan to complete this week.

	Sunday	Monday	Tuesday	Wednesday	Thursday	Friday	Saturday	
Week 1 Weight: Body fat: Cardio: Duration:		226 31% EFX: 5	EFX: 10	EFX: 15	EFX: 20	EFX: 20		Why Too Tired Solution Pace Yourself
Week 2 Weight: Body fat: Weights: Sets: Cardio: Duration:		224 Chest/Back Shoulders: 2x15 EFX: 15 Tread: 15	EFX: 15 Tread: 15	Chest/Back Shoulders: 2x15 EFX: 15 Tread: 15	EFX: 15 Tread: 15	Chest/Back Shoulders: 3x15 EFX: 15 Tread: 15		Why Still to sore from Monday Solution Weight train when recovered
Week 3 Weight: Body fat: Weights: Sets: Cardio: Duration:		222 30% Arms: 2x15 Abs: 2x20 EFX: 15 Tread:R 15	EFX: 15 Tread:R 15	Chest/Back Shoulders: 4x15 EFX: 15 Tread:R 15	Arms: 3x15 Abs: 3x20 EFX: 15 Tread:R 15	EFX: 15 Tread:R 15	EFX: 15 Tread:R 15	Why Worked Over-time Solution Can you make it up another day?
Week 4 Weight: Body fat: Weights: Sets: Cardio: Duration:		220 Legs: 2x20 Stepper: 15 Tread:R 15	Chest/Back Shoulders: 4x15 Stepper: 15 Tread:R 15	Arms: 4x15 Abs: 4x20 Stepper: 15 Tread:R 15	Legs: 3x20 Stepper: 15 Tread:R 15	Stepper: 15 Tread:R 15	Stepper: 15 Tread:R 15	Why Social Event Solution Make it up another day?
Week 5 Weight: Body fat: Weights: Sets: Cardio: Duration:		218 30% Chest/Back Shoulders: 4x15 Cycle: 15 Stepper: 15	Arms: 4x15 Abs: 4x20 Cycle: 15 Stepper: 15	Legs: 4x20 Cycle: 15 Stepper: 15	Chest/Back Shoulders: 4x15 Cycle: 15 Stepper: 15	Cycle: 15 Stepper: 15		

Week 5

Before moving on...

Did you follow through with your plan? If not, cross out what you did not complete on your schedule and write in what you did complete before moving on to the next week.

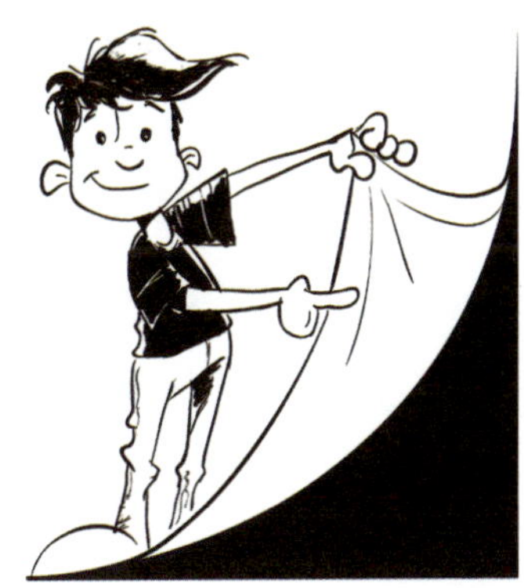

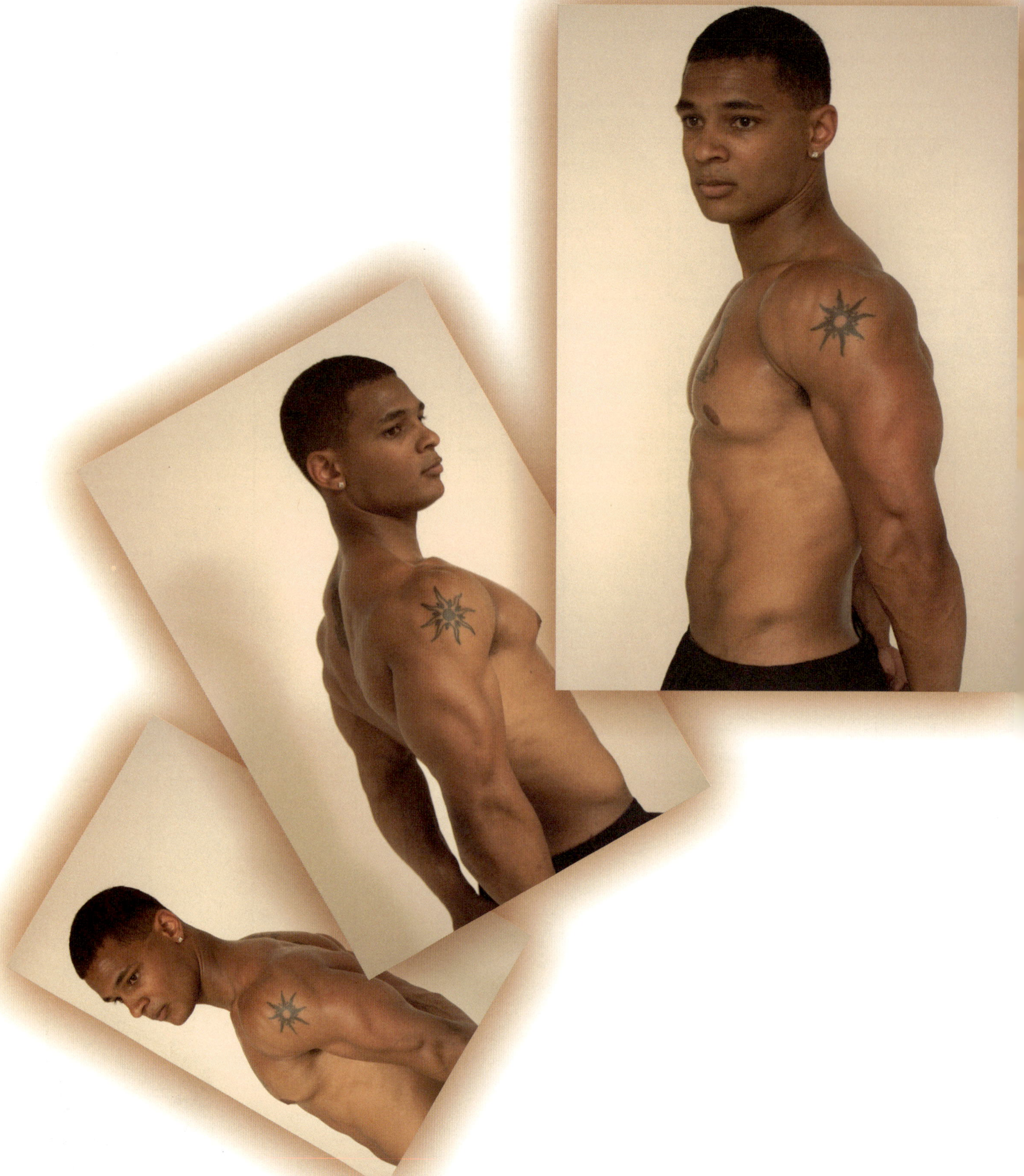

Week 6

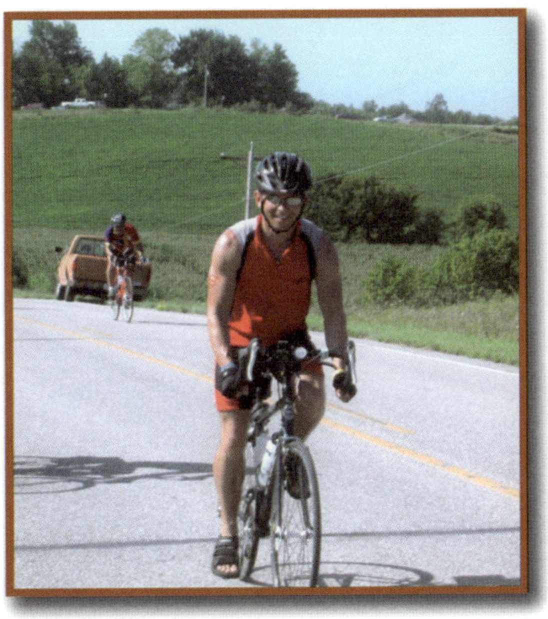

Three years ago, I decided to start living a healthy lifestyle. I was 5′6″ and 175 pounds, overweight, and thought I knew how to workout. I signed up for personal training with Kevin Orr and we met once a week. Every week, Kevin would teach me a new technique for working out as well as review my nutrition for the previous week. This training went on for about six months. I noticed results immediately. I learned that it takes a combination of nutrition, lifestyle, and consistency to really achieve your health goals. Today, three years later, I weigh 152 and am at 14% body fat at the age of 44. Thanks, man!

-Tim Fetters

Goal:

Eat foods that are low on the Glycemic Index.

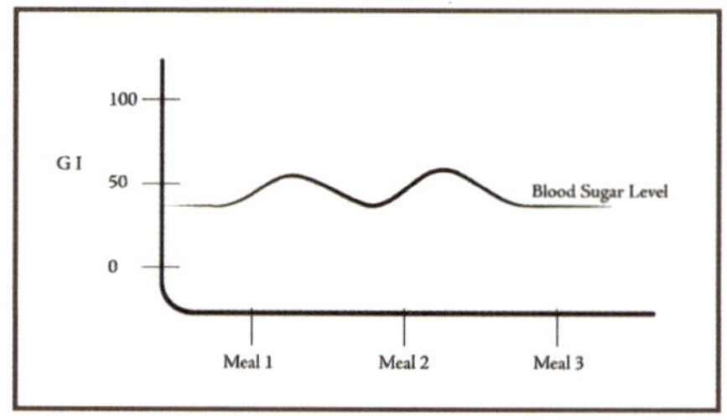

Why?

The Glycemic Index (GI) ranks carbohydrates according to their effect on blood sugar levels. It measures how much your blood sugar increases after eating specific carbohydrates. The faster a food digests, the higher its glycemic level. Foods that have a lower GI take longer to digest and have a lesser effect on your blood sugar level. Eating low glycemic carbohydrates, in combination with good proteins and good fats, assists in stabilizing your blood sugar, as well as, encouraging long-term health benefits. Understanding and using the GI will be a huge advantage to you in building a healthy lifestyle.

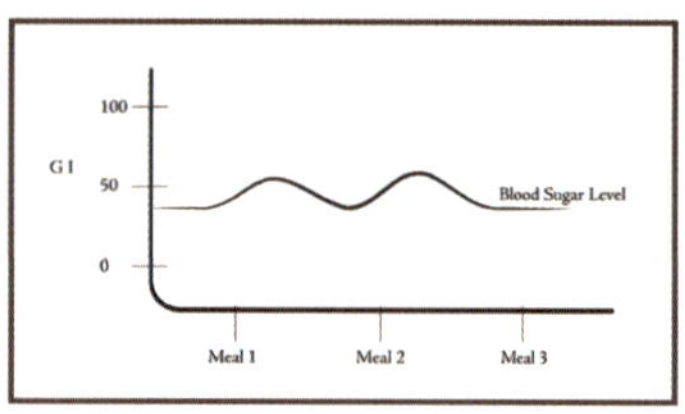

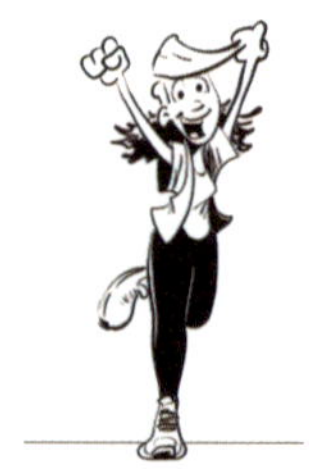

Balanced Blood Sugar = **Optimal Metabolism and Energy**

How?

Carbohydrates are rated from 1 to 100 on the GI: low (less than 55), medium (56-75), or high (76-100).

The key is to eat carbohydrates with a low GI. Foods with a high GI should be avoided, or make up a very small percentage of your total carbohydrates. What's great is that you've already been accomplishing this goal. Avoiding sugars, white flour, and processed foods, as you learned in sessions two, three, and four, nearly guarantees that you are eating low glycemic foods. As you already know, due to their low nutrient and fiber content, most sugars, all white flour, and all processed foods digest very quickly. Remember, the faster a food digest, the higher it is on the Glycemic Index. Essentially, you have already taken the first big step in avoiding high glycemic foods. Using the GI will help you to further fine tune your food choices.

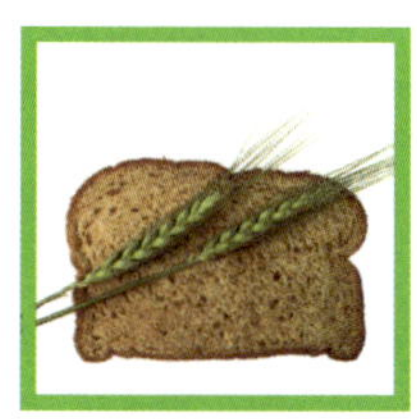

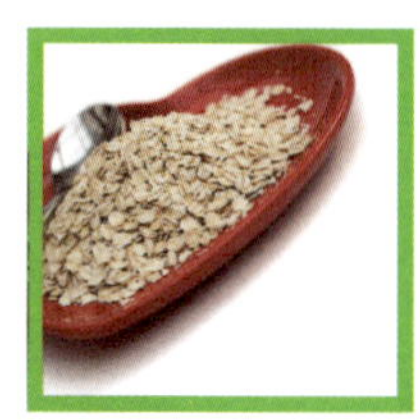

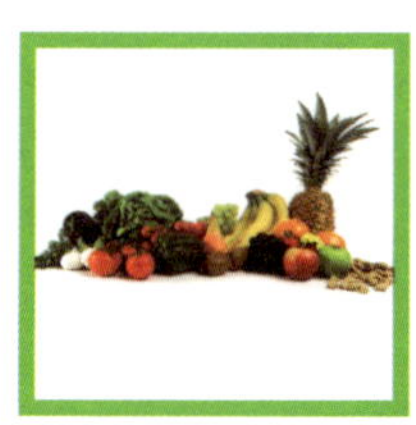

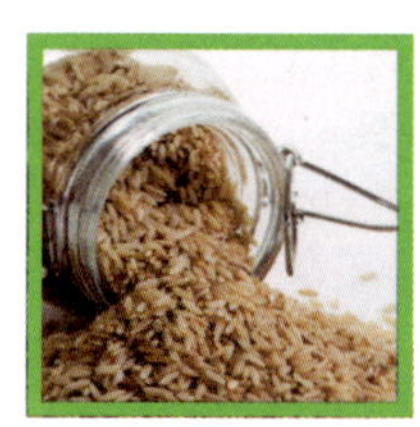

Low glycemic foods assist in stabilizing your blood sugar, so you can feel satiated. This helps with weight control, reduces the risk of heart disease, lowers blood cholesterol levels, prolongs physical endurance, and helps you maintain mental alertness. Diabetics use the GI as a fundamental tool to control their blood sugar levels.

Recommendation: Eat carbohydrates with a low glycemic level in moderation with each meal and snack. See page 256.

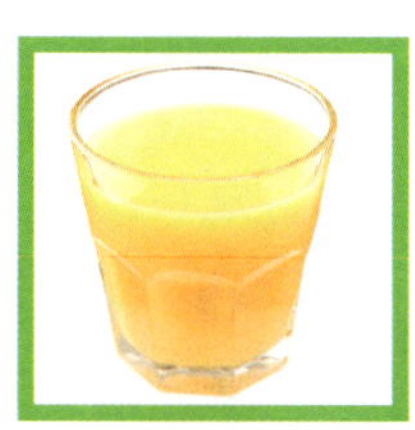

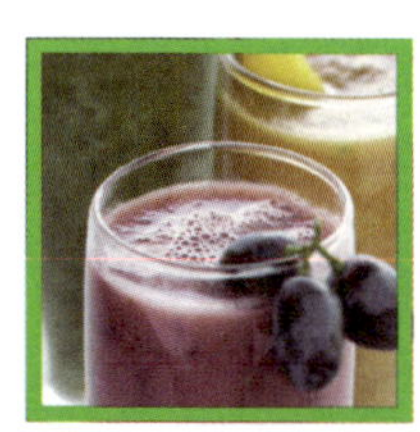

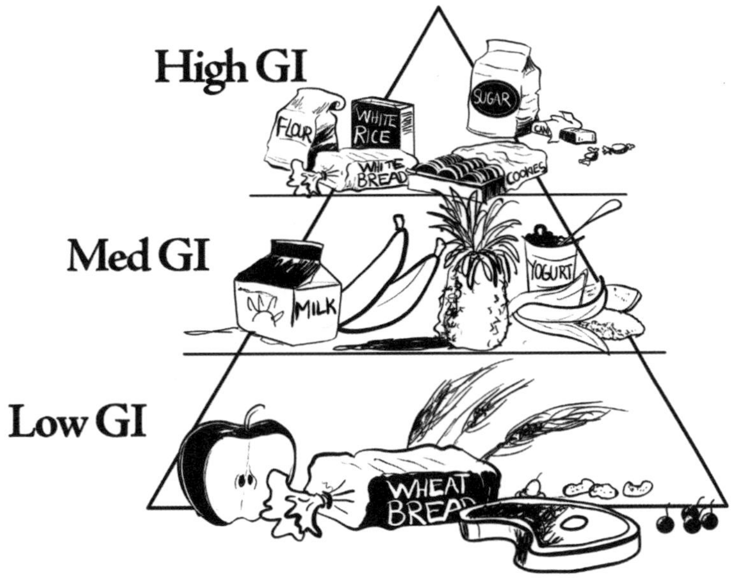

Week 6

Time to review your nutrition log:

1. Check the GI of the foods you are eating. Congratulate yourself on the low GI choices you are already making.

2. If you are eating foods that have a high glycemic level, circle and replace them with low GI alternatives.

3. Keep your "better choice" food selections simple.

4. Continue to record everything you eat and drink in your nutrition log daily.

For Example:

Time	Food and Amount	Substitute
7:00 AM	Cereal	**WW toast**, Adam's® PB, ½ cup cottage cheese
10:00 AM	Carrots	Carrots, swiss cheese, lean meats: turkey, chicken, tuna
12:30 PM	Fruit smoothie	**WW sandwich**
3:00 PM	Banana	**Apple**, string cheese
6:00 PM	Workout	Workout
8:00 PM	Pizza	**WW pasta**, chicken

WW = 100% whole wheat

Questions and Answers

What is the difference between low glycemic and high glycemic food?

Carbohydrate foods that break down quickly during digestion are high glycemic. They require less energy to be converted into glucose and they raise blood sugar to high levels. The low glycemic carbohydrates break down slowly, releasing glucose gradually into the blood stream for less fluctuation in your blood sugar levels. The GI provides a useful tool to help you maintain and control your blood sugar levels.

Why is it so important to keep your blood sugar stable?

High blood sugar levels cause repeated spikes of insulin. Repeated insulin spikes are linked to obesity, diabetes, coronary heart disease, and atherosclerosis. Not only that, but fluctuations in blood sugar also cause fluctuations in energy levels and cause food cravings as well, which make it very difficult to stay on track toward your goals.

What determines the glycemic level?

There are a number of factors that impact the GI of carbohydrates. Cooking, processing, particle size (i.e., whole grains with all layers), the location where the food was grown, its level of ripeness, shelf life, acidity level, enzymes, glycemic load, fiber content, and nutrient-density all influence the glycemic level.

How do I know which carbohydrates are low or high glycemic?

Go to page 256. This will give you a list of the GI of several common foods.

Can I cut out carbohydrates to avoid fluctuations in my blood sugar?

Yes, you **could** cut out carbohydrates to reduce the affect of blood sugar fluctuations. But, eating a diet low in carbohydrates, high in protein, and high in fat for an extended period of time can induce insulin resistance. This means your insulin and blood sugar will be more sensitive to carbohydrates. If your body is not used to using carbohydrates as its preferred source of energy, when you do eat carbohydrates it will cause even bigger spikes in your blood sugar level. And with that comes extreme highs and lows in your energy! This also deprives your body of its primary energy source and sacrifices a variety of nutrients that can be vital to your health. Although, high fat and high protein nutrition plans are low glycemic, they are not appropriate for a healthy lifestyle. Your body needs a balance of proteins, carbohydrates, and fats. Each macronutrient performs a specific function in the body. Cutting out carbohydrates would disrupt these functions and your body wouldn't be able to perform optimally. The key is to balance your blood sugar by eating all three macronutrients together in the appropriate ratios.

What happens if I eat carbohydrates by themselves?

Any time you eat carbohydrates without proteins or fats, it will cause a spike in your blood sugar and insulin level, making it very difficult to maintain a balanced blood sugar.

Can high glycemic carbohydrates cause diabetes?

Remember, repeated insulin spikes have been linked to diabetes. High glycemic carbohydrates digest quickly, require less energy to be converted into glucose and cause high blood sugar levels. This can cause hyperglycemic and hypoglycemic reactions. Consistent high blood sugar levels will cause the repeated spikes of insulin that have been associated with diabetes. It's best to eat low glycemic carbohydrates, which break down slowly releasing glucose gradually into the blood stream causing much less fluctuation in your blood sugar levels.

Is there an easy way to determine the glycemic level of my carbohydrates?

The blood sugar response to a particular food differs from person to person depending on many digestive factors. It's best to carefully monitor your own blood sugar level after eating foods. For example, try eating an apple for one of your snacks and yogurt as another snack. Afterwards, you can generally determine if one or the other is higher or lower glycemic for you by how it makes you feel. The apple may satiate your appetite much longer than yogurt, which is common, despite the fact that both foods are low glycemic and comparable in calorie content. This means the **food that satiates your appetite longer is the one with the lower GI for your body**. The GI is just a tool, but if you find a specific food producing either a high or low, take note of it and use that information in your meal planning.

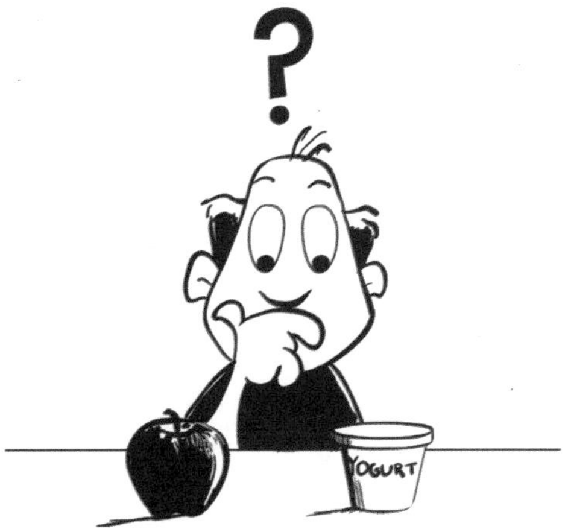

Is it ever okay to eat high glycemic carbohydrates?

The most appropriate times to eat high glycemic carbohydrates are in your pre- and post-workout meals. High glycemic foods in your pre-workout meal prime your muscles and body for maximum endurance, strength, and mental alertness. High glycemic foods in your post-workout replenish your body for maximum recovery. Still, do your best to stay away from refined sugars.

Week 6

Nutrition Log

Date:__________	Sun Mon Tues Wed Thurs Fri Sat	
	Plan	**Actual**
Meal 1	*Food & Amount*	*Food & Amount*
Time:_____		
Meal 2		
Time:_____		
Meal 3		
Time:_____		
Meal 4		
Time:_____		
Meal 5		
Time:_____		
Meal 6		
Time:_____		

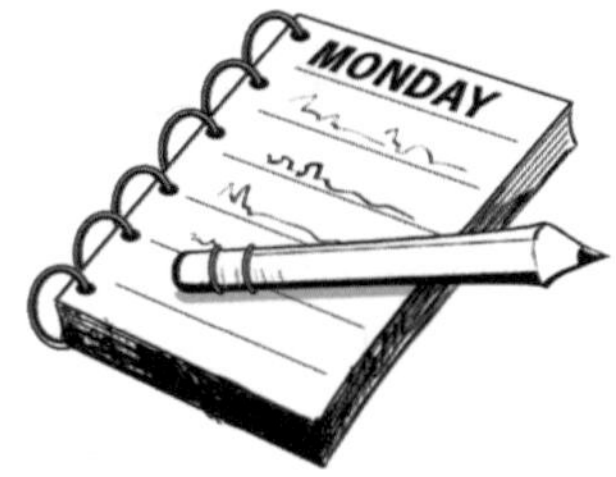

Checklist

Achieved:

- ✓ Consume meal or snack every 3 hours
- ✓ Water every 3 hours
- ✓ Sleep optimal hours
- ✓ Intake multivitamin
- ✓ Weights and cardio
- ✓ Consume PFCs every meal or snack
- ✓ **Foods low on the GI**

Avoided:

- ✓ Sugars
- ✓ White flour
- ✓ Processed foods

Key Points

Week 1
- Eat a small meal or snack once every three hours – five to six meals per day.
- Drink at least 1 cup (8 ounces) of water per meal and at least one cup before, during, and after your workouts.
- Keep a nutrition log.
- Sleep is vital!
- Take a daily multivitamin.

Week 2
- Avoid bad sugars.

Week 3
- Avoid white flour and white rice.

Week 4
- Avoid processed foods.

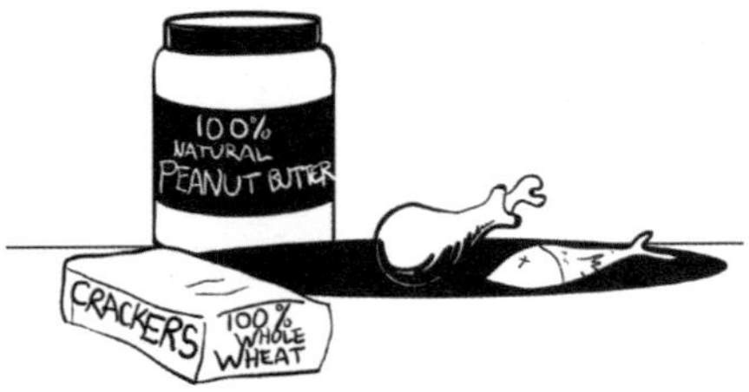

Week 5
- Balance your meals and snacks with a combination of proteins, fats, and carbohydrates.

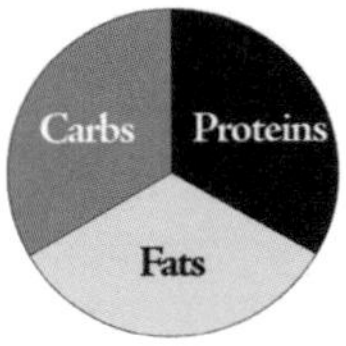

Week 6
- **Eat foods that are low on the Glycemic Index** to further assist in stabilizing your blood sugar and to optimize your energy.

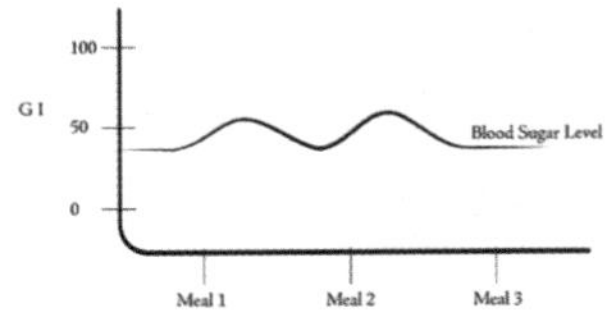

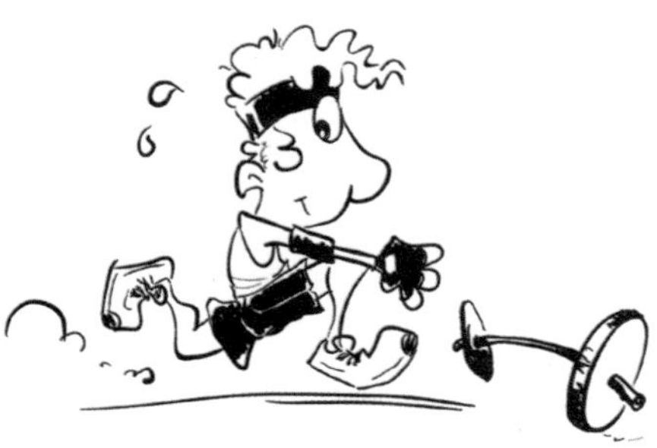

Biceps

Goal:

Complete four sets of 15 reps of the **preacher biceps curls**.

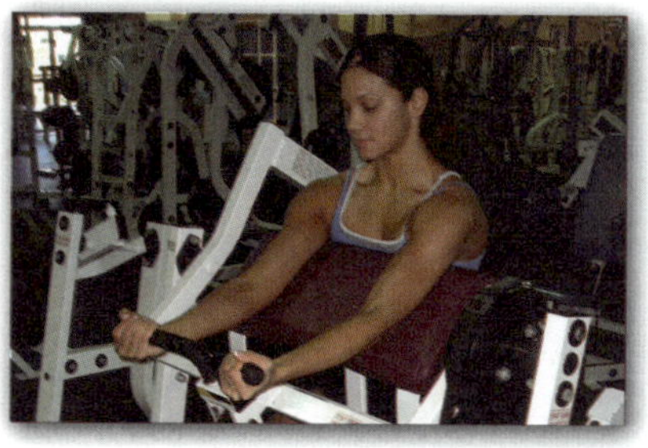

Primary
Biceps

Stabilizers
Shoulders
Forearms
Core

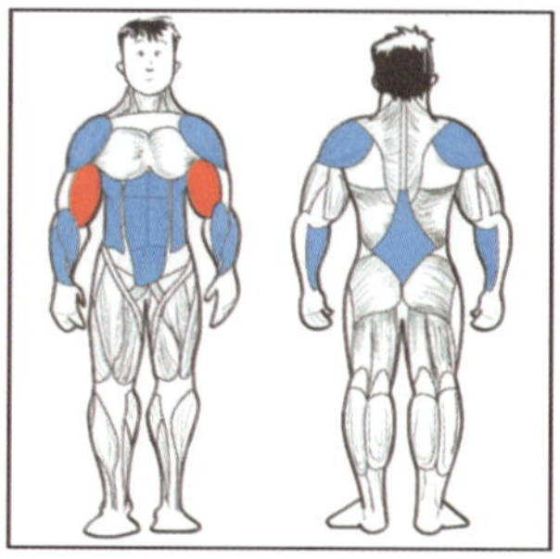

Why?

The preacher biceps curl is a machine exercise targeting your biceps. The muscle stabilizers involved include your shoulders and forearms, as well as the rest of your core. This machine is very effective in reducing overcompensation from other muscles and joints. The preacher pad acts as a stabilizer causing your elbows to become the lever. Compared to dumbbell biceps curls, your biceps muscle must work harder to pull the weight up to your peak contraction. The preacher machine also relieves more joint pressure than free weights, especially in your wrists.

How?

Step 1 - Adjust the seat to make sure you're in a comfortable position, not too high or too low. The best method to determine your seat position is to make sure you have some space between your arm pits and the preacher pad.

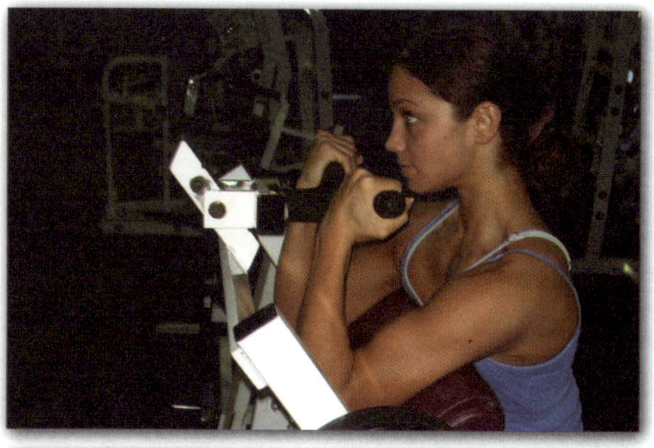

Step 2 - Squeeze your abs to assist the lower back's neutral position.

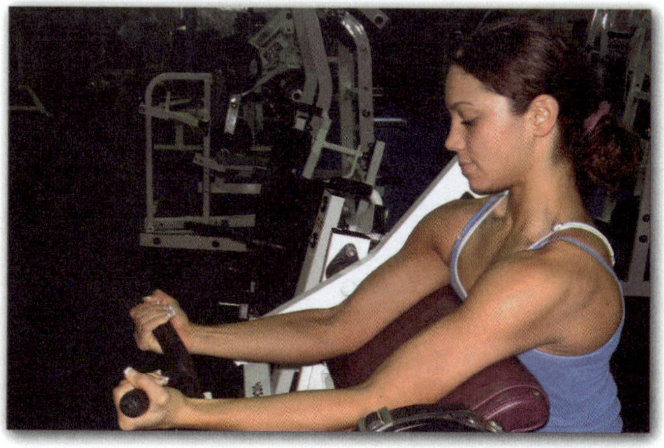

Step 3 - With a light grip, lower your v-bar to a slightly bent-elbow position to maintain tension in your biceps.

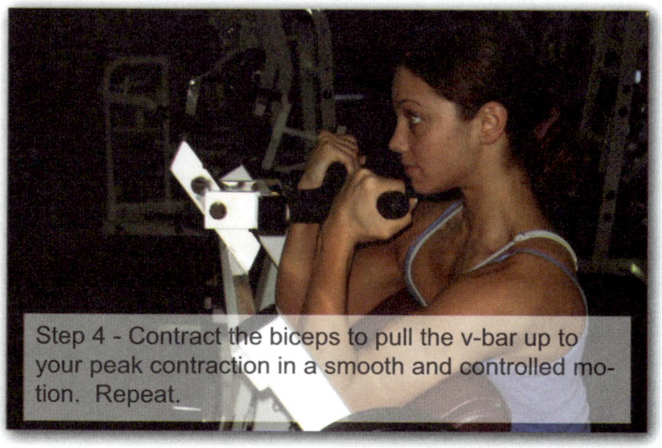

Step 4 - Contract the biceps to pull the v-bar up to your peak contraction in a smooth and controlled motion. Repeat.

Your goal is to complete four sets of 15 (4 x 15).

Range of Motion Techniques

To Maximize Muscle Tension and Minimize Overcompensation

Dos

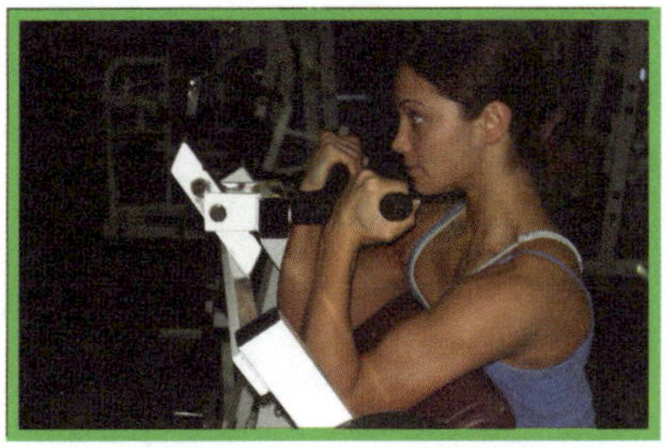

Begin Squeezing Biceps to Peak Contraction

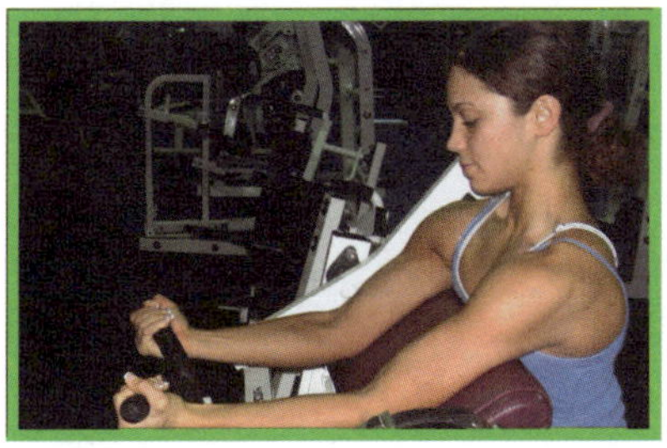

Lower to Resist and Feel Small Stretch in Biceps

Don'ts

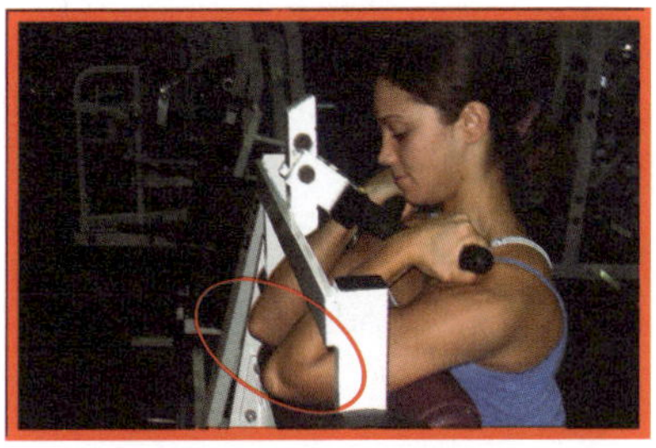

Avoid Exceeding Peak Contraction

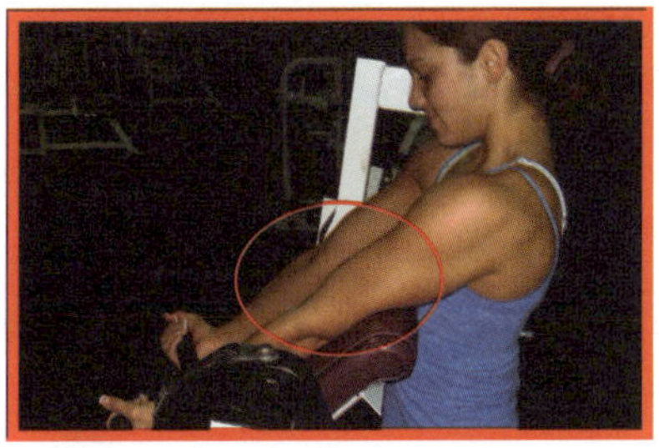

Avoid Locking Out Elbows

Visualize

"Ball Effect"

Squeeze and flex your biceps in your starting position. Resist the preacher bar when lowering it down and curling it up. Imagine curling your biceps into the biggest balls you can curl them into. As you lower the bar, the tight round ball is being pulled and stretched into an oval. Focus on feeling the stretch and tension in your biceps at the bottom of your range of motion. Tighten and squeeze your biceps back into a ball again as you pull the bar up to your starting position.

Repeat the visualization with every rep to maximize the tension in your biceps and minimize overcompensation of your shoulders, forearms, and wrists.

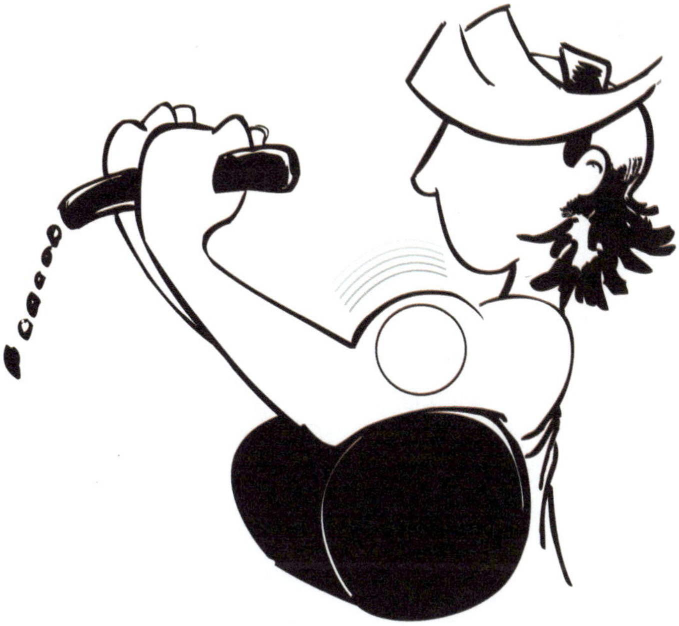

Questions and Answers

Where should I grip the bar?

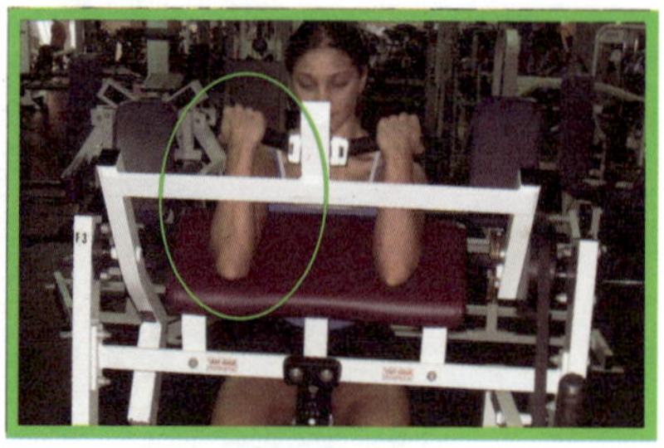

Lightly grip the bar with your hands about shoulder-width apart. Your elbows should be aligned with your shoulders. Elbow placement is very important. If your elbows are in too close or out too far, it will place unnecessary stress in your joints. Also, if your hand grip is too wide, it allows you to overcompensate by placing added stress in your wrists, elbows, and shoulders.

How fast should I perform the reps?

Your tempo should be two seconds down and two seconds up. Expect to have better stability and balance in this exercise than you had when you performed dumbbell biceps curls. Focus on maintaining a smooth and controlled motion. Using proper form increases the effectiveness of the exercise and decreases your risk of injury.

My forearms are burning more than my biceps! Am I doing something wrong?

If your forearms are burning, your grip is probably too tight. Loosen up! Maintaining a light hand grip will help you to avoid forearm overcompensation. If you are still having trouble, try opening your palms when lowering the v-bar and closing them lightly when pulling the bar up. This will help you to avoid forearm overcompensation.

Should I continue if my wrists hurt?

Remember, pain is feedback from your body. If something hurts, your body is trying to warn you that something isn't right. Generally, if you feel discomfort from weight lifting, you need to correct your form and technique. In this case, you can correct your form and continue lifting. Be sure to keep your wrists in a neutral position and keep your hand grip light. Gripping too tightly creates wrist tension. However, if the pain increases as you continue, or you are feeling an intense pain, you may need to stop.

Why do I lock out with dumbbells but not with the preacher curl?

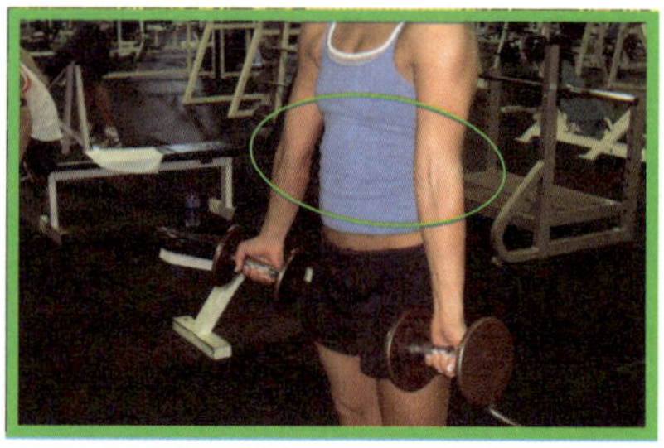

When you lock out your elbows with dumbbells, your biceps stretch. Placing your elbows slightly in front of your body creates tension in your biceps, allowing them to stretch when locked out. Due to the angle of your arm position in the preacher curl, locking out your elbows places excessive tension in your elbow joints. Since your goal is to avoid excessive joint tension, you should not lock out your elbows when performing the preacher curls.

How do I know when I've reached my peak biceps contraction?

Your goal is to keep your elbows on the preacher pad while curling the v-bar up. The moment your elbows lift up, you've reached your peak contraction for your biceps. It is more difficult to maintain this range of motion. If you allow your elbows to lift up, your shoulders and elbows begin to overcompensate. As always, your goal is to avoid overcompensation.

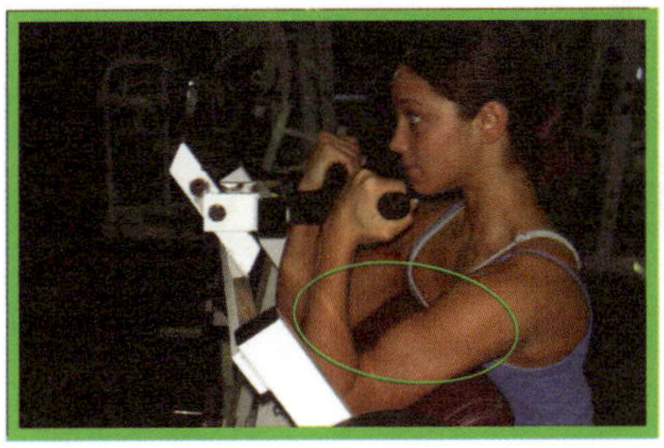

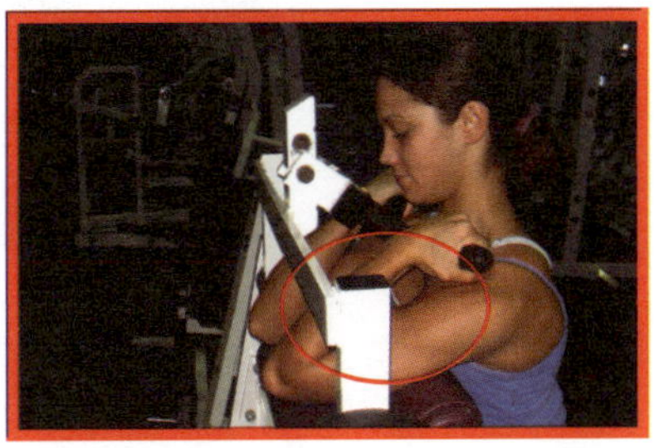

Can I do more than four sets now?

Your goal is to progressively increase the intensity of your workouts. You can perform up to six sets for one exercise per muscle group. If you feel like you could do more than six sets without losing form, you are not working hard enough! You should be fatigued by the end of each set. If you increase the intensity, then four sets should be enough to achieve a pump and/or fatigue. Keep in mind, more is not always better. In fact, the more sets you do to reach a pump, the faster your body plateaus. Furthermore, as you increase the number of sets, you also increase your risk of overuse injuries. Overuse can eventually lead to the onset of arthritis from joint degeneration. Whew, talk about a domino effect! Don't push yourself in the wrong direction. Training correctly results in improved health and wellness.

If I'm comfortable with DB Biceps Curls, can I stay with this exercise?

The preacher biceps curl is a machine exercise targeting your biceps. This machine is very effective in reducing overcompensation from other muscles and joints. Compared to dumbbell biceps curls, your biceps muscle must work harder to pull the weight up to your peak contraction. The preacher machine also relieves more joint pressure than free weights, especially in your wrists. Variety is the key to reduce the risk of injuries.

Triceps

Goal:

Complete four sets of 15 reps of **dumbbell flat triceps extension**.

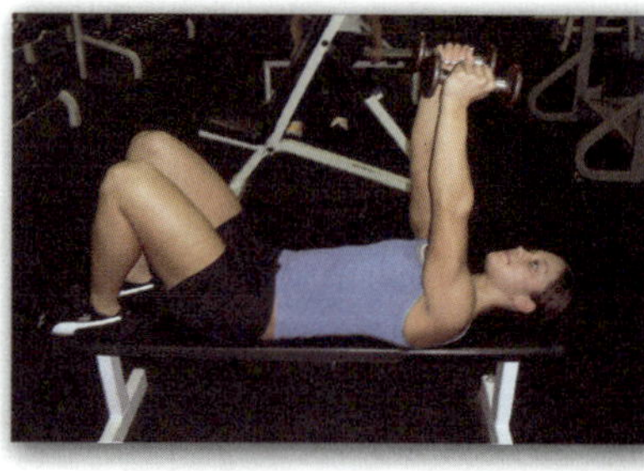

Primary
Triceps

Stabilizers
Shoulders
Forearms
Core

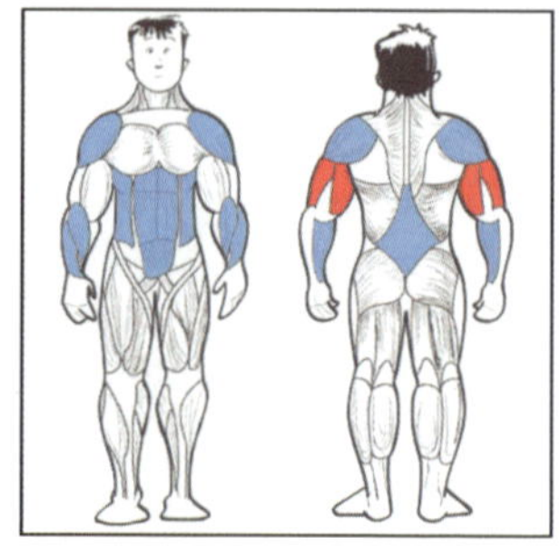

Why?

The dumbbell triceps extension is a free weight exercise targeting your triceps. The muscle stabilizers include your shoulders and forearms, as well as the rest of your core. In comparison to other triceps exercises, dumbbell triceps extension use more stabilizers to maintain the motion. This assists in improved stability and balance and leads to a greater foundation of strength and conditioning.

How?

Step 1 - Grab the dumbbells and lay down with your feet on the bench and your dumbbells directly above your chest.

Step 2 - Squeeze your abs to push your lower back into a neutral position.

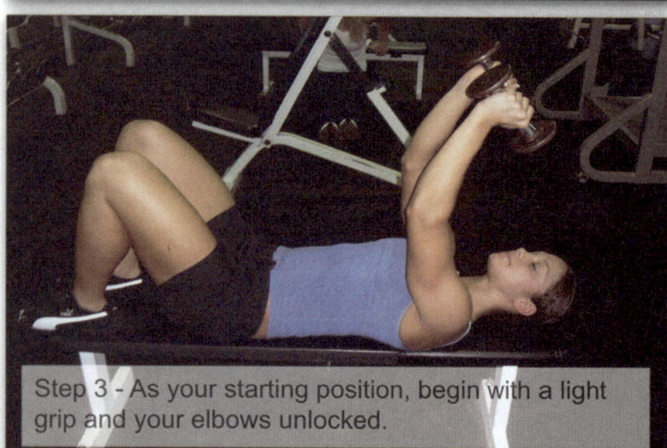

Step 3 - As your starting position, begin with a light grip and your elbows unlocked.

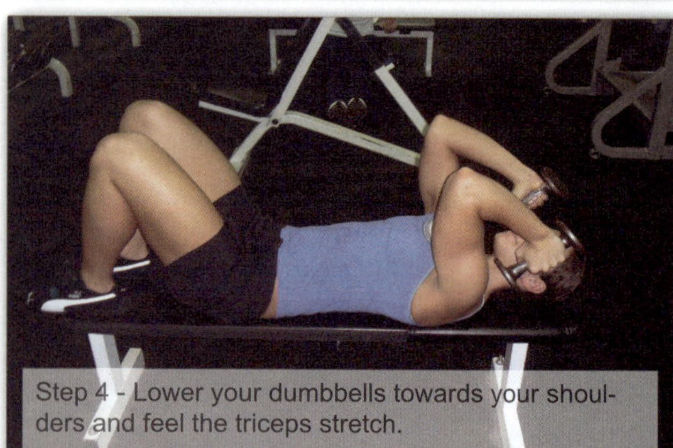

Step 4 - Lower your dumbbells towards your shoulders and feel the triceps stretch.

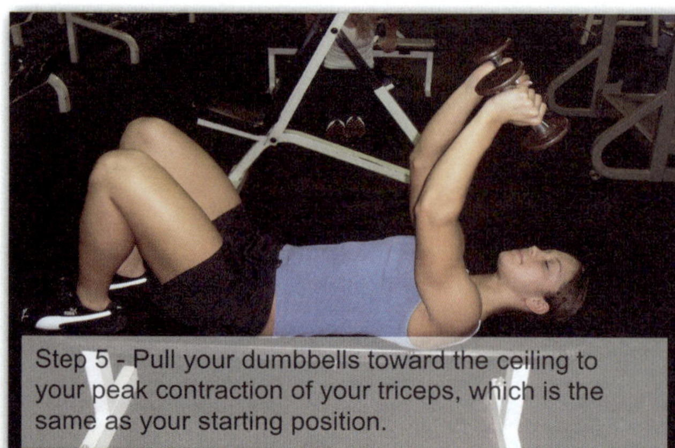

Step 5 - Pull your dumbbells toward the ceiling to your peak contraction of your triceps, which is the same as your starting position.

Step 6 - Repeat with a smooth and controlled motion to maximize the tension in your triceps.

Your goal is to complete four sets of 15 (4 x 15).

Range of Motion Techniques

To Maximize Muscle Tension and Minimize Overcompensation

Dos	**Don'ts**
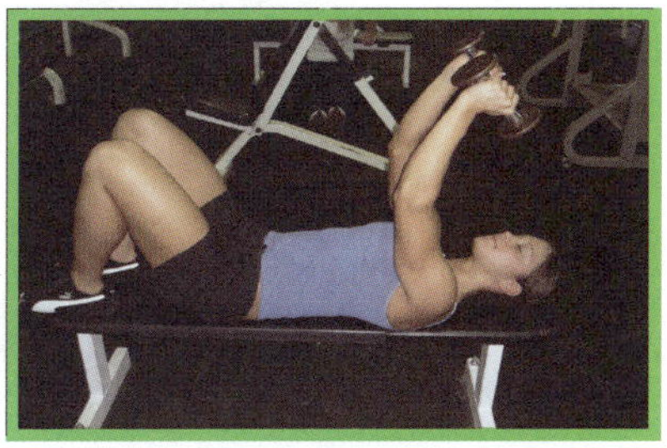 Begin with Elbows Bent	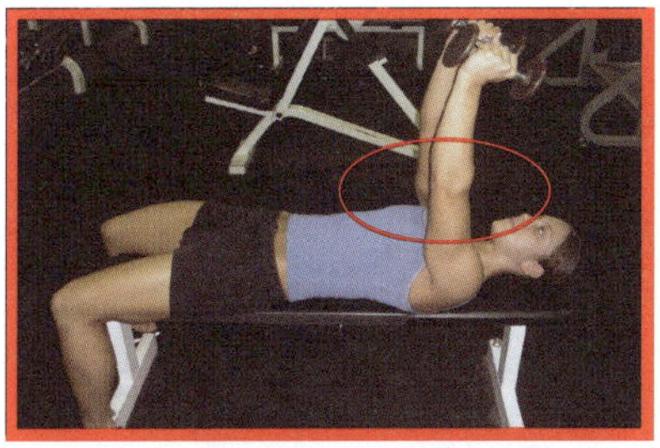 Avoid Locking Out Elbows and Arching Lower Back
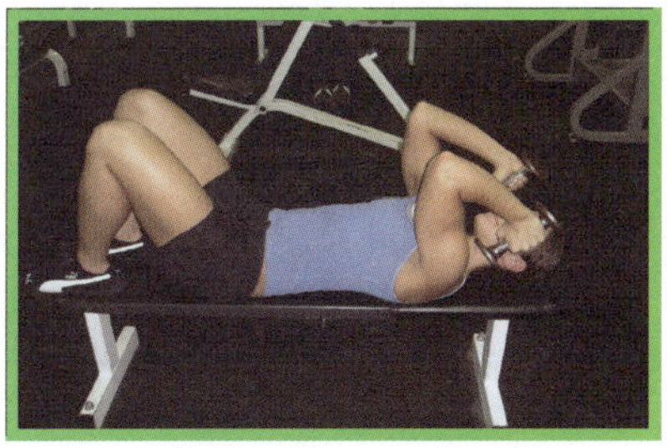 Stretch Triceps to Resist at Bottom	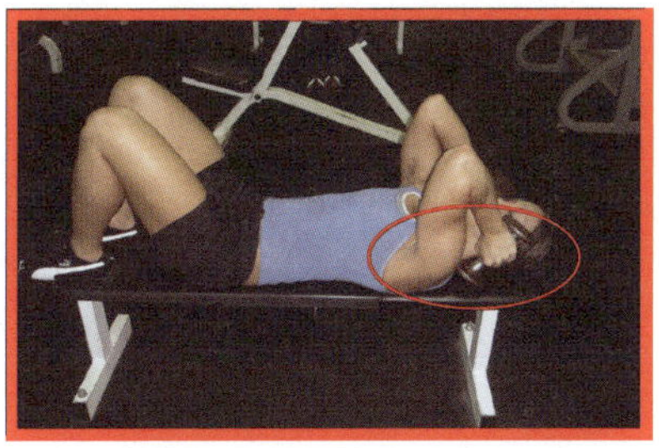 Avoid Coming Down too Low

Visualize

"Cable and Rubber Band Effect"

While lying on a bench with your elbows tucked in, imagine cables pulling them straight up towards the ceiling. Resist the dumbbells as you lower them down and as you push them back up.

Focus on feeling a stretch in your triceps as you lower the dumbbells. Visualize your triceps as a rubber band, lengthening and stretching as you resist the weight. Your triceps, as the "rubber band," tighten so much that it pulls your dumbbells up to your starting position.

Continue to visualize your elbows tucked in and pulled up by a cable. Repeat the visualizations and stay within the proper range of motion. This will maximize the tension in your triceps and minimize overcompensation of your shoulders, elbows, and wrists.

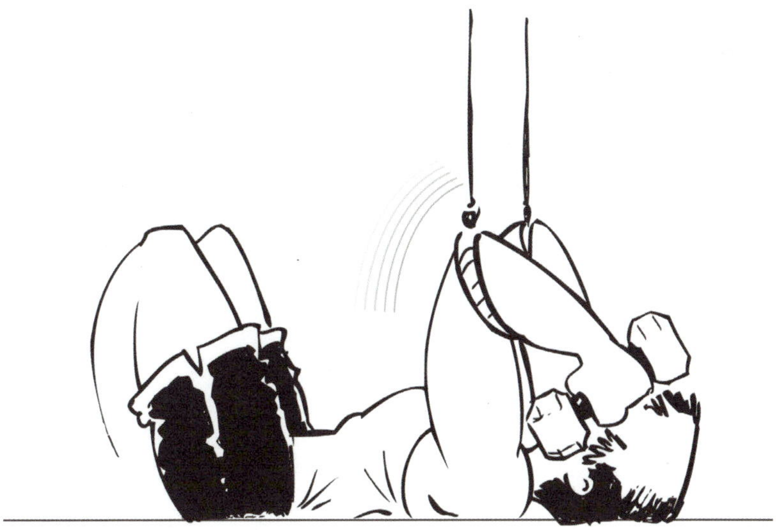

Questions and Answers

What if I feel my elbows?

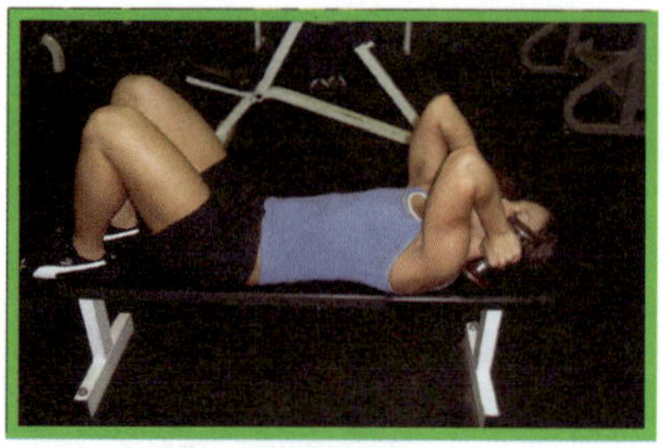

If you are feeling your elbows, you may need to adjust your form. Squeeze your abs to keep your lower back in a neutral position. Tuck your elbows in, pull them straight up towards the ceiling, and visualize! Proper form decreases joint tension and maximizes muscle tension.

What if I feel my wrists again?

If you are feeling your wrists, check your grip. Remember to hold the dumbbells lightly. Your thumbs should wrap around the bar to secure your wrists. This will help to keep your wrists strong. Gripping too tightly leads to injury by increasing wrist joint tension and allowing your forearms and other stabilizers to overcompensate.

What if my lower back won't stay flat?

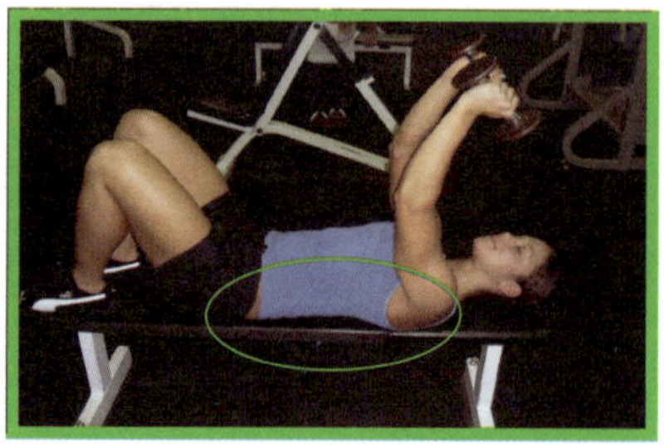

It's important to keep your lower back flat. This relieves the pressure in your lower back, keeps it from overcompensating, and forces your triceps to do the work. Squeeze your abs and try placing your feet on the bench instead of the floor.

Why do I need to feel my triceps stretch every rep?

Feeling a stretch in your triceps ensures that your triceps are doing the work. If the triceps are doing the work, you can be sure no other muscle groups are overcompensating.

I have always struggled to find my exercise niche. Nothing worked because I didn't have a good foundation; I didn't know what weights to use, how to use them, or what other exercise would be effective, let alone what to eat. Through my work with Kevin, I was able to establish a nutrition and exercise schedule to fit my busy life. Because of Kevin's positive feedback and support, I have continued to lose weight, and I exercise on a regular basis. The success for me has been creating an exercise routine and eating schedule that is flexible but easy to follow. I take it one day at a time, otherwise, it's too overwhelming. The only person accountable for my health and fitness is ME. It's my responsibility to incorporate good eating habits and exercise into my life. It is the decision and commitment I made to be a healthier wife, mother, sister, daughter, and friend.

- Meriza Rodrigues

At 50 years of age and active in snowboarding and backpacking, I need to maintain a significant level of fitness for these activities to be enjoyable and injury free. My physical interests are contrasted by my eight-10-hour a day desk job. These two factors combined with limited time for workouts led me to a two year relationship with Kevin and first hand experience with his methods. In short, they work and I remain in good health, injury free, and able to fully participate in any physical activity I choose. I largely owe my ability to enjoy this active lifestyle to Kevin and I am glad to see him sharing his knowledge and experience with this fabulous book which I highly recommend.

- Mike Halladay

Abs

Goal:

Complete four sets of 20 reps of **reverse crunches.**

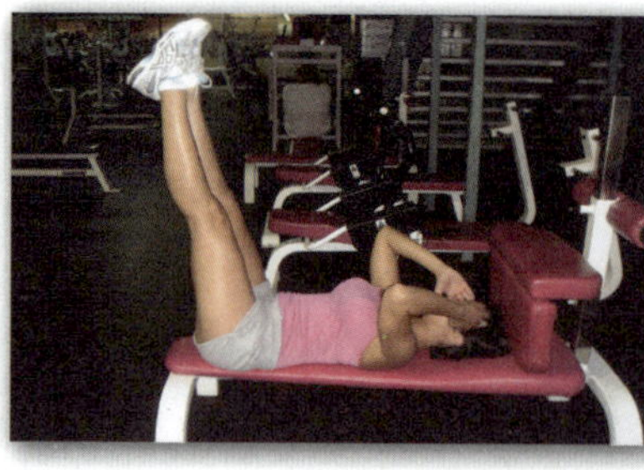

Primary
Abs

Stabilizers
Lower Back
Core
Hip Flexors
Quads
Neck

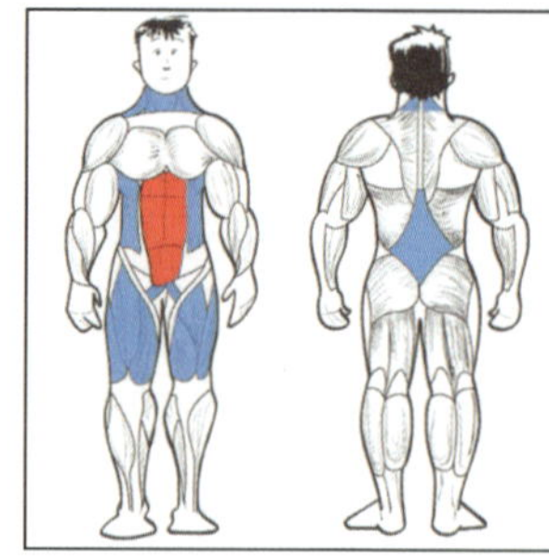

Why?

Reverse crunches are an excellent exercise targeting the entire region of your abs. Your abdominal muscles are one of the biggest stabilizers of your core. They help to maintain proper posture and exercise technique. The stabilizing muscles include your lower back, hip flexors, quads, neck, and a number of little muscles that make up your core. Reverse crunches are great for training variety.

How?

Step 1 - Lay flat on your back either on the floor or bench with your legs lifted straight up.

Step 2 - Squeeze your abs to push your lower back into a neutral position against the bench.

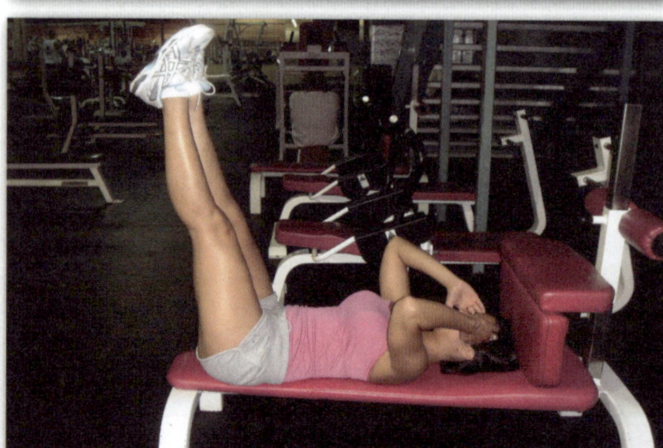

Step 3 - Place your hands at the temple of your head.

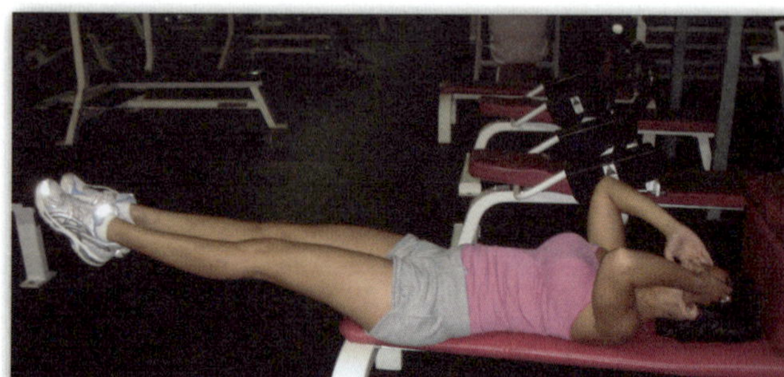

Step 4 - Lower your legs halfway while keeping your lower back flat. You should feel a slight stretch in the lower region of your abs.

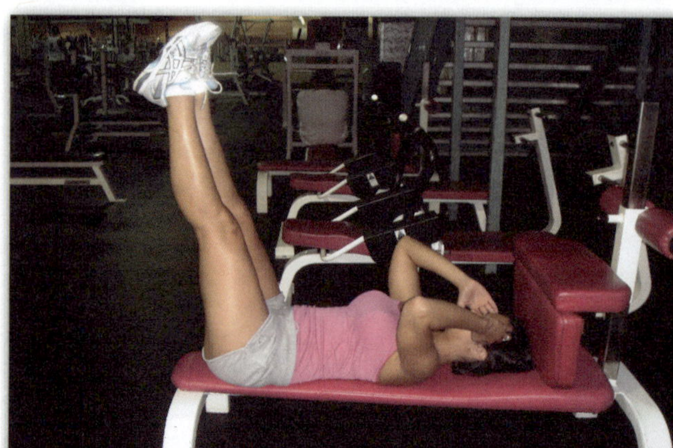

Step 5 - Roll your glutes and hips to pull your legs back up to your starting position. Repeat.

Your goal is to complete four sets of 20 (4 x 20).

Range of Motion Techniques
To Maximize Muscle Tension and Minimize Overcompensation

Dos

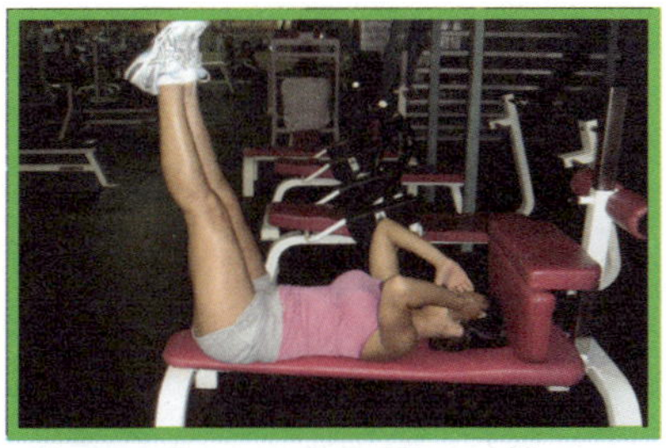

Begin Squeezing Your Abs at Top

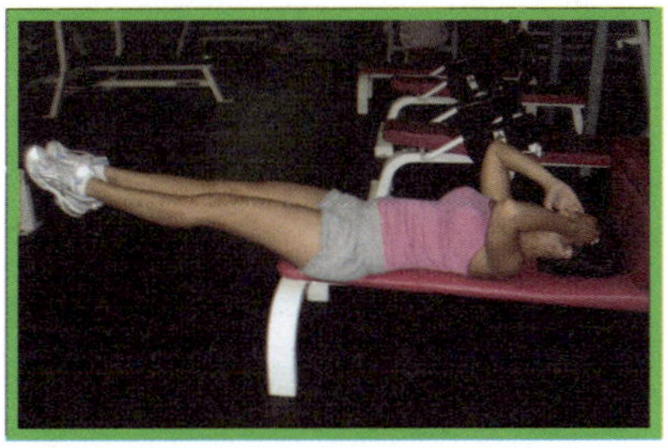

Lower Legs to Resist and Feel Abs Stretch

Don'ts

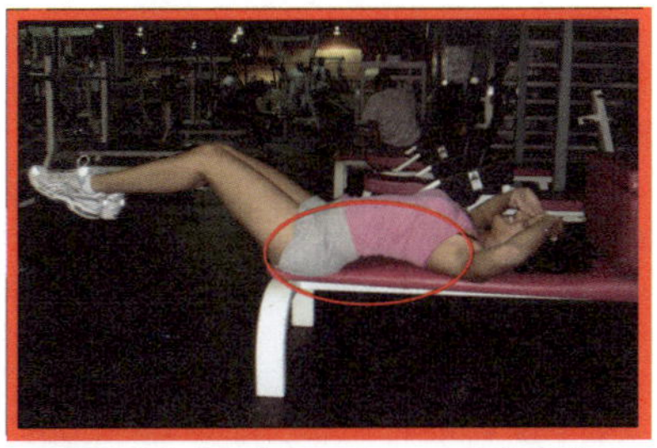

Avoid Arching Lower Back

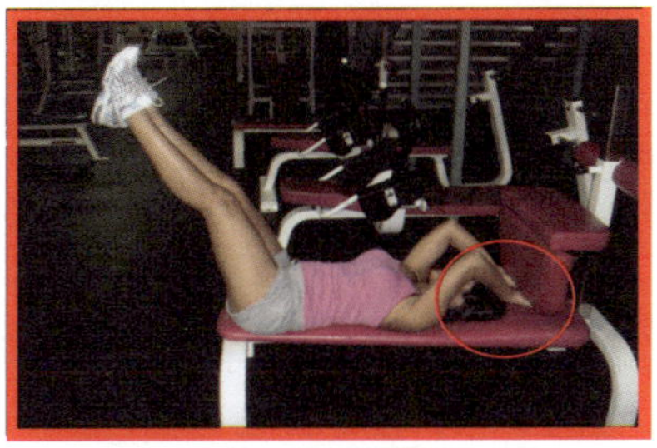

Avoid Overcompensation with Upper Body

Visualize

"Rubber Band Effect"

While lying on a bench, tightly squeeze your abs as you lower your legs and raise them back up. Imagine that your abs are a rubber band. As you lower your legs, visualize the rubber band stretching and lengthening your abs. As your legs lower, the tension increases so much that the rubber band tightens, pulling your legs back up to your peak contraction. Focus on maintaining the tension in your abs as the rubber band stretches and tightens, moving your legs down and up.

Visualize every rep and stay within the proper range of motion. This will maximize the tension in your abs and minimize overcompensations.

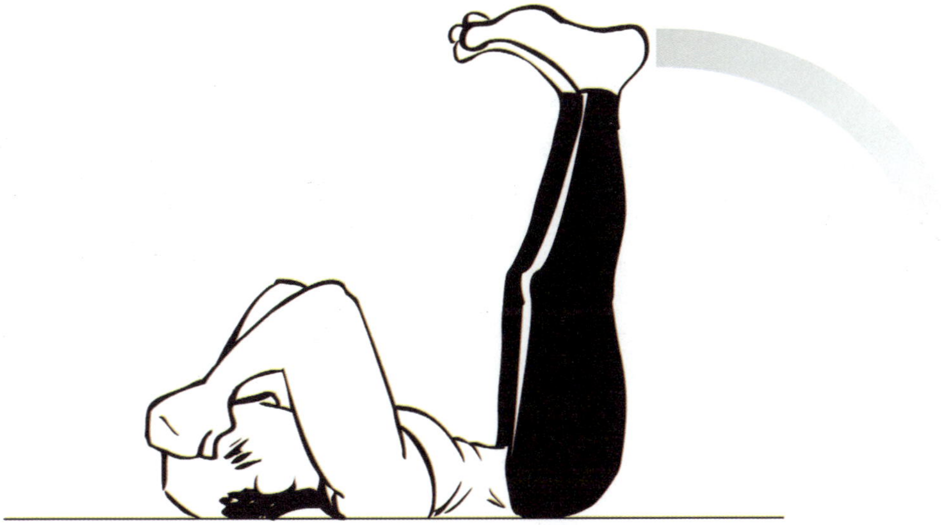

Questions and Answers

What should I do if I feel burning in my lower back?

By now you should know the difference between good pain and bad pain. Good pain leads to increased strength and conditioning, and bad pain leads to injury. If you are experiencing a light burning sensation in your lower back, that is great! Your muscles are fatigued! Muscle fatigue leads to strengthening and conditioning. However, if you're feeling pain in your lower back while performing crunches, you may be arching too much. Focus on squeezing your abs to push your lower back into a neutral position against the bench. This relieves the pressure in your lower back and forces your abs to do the muscle work.

Why do I need to feel a stretch in my abs?

You should feel a slight stretch in the lower region of your abs as you lower your legs. The stretch ensures that your abs are resisting the weight of your legs. If you can't feel the stretch, you may be overcompensating with your hip flexors or lower back.

What if I can't stay balanced?

Place your hands at your temples for maximum tension in your abs. If you can't stay balanced with your hands at your temples, then it is OK to lightly grab onto the bench behind your head until you increase the strength in your abs.

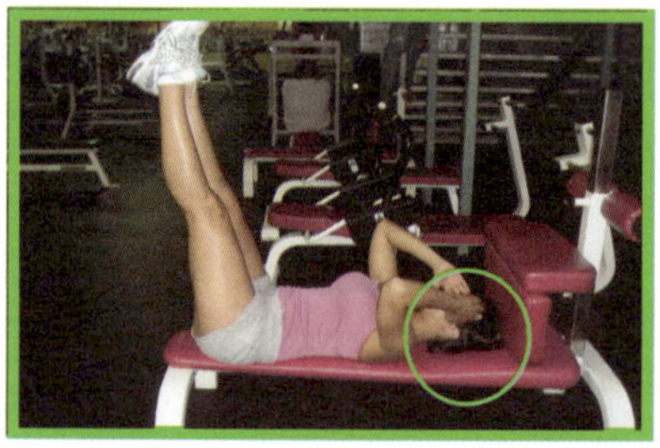

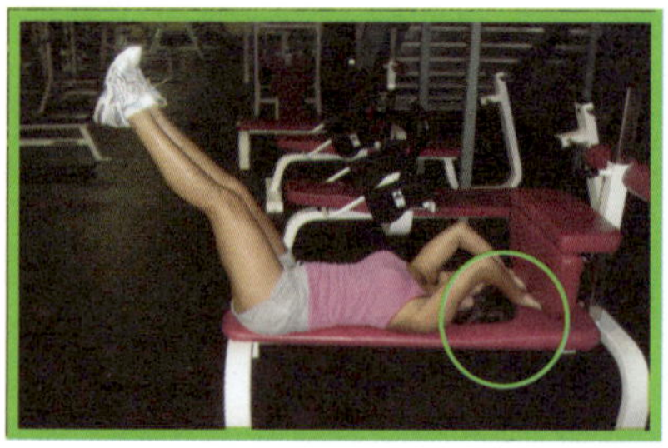

Can I lower my legs further than halfway?

Yes, lower your legs as far as possible. As long as you can maintain a flat lower back position, it is OK to lower your legs farther for a deeper, more intense stretch. If your lower back arches, you've lost form. Lower your legs until your lower back is about to arch and then raise them up. This maximizes the resistance, strength, and tension in your abs. Just be sure to avoid using your lower back, hip flexors, or quads. If you can feel them, you're overcompensating!

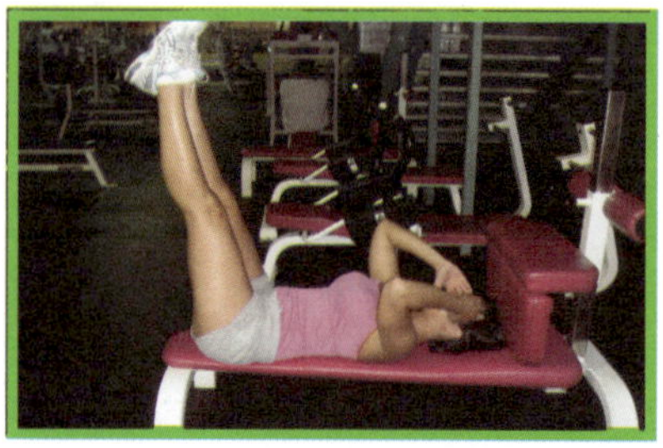

Starting Position

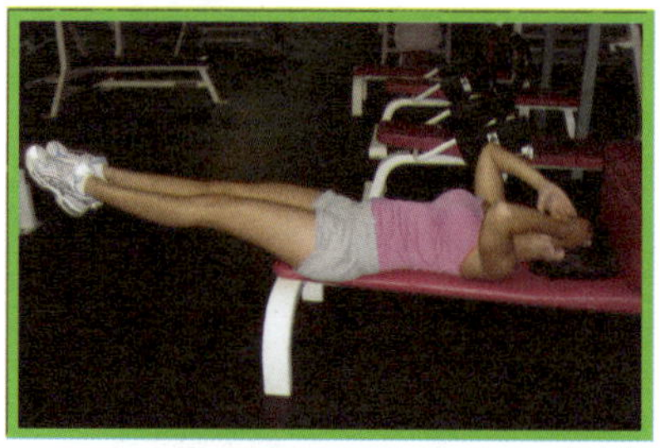

Lower Your Legs

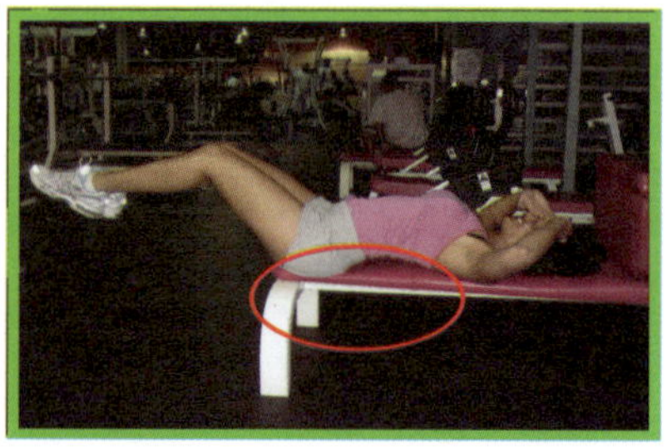

Minimize Arching Your Lower Back

What if I feel my leg muscles burn?

If you are feeling your legs, you are overcompensating. When your abs are fatigued, other muscle groups kick in to complete the motion. Your legs, specifically your quad muscles and your hip flexors, will overcompensate for the lack of strength in your abs. The moment you feel your legs, you're done with that set. If you continue to overcompensate with your legs, you will train less of your abs. Save your legs for leg day and focus on your abs!

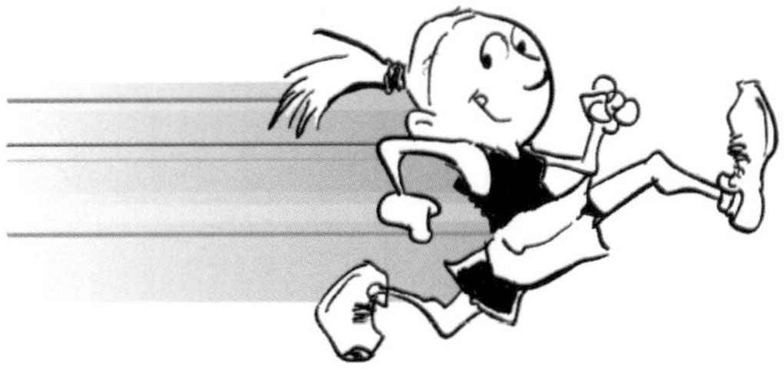

Cardio

Goal:

Complete 15 minutes on the **stairs** and 15 minutes on the stationary bike.

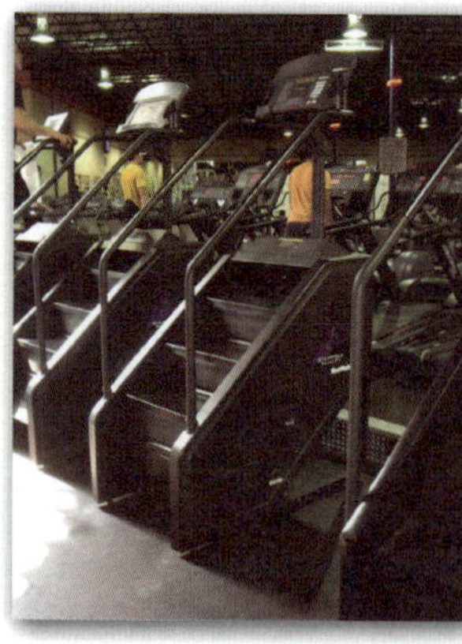

Primary
Quads
Glutes
Hamstrings

Stabilizers
Lower Back
Core
Calves
Shins

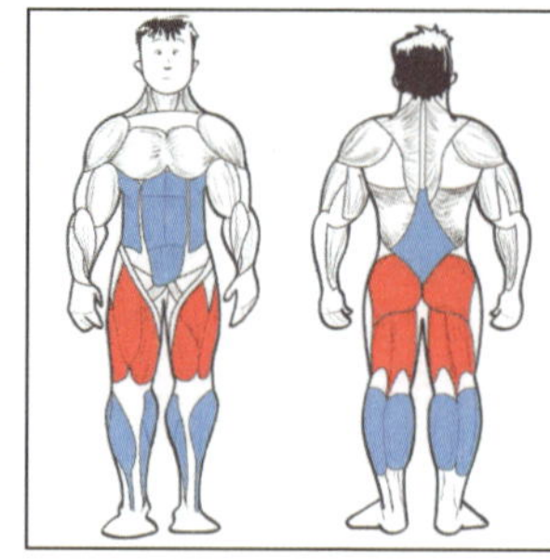

Why?

The stairs are a high-intensity cardio machine targeting the major muscle groups of your legs. It strengthens and conditions your quads, glutes, and hamstrings as well as your lower back, shins, calves, and core. This climbing machine is similar to the stair stepper. The stairs are more difficult than the stair steppers. It takes more energy to lift your legs up than it does to push down to take a step. This can be a very challenging exercise! It is another step up in cardiovascular conditioning since it requires a higher energy output and increased lung capacity.

How?

Step 1 - Step onto the stairs and press a program showing gradual up and down hills such as **CROSS COUNTRY** or **HILLS**.

Step 2 - Depending on your physical condition, choose your intensity level from 1 up to 10.

Step 3 - Enter 15 minutes and begin climbing the steps.

Step 4 - Keep your hands in a neutral position, about level with your waist.

Step 5 - Your glutes should be pushed back as if you're about to sit down. This helps maintain proper posture.

Step 6 - Step onto the steps as softly as possible with the most pressure in the center of your feet.

Step 7 - Your goal is to pace yourself for 15 minutes at medium intensity in addition to completing 15 minutes on the bike.

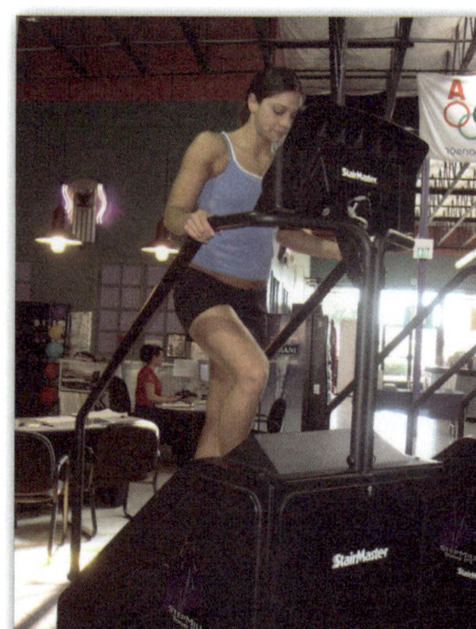

Range of Motion Techniques

To Maximize Muscle Tension and Minimize Overcompensation

Dos

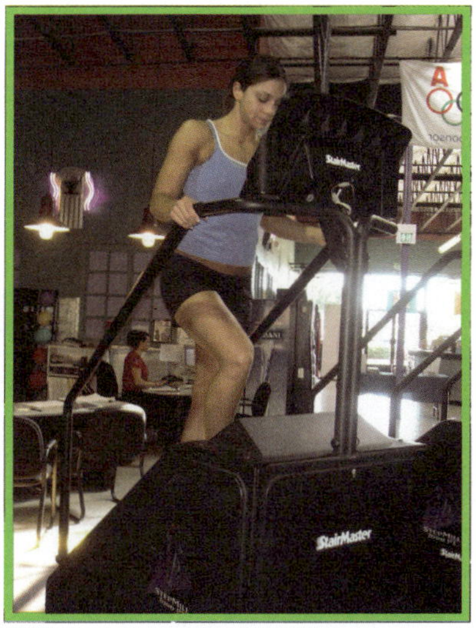

Begin with Proper Posture: Glutes Back, Knees Bent, Lean Slightly Forward

Don'ts

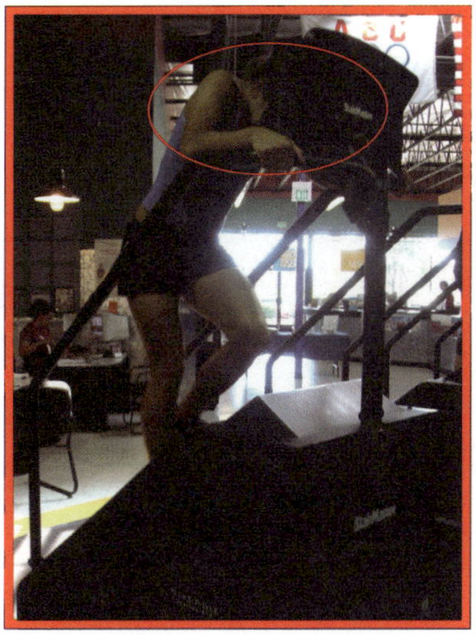

Avoid Swinging Sideways or 'Hanging On'

Visualize

"Hill and Balloon Effect"

Imagine yourself climbing a steep hill. Take large steps with balloons beneath your feet. Step as softly as possible to avoid "popping" the balloons.

This visualization technique assists in correcting your posture. It puts your body in the best position to maximize the use of your glutes, quads, hamstrings, and calves, while minimizing joint overcompensation.

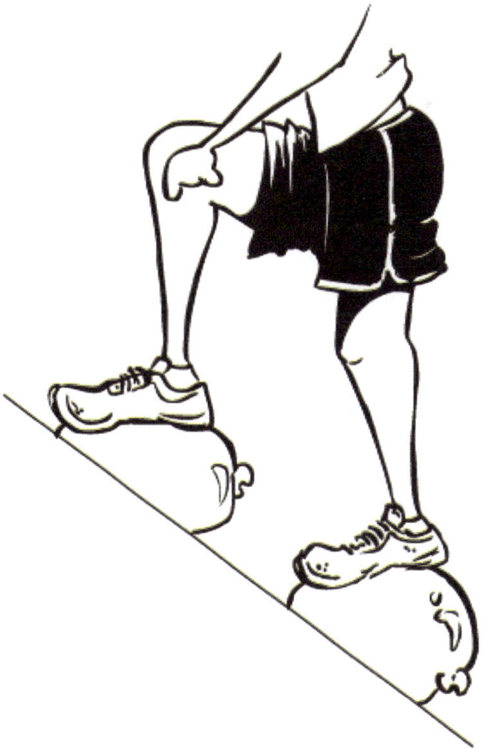

Questions and Answers

Can I hold on?

This is one of the most common questions in the gym. Eventually, you'll be able to place your hands on your hips or let them hang naturally in motion at your sides. But, until then, you can lightly hold the handles at shoulder height. If you feel the need to grip tightly or to "hang on" to the bar, you are probably stepping too fast. Decrease your speed just enough to step up and down using a light grip.

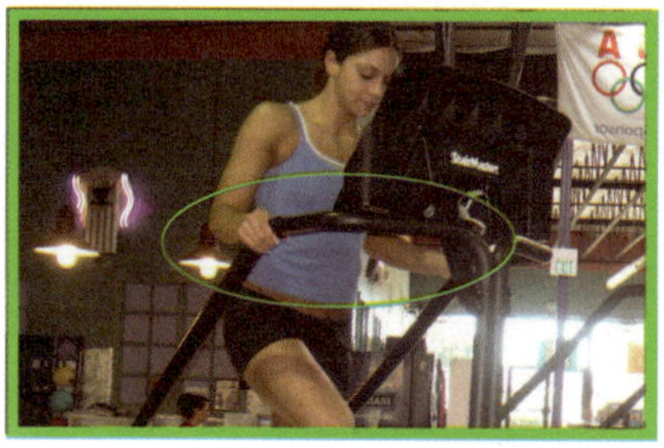

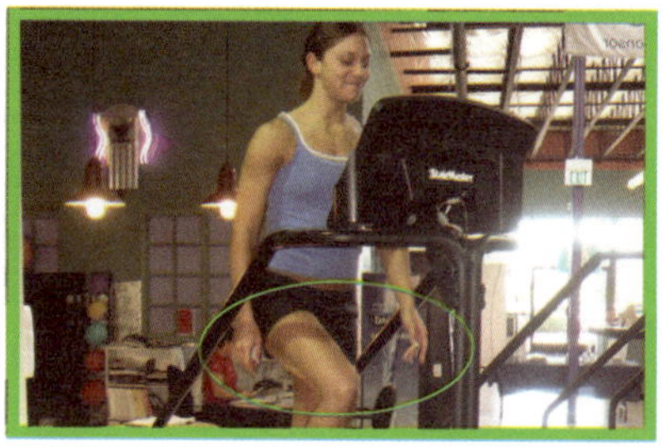

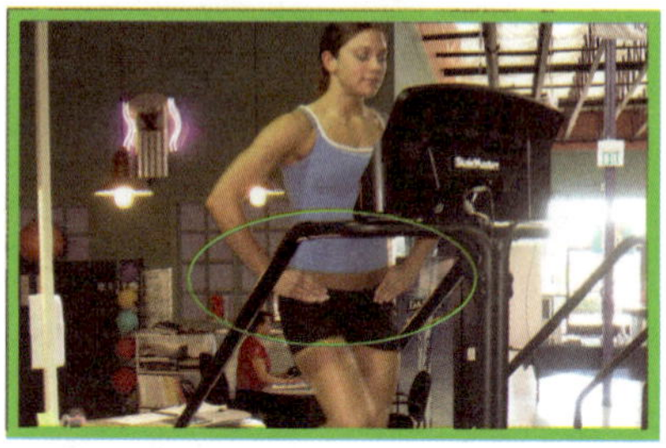

My knees hurt! Should I keep going?

That depends on your definition of hurt. Some people view a burning sensation or slight tension as painful, while others view it as a positive burn. If you feel actual knee pain, you need to reduce your intensity. Most knee pain is a result of improper form and technique. In this case, your glutes may not be far back enough. If your hips are back and your glutes are out, shift your weight to your heels and point your toes up. This relieves the pressure in your knees and allows your quads and glutes to do the work. If you continue to experience pain, you will need to stop.

My lower back hurts! Should I keep going?

It's OK to feel a light burning sensation or tightness in your lower back muscles, but feeling pain is a different story. Slow down and make sure you are using proper form. Your glutes should be pushed back and your weight should be on your heels. Never allow your knees to travel beyond your toes. Proper technique minimizes joint and ligament pressure in your knees and lower back, which ultimately decreases the risk of injury. Most muscle and joint pains are due to a lack of activity, cardio, and strength training. If you continue to feel pain in your lower back, then you may need to stop to avoid antagonizing your pain. In this case, go back to the treadmill or EFX until you strengthen a little more.

I sound like I'm stomping! How can I step quietly?

Step as softly as possible. Place most of the pressure in the center of your feet. As you step, visualize yourself quietly sneaking up on a friend who is resting peacefully at the top of the hill. If you are still pounding the stairs, decrease the intensity enough to control the pounding. Pounding is high impact and creates excessive joint tension. If you cannot step quietly, you may not be ready for the stairs. Continue to train on the EFX or Treadmill until you have developed a better foundation of conditioning. Keep up the hard work and you will be ready for the stairs in no time!

Can I skip a stair and take larger steps?

You bet! Take the largest steps possible. Taking large steps is the most effective way of using the stairs. The bigger your steps, the better the workout. If you skip every other stair you will get a better workout than if you step on every stair. But remember that maintaining proper form is your number one priority. No stomping! Keep the intensity low enough to maintain control of your steps. If you are ready to bump up the intensity, try taking two steps at a time.

Do I need to continue stretching?

Yes. Don't forget to stretch your hamstrings, quads, and calves after your cardio training!

Hamstrings

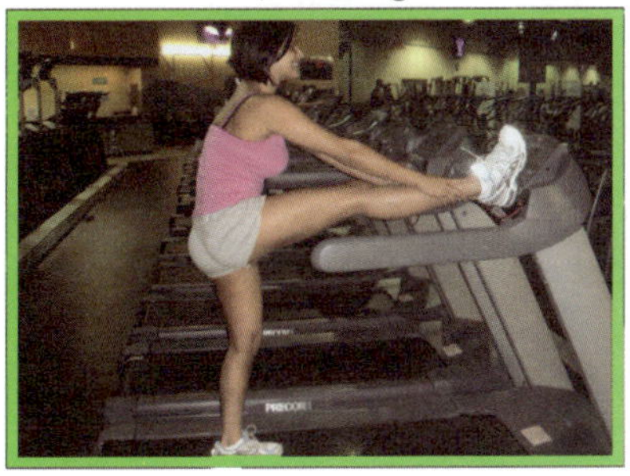

Quads

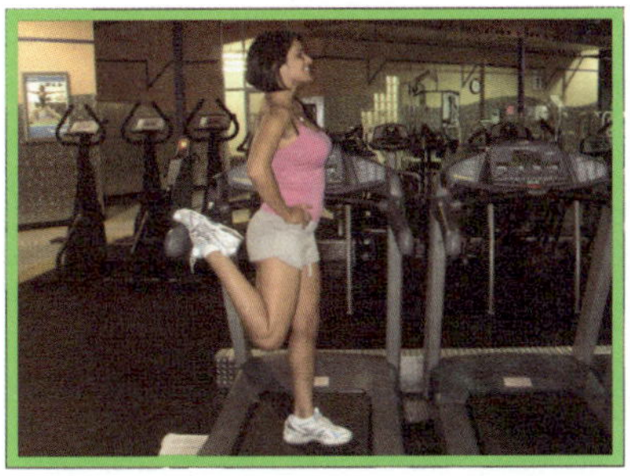

Calves

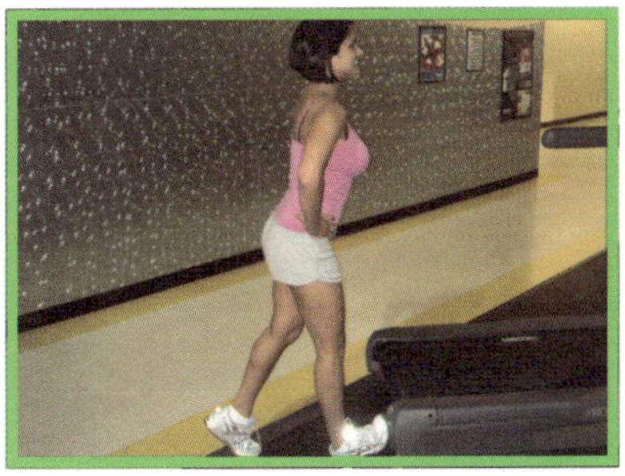

The Secrets to Success!

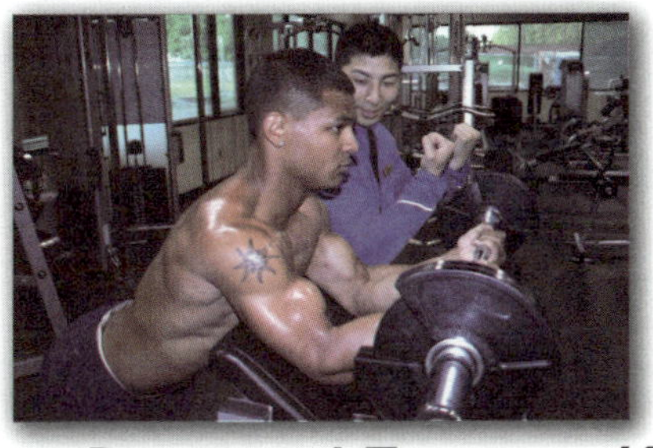

From Your Personal Trainer, Kevin Orr

Compared to changing your eating habits, which can be a challenge for many people, staying the course with your workouts will be easier for you as you work to achieve your health and fitness goals. However, you may feel aches and pains from weight training that might make you want to stop. Don't! Minor aches and pains come with weight training, but when you're working out correctly, the benefits far outweigh that slight discomfort. Weight training does carry some risk, though. Here are some of the most important techniques to muscles to do the work and minimize your risk of injury:

a. First and foremost, maintain proper posture. Abs should be firm while your lower back and shoulders should be neutral.
b. Visualize your muscles contracting and squeezing while performing the exercise.
c. Perform the exercise within its range of motion. This decreases joint tension.
d. Perform your exercise motion in a smooth and controlled manner. Jerky movements are definitely harder on your joints.
e. Relax your hand grip. A tight hand grip increases joint tension.
f. Your first set is a light warm up. Before increasing intensity, your muscles need more blood flow while your joints and tendons need to be more lubricated.

If you still feel pain while performing an exercise, stop. Avoid anything that may be causing your pain. If you do injure yourself, you won't heal and recover if you are constantly antagonizing the joint or muscle. Make sure that you absolutely avoid antagonizing any injuries, aches, or pains. That is the secret! If a pain persists, you may need to consult your physician.

Example Weight & Cardio Routine

Continue to choose a workout routine based on your level of fitness and your schedule before progressing to Week Seven. Write it down in your schedule, on page 249. If none of the example routines work for you, configure a routine that fits your needs, and write it down. Planning ahead will help you set yourself up for success.

Weight Routine 1

Sunday	Monday	Tuesday	Wednesday	Thursday	Friday	Saturday
	Arms: 4x15 Abs: 4x20		Legs: 4x20 Chest/Back/ Shoulders 4x15		Arms: 4x15 Abs: 4x20	

Weight Routine 2

Sunday	Monday	Tuesday	Wednesday	Thursday	Friday	Saturday
		Arms: 4x15 Abs: 4x20	Legs 4x20	Chest/Back/ Shoulders 4x15		Arms: 4x15 Abs: 4x20

Weight Routine 3

Sunday	Monday	Tuesday	Wednesday	Thursday	Friday	Saturday
	Arms: 4x15 Abs: 4x20	Legs 4x20	Chest/Back/ Shoulders 4x15	Arms: 4x15 Abs: 4x20		

Continue to choose routine 1, 2, or 3 to begin your weekly cardio routine, or rearrange your cardio training to best fit you.

Cardio Routine 1

Sunday	Monday	Tuesday	Wednesday	Thursday	Friday	Saturday
	Stairs: 15 Cycle: 15		Stairs: 15 Cycle: 15		Stairs: 15 Cycle: 15	

Cardio Routine 2

Sunday	Monday	Tuesday	Wednesday	Thursday	Friday	Saturday
		Stairs: 15 Cycle: 15	Stairs: 15 Cycle: 15	Stairs: 15 Cycle: 15		Stairs: 15 Cycle: 15

Cardio Routine 3

Sunday	Monday	Tuesday	Wednesday	Thursday	Friday	Saturday
	Stairs: 15 Cycle: 15	Stairs: 15 Cycle: 15	Stairs: 15 Cycle: 15	Stairs: 15 Cycle: 15	Stairs: 15 Cycle: 15	

Example Schedule

On your schedule, page 249, continue to write down which cardio machines along with the duration you plan to complete this week.

	Sunday	Monday	Tuesday	Wednesday	Thursday	Friday	Saturday	
Week 5 Weight: Body fat: Cardio: Duration:		*218* *30%* *Chest/Back* *Shoulders: 4x15* *Cycle: 15* *Stepper: 15*	*Arms: 4x15* *Abs: 4x20* *Cycle: 15* *Stepper: 15*	*Legs: 4x20* *Cycle: 15* *Stepper: 15*	*Chest/Back* *Shoulders: 4x15* *Cycle: 15* *Stepper: 15*	*Legs: 4x20* *Cycle: 15* *Stepper: 15*	*Chest/Back* *Shoulders: 4x15* *Cycle:* *Stepper:*	Why *Sick!* Solution *Make it up another day when feeling better*
Week 6 Weight: Body fat: Weights: Sets: Cardio: Duration:		*216* *Arms: 4x15* *Abs: 4x20* *Stairs: 15* *Cycle: 15*	*Legs: 4x20* *Stairs: 15* *Cycle: 15*	*Chest/Back* *Shoulders: 4x15* *Stairs: 15* *Cycle: 15*	*Arms: 4x15* *Abs: 4x20* *Stairs: 15* *Cycle: 15*	*Stairs: 15* *Cycle: 15*		

Before moving on...

Did you follow through with your plan? If not, cross out what you did not complete on your schedule and write in what you did complete before moving on to the next week.

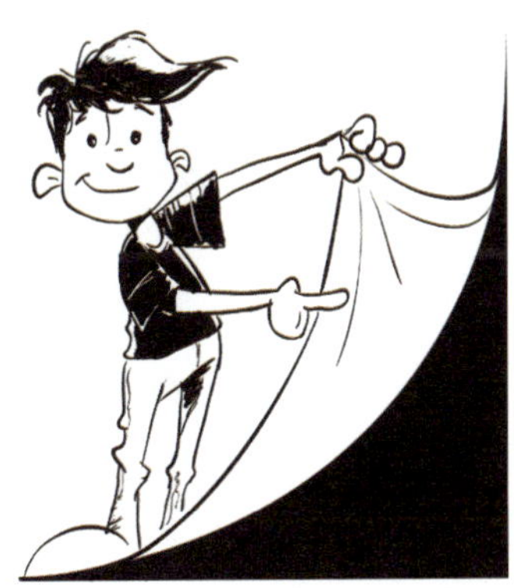

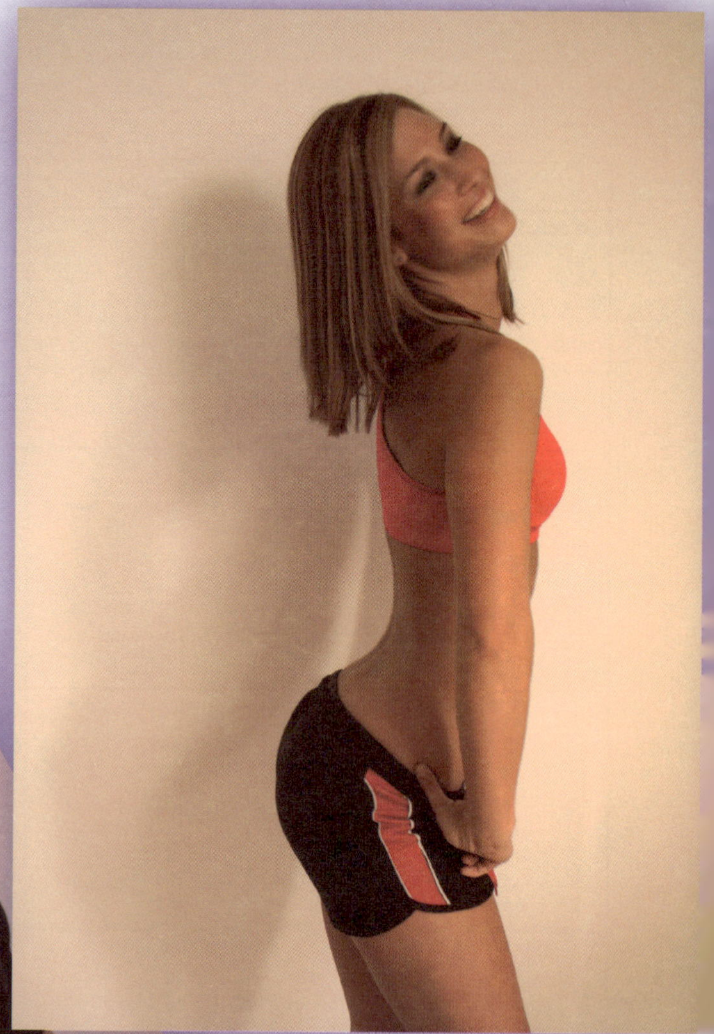

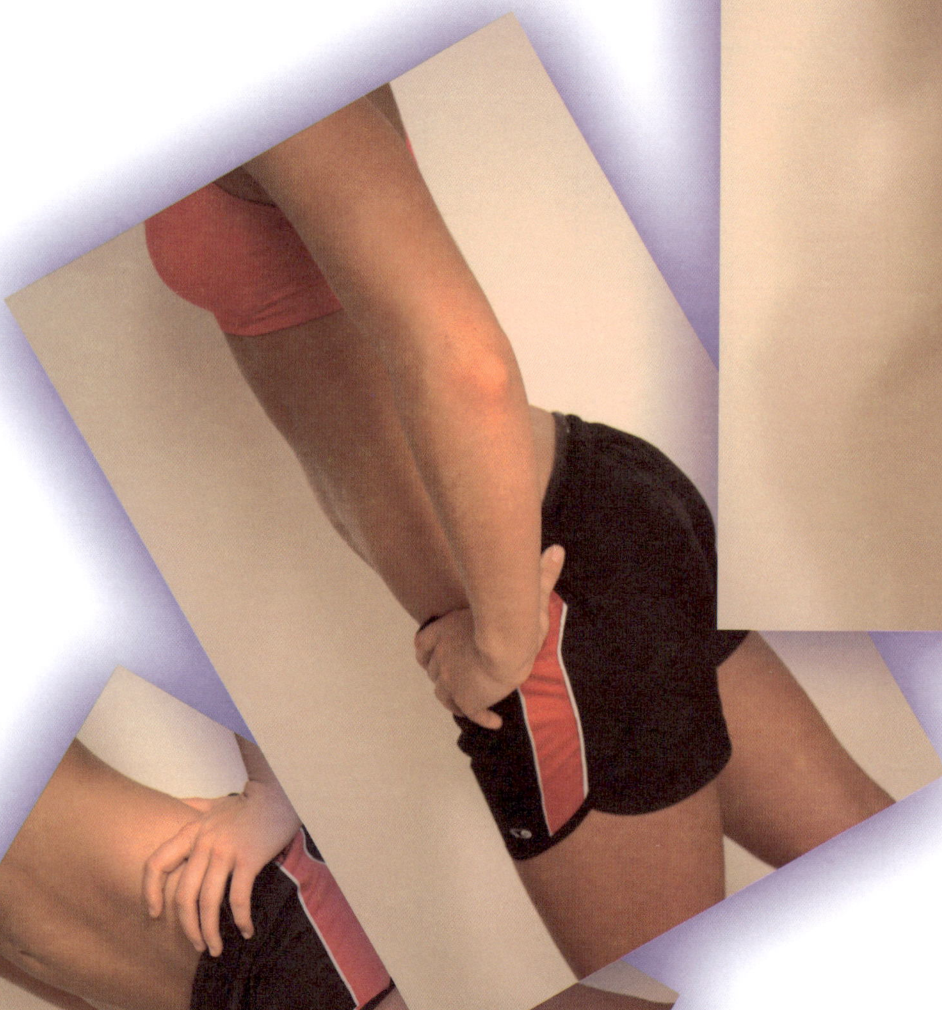

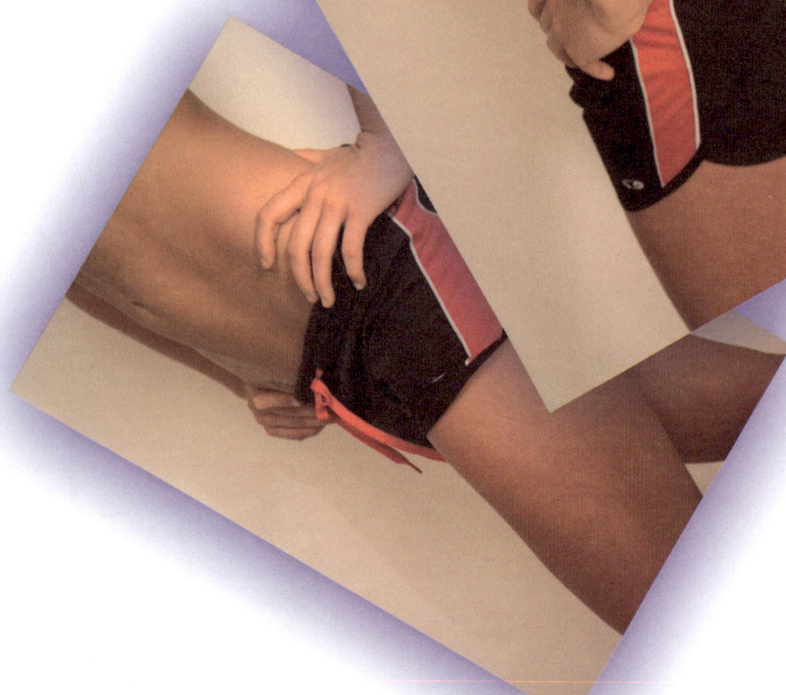

Week 7

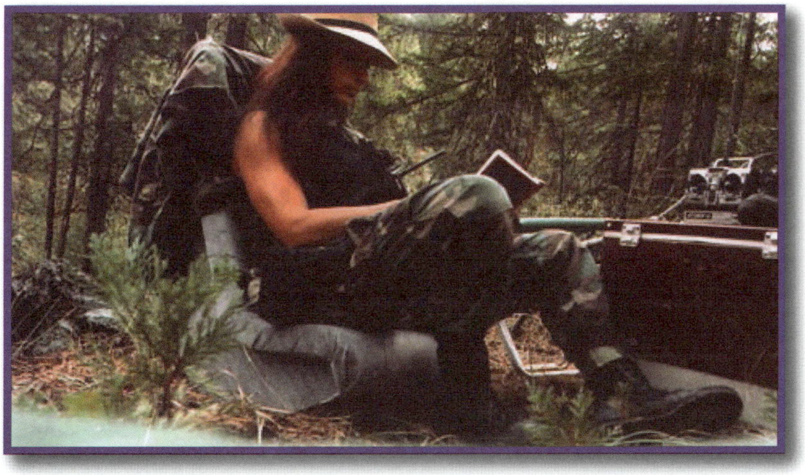

I knew, or thought I knew, a great deal about nutrition, but actually had no clue about my own body and metabolism or how anything affected that. I was slightly overweight, well beneath a realistic fitness goal, and my workouts were sorely inefficient. I had a great deal of work to do both mentally and physically. I can say without hesitation that the knowledge I gained from working with Kevin forever changed my whole approach to fitness, nutrition, and lifestyle. Kevin's approach to everything was always easy to follow because he keeps things in simple perspective. To this day, I have one of Kevin's mottos posted on my bulletin board at the office: If things aren't going right for you, fix it!

-Sherene Jennings

Goal:

Balance your meals and snacks with a specific ratio of proteins, fats, and carbohydrates (PFCs).

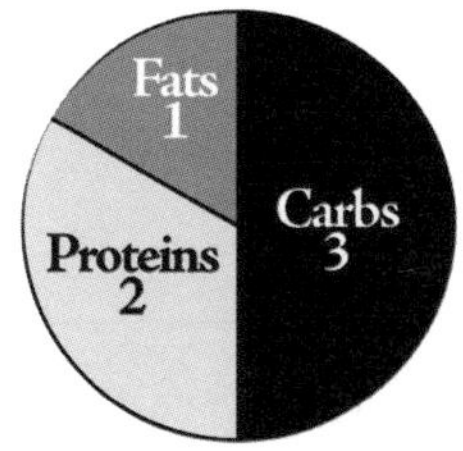

Why?

If you're ready to go to the next level in balancing blood sugar and gaining optimal energy, then it is time to count the number of PFC grams in each meal. Consuming the three macronutrients, proteins, good fats, and good carbohydrates, in moderation, is a great way to continue to build your positive nutrition habits. Carefully balancing the ratio of the proteins, fats, and carbohydrates you eat is a more precise method of fine tuning your nutrition. This will help you:

- Pinpoint exactly how to maintain the balance of your blood sugar levels throughout the day
- Eliminate the guess work when measuring serving sizes
- Gain more energy, strength, and endurance
- Break your body fat loss and strength plateaus

Calculating PFCs will lead to greater results!

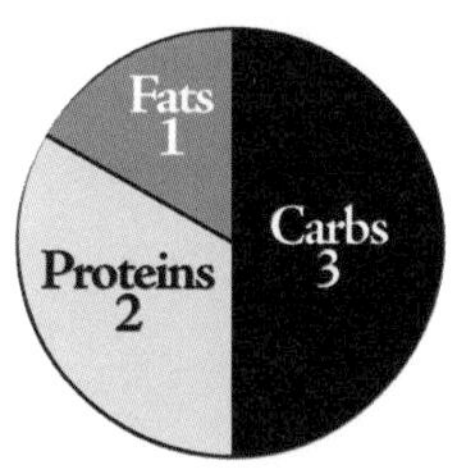

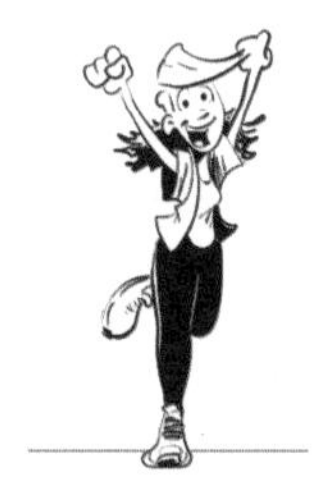

Balanced Blood Sugar = Optimal Metabolism and Energy

How?

Check your nutrition log and determine the number of PFCs in your current meals.

- Find the information you need on the nutrition facts label of the foods in your meals and snacks for the past week.

- For fresh meats and produce, you can go to www.makeyouhappen.com and search the Nutrition Log for all foods. The nutrition information is based on the U.S. Department of Agriculture (USDA) nutrition facts database.

Nutrition Facts

Serving Size 3 oz. (85g)

Amount Per Serving	As Served
Calories 38	**Calories from Fat** 0
	% Daily Value
Total Fat 0g	0%
Saturated Fat 0g	0%
Cholesterol 0g	0%
Sodium 0g	2%
Total Carbohydrate 0g	3%
Dietary Fiber 0g	8%
Sugars 0g	
Protein 0g	
Vitamin A 270% • **Vitamin C** 10%	
Calcium 2% • **Iron** 0%	

Percent Daily Values are based on a 2,000 calorie diet. Your daily values may be higher or lower depending on your calorie needs:

	Calories	2,000	2,500
Total Fat	Less than	65g	80g
Sat Fat	Less than	20g	80g
Cholesterol	Less than	300mg	300mg
Sodium	Less than	2,400mg	2,400mg
Total Carbohydrate		300g	375g
Dietary Fiber		25g	30g

PFC 1-2-3 Method

For every gram of fat you eat, you will need to consume two grams of protein and three grams of carbohydrates.

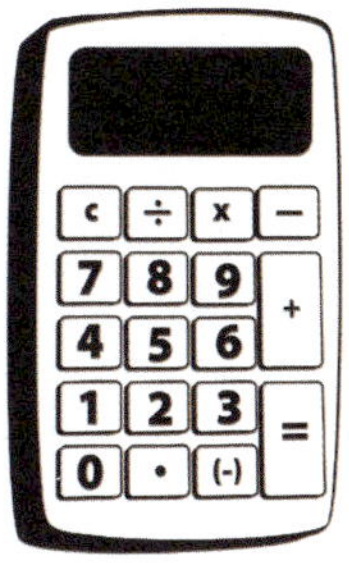

1-2-3 Method

1	-	2	-	3
Fat		Protein		Carbohydrates

Formula:	**Example:**
5 grams of fat 10 grams of protein 15 grams of carbohydrates	1 string cheese 1 small apple
10 grams of fat 20 grams of protein 30 grams of carbohydrates	1 cup of cottage cheese 2 small apples
15 grams of fat 30 grams of protein 45 grams of carbohydrates	1 slice of cheese 3 oz chicken 2 slices of WW bread

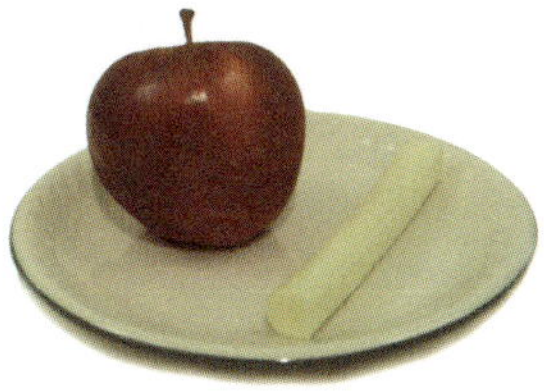

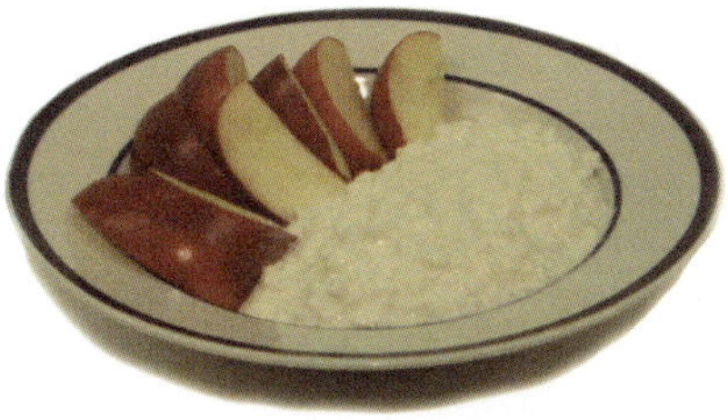

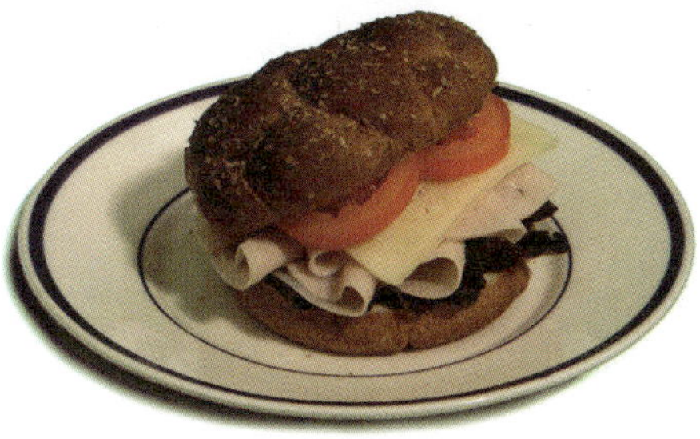

PFC Ratio Method

Protein requirements are typically, a minimum of one gram per pound of weight. The maximum amount of protein grams your body can digest and utilize is approximately 30 grams per meal every three hours. Your minimum intake should be 15 grams per meal.
Recommendation: Average your daily protein intake and divide it by the number of meals and snacks you eat to determine your current protein intake per meal. Next, divide your current body weight by the number of meals you eat to determine what your protein intake should be according to the PFC ratio.

Min = 15 grams per meal every three hours	Max = 30 grams per meal every three hours

Fat requirements are based on your protein intake. The maximum amount of your fat intake is half your protein intake. Your minimum intake should be 5 grams per meal, no matter how many grams of protein you're intaking. The maximum is 30 grams of fat.
Recommendation: Calculate your fat intake based on your protein intake.

Min = 5 grams per meal every three hours	Max = protein intake / 2

Carbohydrate requirements are also based on your protein intake. The maximum amount of carbohydrate grams is two times your protein intake. The minimum is the same amount of protein grams consumed.
Recommendation: Calculate your carbohydrate intake based on your protein intake.

Min = protein intake equals carb	Max = protein intake x 2

Select the ratio you want to use and review your nutrition log.

1. Calculate proteins, fats, and carbohydrates for each meal and snack.

2. Calculate the amount of PFC you need to add or delete to balance each meal and snack in the proper ratio.

3. Continue to write down what you eat and drink. Begin calculating the PFC grams in each meal and snack.

For Example, based on the PFC 1-2-3 Method:

Time	Food and Amount	P	F	C
7:00 AM	2 slices WW Toast, 1 Tbsp Adam's® PB	12	10	44
	PFC 1-2-3 method	**20**	**10**	**30**
	1 WW Toast	4	1.5	20
	1 Tbsp Adam's® PB	4	8	3
	½ cup of low-fat cottage cheese	12	2.5	4

WW = 100% whole wheat

Here's a quick reference for calculating your PFCs. An expanded reference can be found on www.makeyouhappen.com under Nutrition Log.

Proteins (4 oz)			
	P	F	C
Chicken	20	3	0
Turkey	20	3	0
Fish	20	20	0
Ham	20	5	0
Steak	20	10-20	0
Hamburger	20	20	0
Salmon	20	10-20	0
White Cheese (1oz)	8	7	0
Cottage Cheese (1/2 cup)	15	5	5
Milk (1 cup)	7	5	15

Fats (2 tbsp)			
	P	F	C
Olive Oil	0	15	0
Flax Oil	0	15	0
Avocado	1	6	4
Olives (4)	0	2	1
White Cheese (1 oz)	8	7	0
Adams PB	8	16	6

Carbohydrates (1 cup)			
	P	F	C
Wheat Bread (1 slice)	4	2	20
Wheat tortilla (1)	2	1	15
Wheat Pasta	12	4	60
Wheat Crackers	2	4	10
Wheat Bagel (1)	7	3	41
Wheat English Muffin (1)	1	6	27
Brown Rice	5	2	46
Wild Rice	7	1	35
Fruits			
Apple	0	0	20
Orange	2	0	25
Water-melon	1	0	11
Banana	1	1	35
Grapes	1	0	30
Fruit Juice	0	0	34
Vegetables			
Broccoli	2	0	5
Cauliflower	2	0	5
Lettuce	1	0	1
Carrots	1	0	13
Tomato	1	0	9
Corn	5	2	40

*Nutrition facts may vary depending on type, location grown, weather, storage, shelf-life, transportation, and seasonal patterns.

Questions and Answers

How do I know how many grams of protein I'm supposed to eat per meal?

As a rule of thumb, divide your current body weight by the number of meals you are eating each day. That is your average protein requirement per meal.

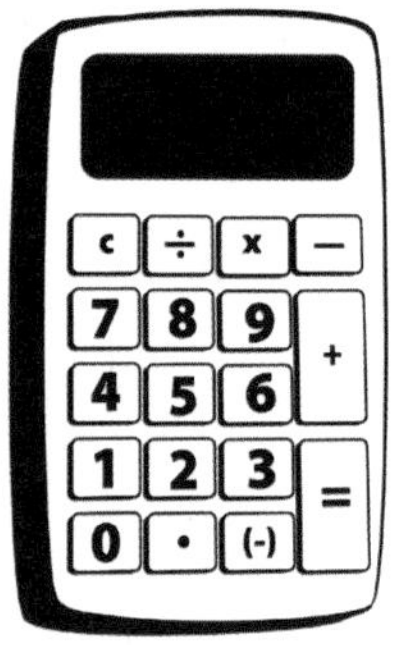

Daily Protein Grams
150 lbs ÷ 5 meals = 30 grams per meal or snack

If you are still hungry after you have calculated your protein requirement, then increase your protein. This also allows you to increase your fats and carbohydrates according to your ratio methods.

Do I eat that many grams of protein for snacks, too?

You can; however, you may get too full for your next meal. You should cut your regular meal in half or maybe in thirds to be considered a snack. A snack is simply a small meal to curb your hunger between meals.

If your body can only use 30 grams of protein every three hours, why does the average protein shake have more than 40 grams of protein?

Meal replacement powders, commonly known as protein shakes, should be used for post-workout meals only. Your body is screaming for nutrients and calories for optimal muscle and energy recovery after you have worked out. It has the ability to utilize more calories in the liquid form of protein and carbohydrates to refuel. If you really have to drink a protein drink at another time besides your post-workout meal, make sure the protein content meets your protein requirements for your ratio method.

I'm hungry! I'm an endurance athlete. Do I need more calories?

As an endurance athlete, your body does require more calories for fuel. The best way to meet this need is to increase your carbohydrates. It's OK to increase your carbohydrates beyond the recommended limit of twice the amount of your protein as long as you're hungry within three hours.

Do I need more protein if I'm a strength athlete focusing on building muscle?

Building muscle does require protein to repair damaged muscle tissue from weight training or high intensity activity. Your body, however, can only utilize a maximum amount of grams of protein per meal. For your strength and high intensity goals, it is safe to calculate one gram of protein per pound of your body weight for your total grams of protein required daily.

FORMULA:

175 lbs = 175 grams of protein divided by 6 meals per day = 29 grams of protein per meal

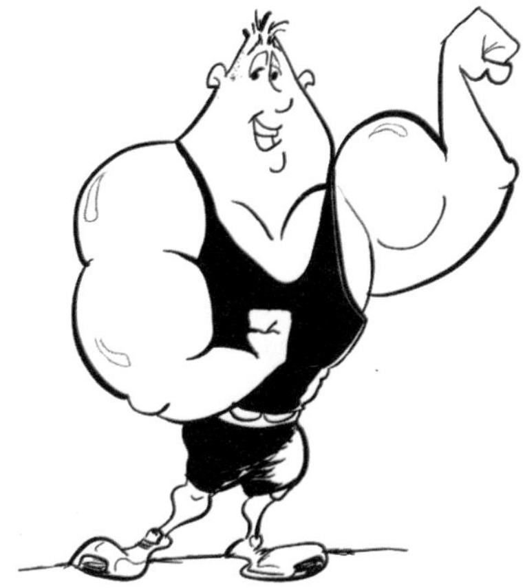

Don't forget, as a strength athlete, you may be required to eat more carbohydrates, more than twice your protein intake, to prepare for and recover from your strength or high intensity activity. Make sure you continue to follow your principle of eating a meal every three hours. If you're starving and your blood sugar is dipping, then your body requires more carbohydrates than the PFC Ratio Method.

If I were to eat 30 grams of protein six times in one day, I would eat 180 grams of protein. However, I weigh more than 180 pounds. Do I eat more protein per meal?

If you weigh more than 180 pounds due to higher body fat, then you do *not* need to eat more than your weight. Your goal is to eat 1 gram of protein per pound of lean muscle for optimal recovery and to maintain the muscle you have gained from your strength training workouts. What's considered lean muscle is weight minus the weight of bones, water, body fluids, food, and body fat. That said, it is not necessary to calculate your lean muscle to find success at this point. Use 1 gram of protein per pound of total weight as the rule of thumb for determining your protein requirement.

This seems like a lot of calories. Will I gain weight?

When your PFCs are moderate and balanced by using either the PFC 1-2-3 Method or the PFC Ratio Method and if you're slightly hungry for every meal every three hours, then no, you should not be gaining weight.

Why don't I just count calories or points?

Counting calories and/or points is a very simple method for making food choices for losing weight. Calories and points do not, by themselves, help you make nutritional decisions that positively impact homeostasis, the hormonal balance, that affects your metabolism, blood sugar, energy, strength and overall health. Eating PFCs in the optimal ratios does impact homeostasis. PFCs allow you to make informed nutritional decisions about what you are eating beyond calorie or point values.

Calculating PFC grams is too hard and it takes too much time. Isn't there an easier method?

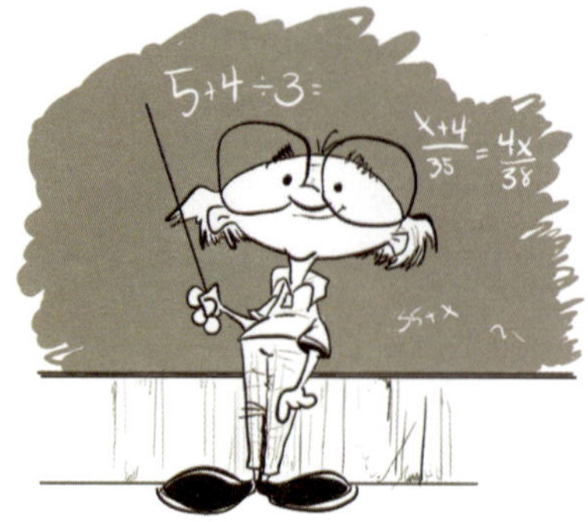

Unfortunately, there is not an easier method. Calculating your PFCs truly helps you determine how many calories your body really needs. If you were satisfied with your previous method of balancing your proteins, fats, and carbohydrates, and you were experiencing the results you want, then you should stick with it. But, if you really want to fine tune your nutrition and create long term results, then calculating your PFCs is the best approach!

I have more energy with the PFC 1-2-3 Method than I do with the PFC Ratio Method. Am I calculating something wrong in the PFC Ratio Method?

The PFC 1-2-3 Method is a simple ratio calculation for those who want to maintain their body fat loss or strength gains. It's also a great tool for maintaining a healthy blood sugar balance and optimal energy. If you have more energy with the PFC 1-2-3 Method, then it is perfect for you. If you have less energy with the PFC 1-2-3 Method, then you're probably eating too many or not enough carbohydrates to support your individual activity level and metabolic needs, which leads to blood sugar lows. The PFC Ratio Method provides more flexiblity for those requiring more or less carbohydrates to fit their lifestyle activity and workout intensity.

PFC Methods	Lifestyle Activity		Workout Intensity	
PFC 1-2-3 Method	Moderate:	10/20/30	Moderate:	10/20/30
PFC Ratio Method	Low:	10/20/20	Low:	10/20/20
	High:	10/20/40	High:	10/20/40

Which method of determining PFCs works best for body fat loss?

The PFC Ratio Method is typically best due to the flexibility it allows for increasing or decreasing carbohydrates as needed.

1. First, decrease your carbohydrates to equal your protein intake, which is the minimum requirement of carbohydrate intake.

2. Secondly, increase your fat intake close to your maximum amount, which is half the protein intake.

If you're slightly hungry three hours later, then this body fat loss ratio works the best. If you're too hungry, then increase your protein a little allowing you to increase your fats and carbohydrates. If you're at your maximum number of protein grams and you're still hungry, then increase your carbohydrates slightly higher but not beyond your maximum number of carbohydrates based on your protein intake.

Starting Point Per Meal	I'm Hungry! Per Meal	I'm Still Hungry! Per Meal
20 grams of protein	25 grams of protein	30 grams of protein
10 grams of fat	12 grams of fat	15 grams of fat
20 grams of carbohydrates	25 grams of carbohydrates	40 grams of carbohydrates

How do I calculate calories per meal?

If your goal is calorie-driven to further fine tune your results, then you will need to calculate calories.

Macronutrient	Calories
Protein	4
Fat	9
Carbohydrate	4
Alcohol	7

The PFC 1-2-3 and Ratio Method are lifestyle-driven. They are easier methods for eating balanced, hunger-controlling meals and snacks than the time-consuming method of calculating calories.

How do I break down PFCs when I'm eating out?

After you are familiar with calculating your PFCs, you will have a better *eye* for it in how much proteins, fats, and carbohydrates will be in food portions.

Is there a nutrition log that is easy to use for recording my calculated PFC Ratios?

Yes, you can make copies of the nutrition log on the next page.

Nutrition Log

Date:__________	Sun Mon Tues Wed Thurs Fri Sat					
	Plan			**Actual**		
Meal 1	P	F	C	P	F	C
Time:_____						
Meal 2	P	F	C	P	F	C
Time:_____						
Meal 3	P	F	C	P	F	C
Time:_____						
Meal 4	P	F	C	P	F	C
Time:_____						
Meal 5	P	F	C	P	F	C
Time:_____						
Meal 6	P	F	C	P	F	C
Time:_____						

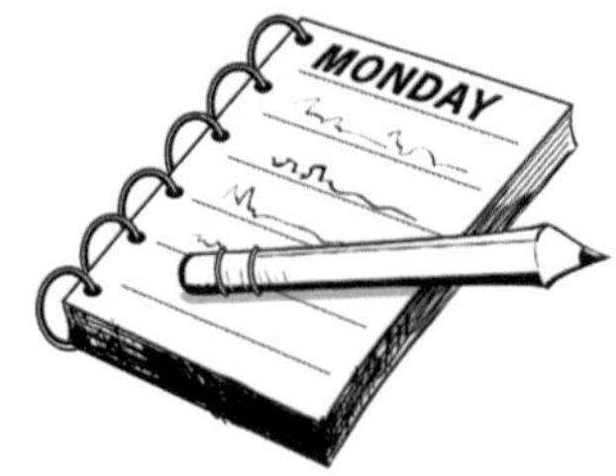

Checklist

Achieved:

- ✓ Consume meal or snack every 3 hours
- ✓ Water every 3 hours
- ✓ Sleep optimal hours
- ✓ Intake multivitamin
- ✓ Weights and cardio
- ✓ Consume PFCs everymeal or snack
- ✓ Foods low on the GI
- ✓ **PFC ratio balance**

Avoided:

- ✓ Sugars
- ✓ White flour
- ✓ Processed foods

Key Points

Week 1
- Eat a small meal or snack once every three hours – five to six meals per day.
- Drink at least 1 cup (8 ounces) of water per meal and at least one cup before, during, and after your workouts.
- Keep a nutrition log.
- Sleep is vital!
- Take a daily multivitamin.

Week 2
- Avoid bad sugars.

Week 3
- Avoid white flour and white rice.

Week 4
- Avoid processed foods.

Week 5
- Balance your meals and snacks with a combination of proteins, fats, and carbohydrates.

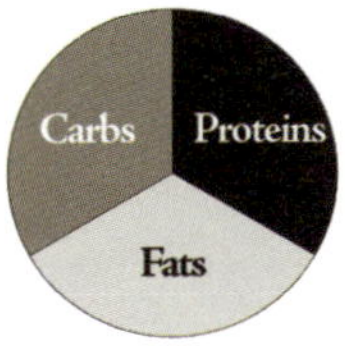

Week 6
- Eat foods that are low on the Glycemic Index.

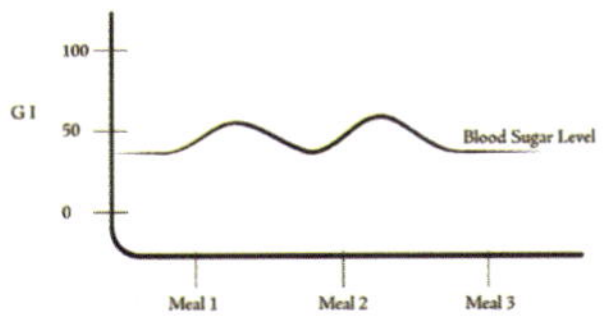

Week 7
- **Balance your meals and snacks with a specific ratio of proteins, fats, and carbohydrates** to fine tune your nutrition for optimal energy.

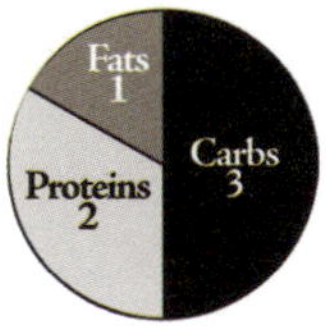

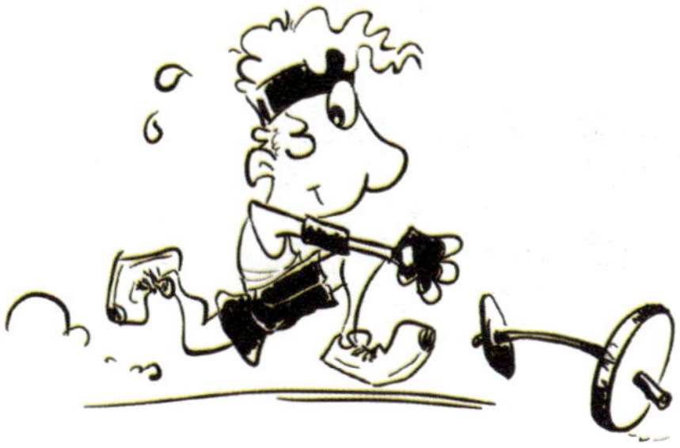

Legs

Goal:

Complete three sets of 20 **lunges**.

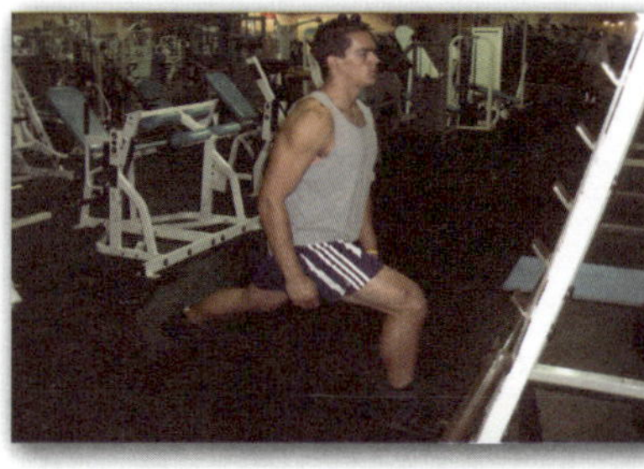

Primary
Glutes
Quads
Hamstrings

Stabilizers
Lower Back
Core
Calves
Shins

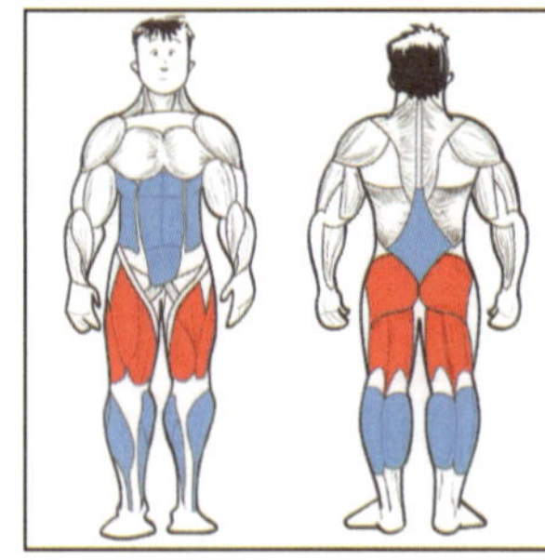

Why?

Lunges are a free weight exercise targeting the major muscle groups of your legs. In fact, they are one of the best leg exercises for strength and conditioning in your quads, glutes, and hamstrings. Your body has to work very hard, both physically and cardiovascularly, just to maintain and stabilize the lunge motion. The muscle stabilizers include your lower back and calves, as well as numerous stabilizers throughout your entire body.

How?

Step 1 - Stand in front of a mirror to monitor your position and technique.

Step 2 - Squeeze your abs to maintain proper posture.

Step 3 - Lengthen your legs into a lunge position.

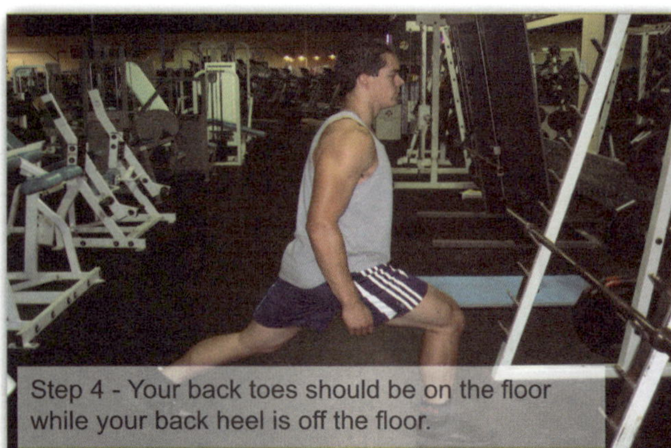

Step 4 - Your back toes should be on the floor while your back heel is off the floor.

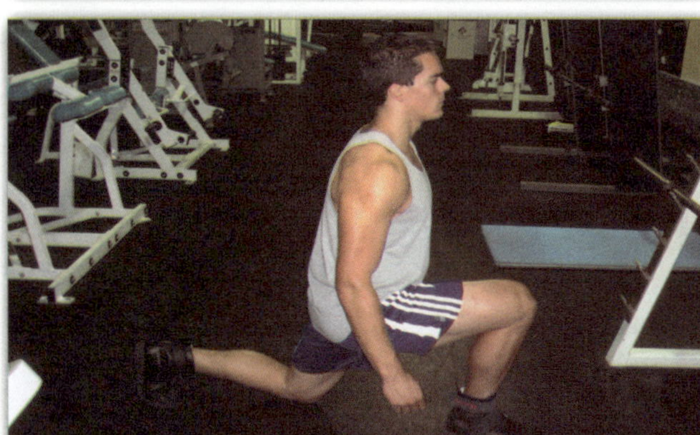

Step 5 - Slowly lower yourself to nearly touching the floor with your back knee.

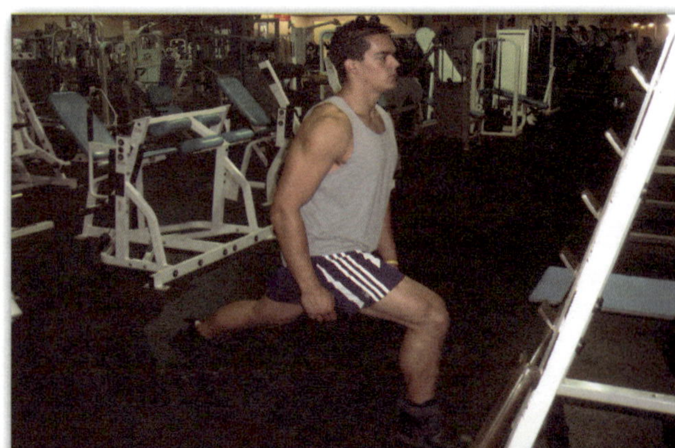

Step 6 - Push up to your starting position. Repeat for 20 reps, then switch legs.

Your goal is to complete three sets of 20 (3 x 20).

Range of Motion Techniques

To Maximize Muscle Tension and Minimize Overcompensation

Dos

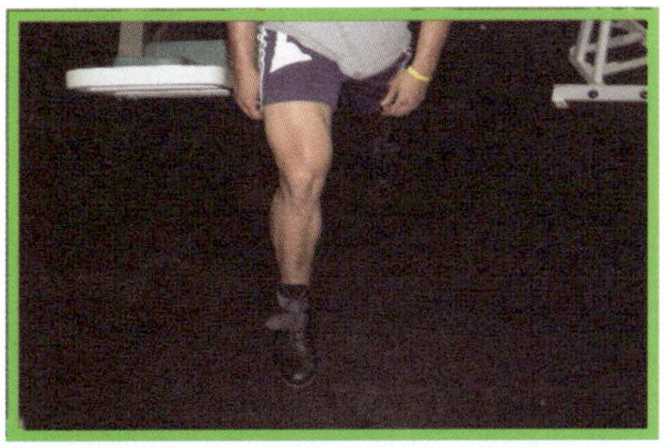

Begin with a Shoulder-Width Stance and Knees Bent

Don'ts

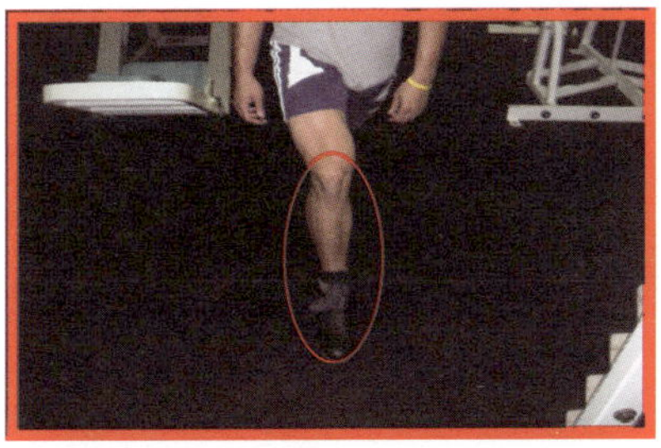

Avoid Standing on One Line With Both Feet

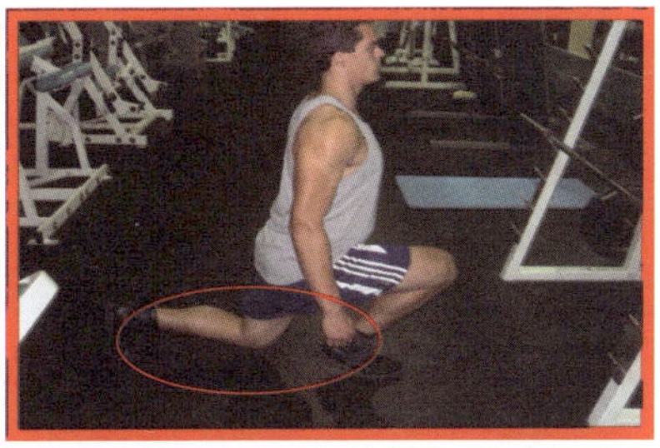

Avoid Shortening Your Stance

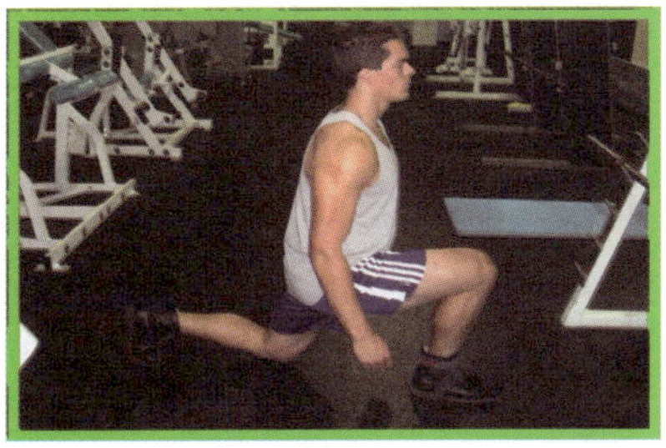

Front Upper Thigh Should Almost be Parallel With Floor

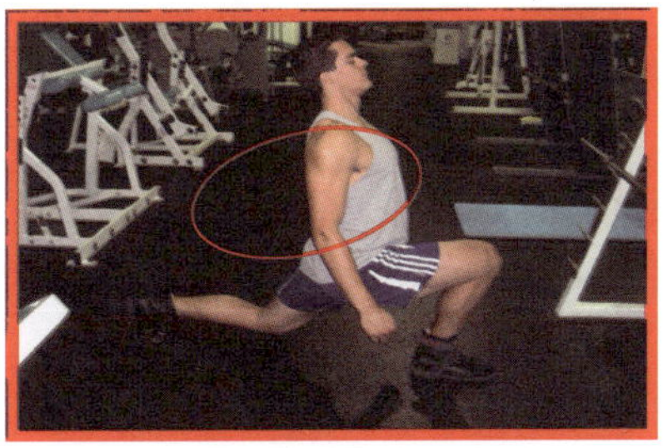

Avoid Leaning Too Far Back or Staying Straight up

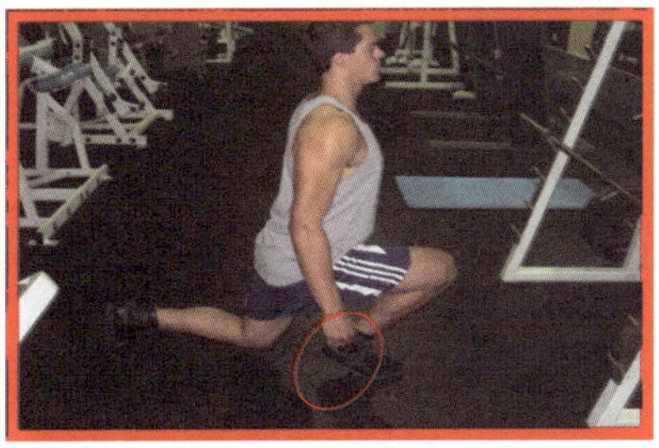

Avoid Lifting Your Front Heel off the Floor

Visualize

"Cable and Balloon Effect"

Imagine yourself lunging down and up with balloons beneath your feet. You have cables attached to your shoulders guiding you through the lunge motion. The cables lower you down and pull you straight up toward the ceiling in a smooth, controlled motion. There is another cable attached to your front knee, pulling it straight forward as you lunge down. Visualize the cables working together to pull your knee straight forward and smoothly lower you down and pull you up, without popping the balloons beneath your feet.

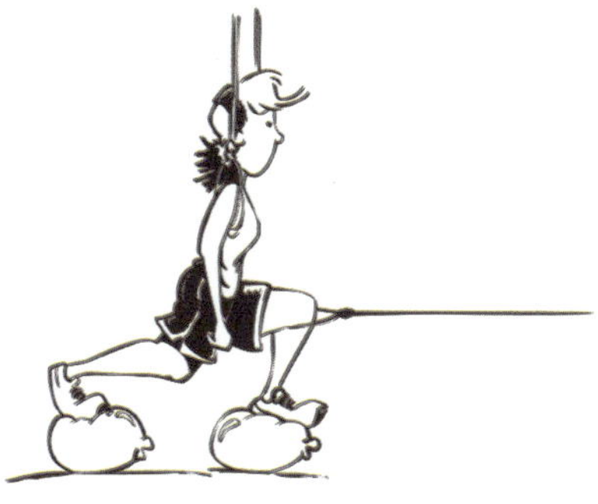

As the shoulder cables guide you through the lunge motion, the balloons help to decrease the tension in your knees and toes by reducing the amount of pressure placed on the floor. The cable attached to your front knee provides knee stabilization, places you in proper alignment, and forces your leg muscles to do the work.

Due to the strength requirements of the lunge, you may need to develop more leg strength before you will be able to visualize correctly. The good news is that lunges are one of the most effective strength building leg exercises you can perform.

Week 7

Questions and Answers

Lunges are too difficult. Is there anything I can do for my balance?

If you need increased stability or balance, you can hold onto a post or bar until your strength increases and your balance improves.

Why do I have to feel like I'm leaning forward?

Leaning forward slightly decreases tension in your lower back joint and maximizes the tension in your legs allowing you to get the most effective workout.

Why do I need my weight on my front heel?

As you move through the lunge motion, it is easy to allow your weight to shift to your knees. Unfortunately, pressure in your knees will lead to unwanted injuries. By placing your weight on your front heel, you are able to keep the weight off your knees. When your weight is on your heel, the heel of your shoe will be flat on the floor. If your heel picks up, your weight has shifted to your knees. The best way to ensure your front heel stays flat on the floor is to lift your toes up inside of your shoe. You can imagine a cable is pulling your toes up to the ceiling. Be sure your knee stays above or behind your toes.

I can't lunge down low enough. What can I do to improve my form?

If you've been performing squats with no trouble, you should be able to perform lunges. However, you may need to work up to proper lunge form. Try limiting your range of motion and limit the number of reps. This will strengthen and condition your legs for proper lunge form and technique.

Can I perform more than three sets of 20 reps?

Yes, if you are ready, you can perform up to six sets of 20 reps! But, if it is your first time performing lunges, you should do the minimal amount of sets and reps to ease into lunges. Otherwise, you might become extremely sore.

What should I feel after performing lunges?

You should feel a burning sensation in your legs by the end of each set. When you're finished, you should have a slight pump and/or a "wobble" effect in your legs. When you're pumped, your legs will feel full or swollen. People often describe it as feeling like jello. However you describe it, the feeling is very positive; your body is telling you that you're training at optimal intensity.

What if I feel pain in my knees when lunging?

Knee pain is typically associated with bad form. Do your best to use proper form.

1. Make sure your knees never go beyond your toes.
2. Keep your weight in your front heel flat on the floor.
3. Always keep your back leg at an angle, not straight up and down.

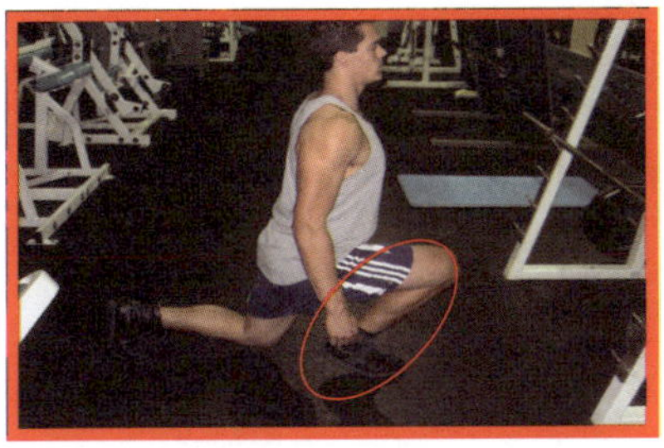

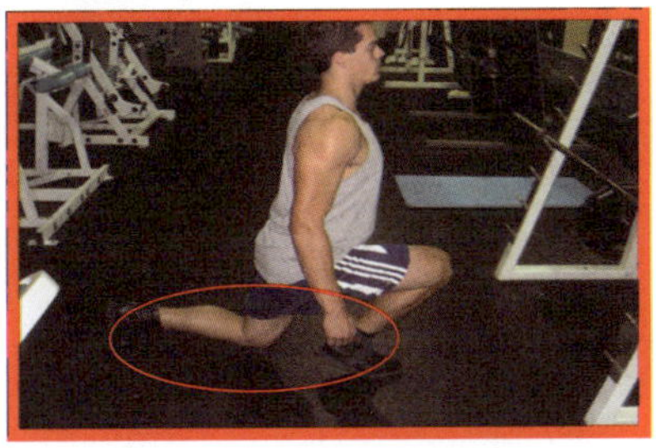

If you continue to feel pain in your knees then stop! Go back to performing squats or exercises that you do not cause pain.

Why are my back quads stretching and burning?

If your back quads are stretching or burning, it is due to inflexibility. The good news is that the burning sensation is positive muscle tension. You may need to limit the number of reps you complete. You should reach a slight burning sensation, but avoid pushing beyond the burning sensation. Otherwise, you may be too sore to walk tomorrow.

Calves

Goal:

Complete four sets of 20 reps on the **single calf raises**.

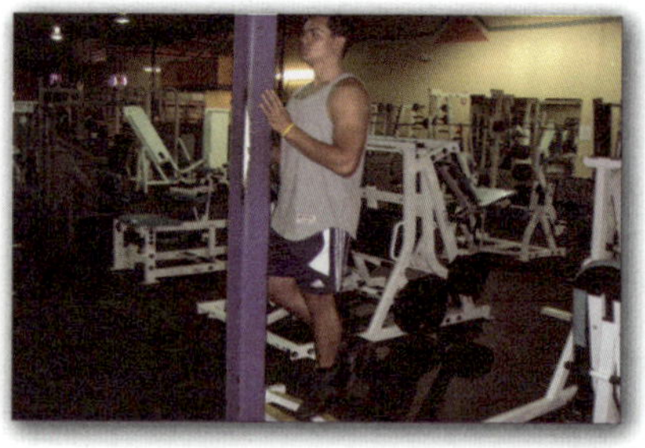

Primary
Calves

Stabilizers
Quads
Hamstrings
Core

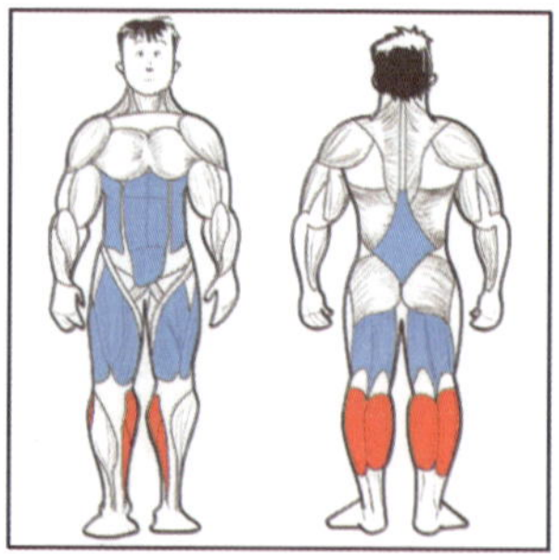

Why?

Single calf raises are a high intensity exercise targeting your calves. Training each calf independently increases the intensity of the exercise. Your quads, hamstrings, and core muscles all work together to stabilize the motion.

How?

Step 1 - Stand on the edge of a calf stand. Place your weight on the ball of your feet .

Step 2 - Squeeze your abs to push your lower back into a neutral position.

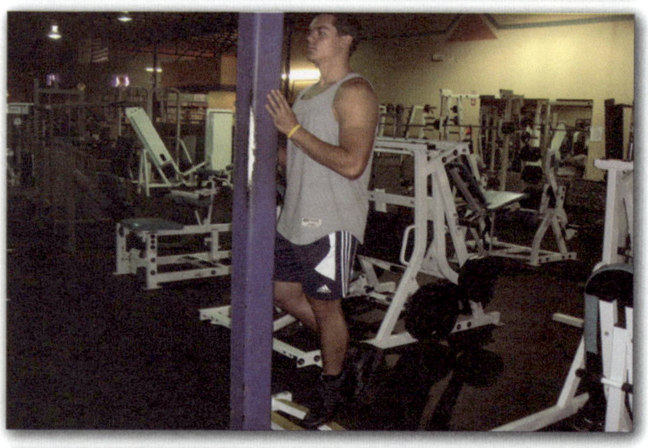

Step 3 - Pull your hips slightly back and lean slightly forward.

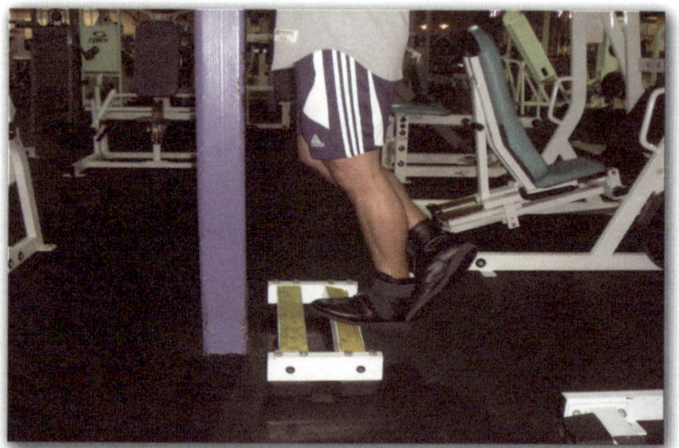

Step 4 - Lower your heel to the point of feeling a slight stretch in your calf.

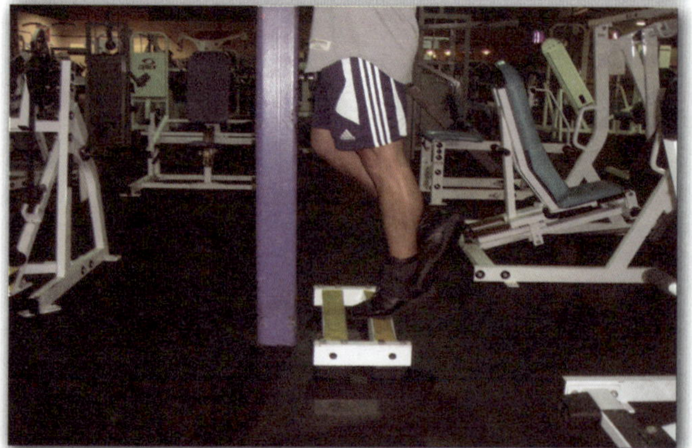

Step 5 - Lift and squeeze up to the peak contraction of your calf raise. Switch legs and repeat.

Your goal is to complete four sets of 20 (4 x 20).

Range of Motion Techniques

To Maximize Muscle Tension and Minimize Overcompensation

Dos

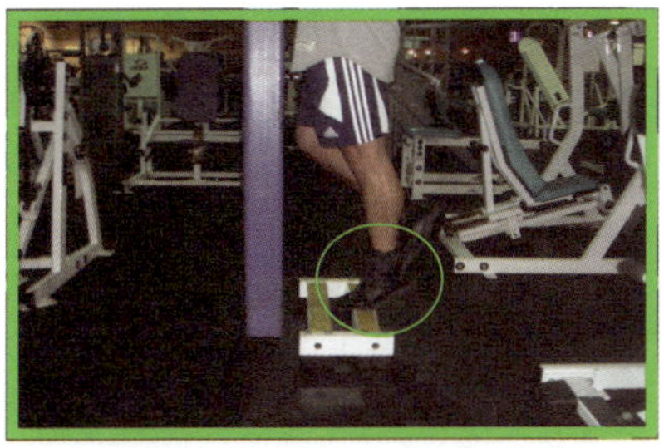

Begin With Squeezing Calves at Top

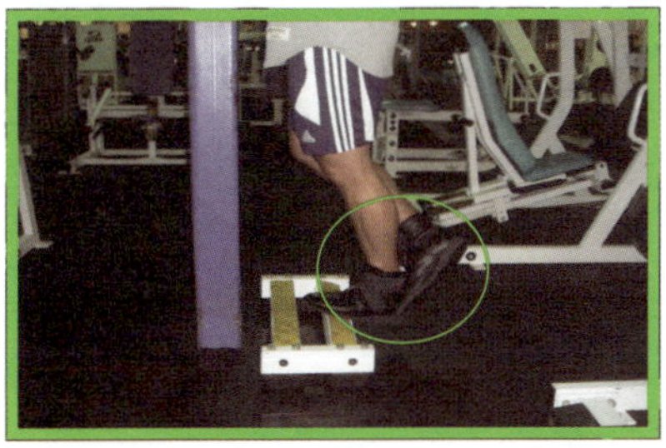

Lower Heels to Resist and Feel Calves Stretching

Don'ts

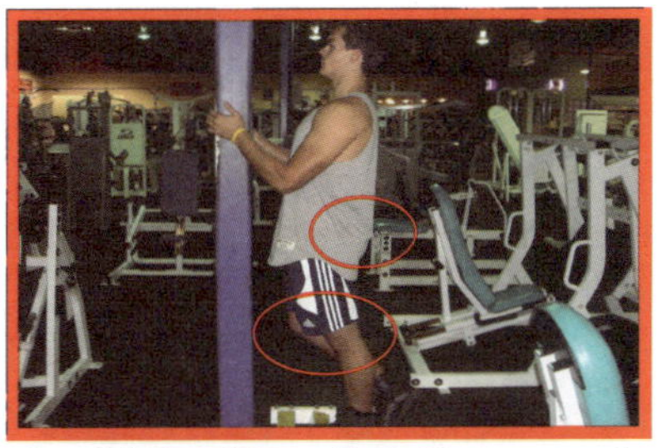

Avoid Locking Out Knees and Arching Lower Back

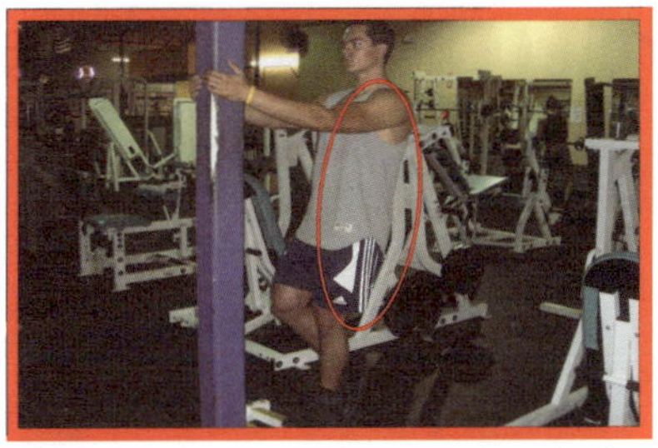

Avoid Leaning Too Far Back Or Using Arms For Help

Visualize

"Balloon Effect"

When performing calf raises on one leg, imagine yourself standing on a balloon. Using a smooth and controlled motion, lower yourself down softly and push yourself up without popping the balloon. Resist your weight as you lower your heel toward the ground. Focus on feeling a stretch in your calf at the bottom of the range of motion. Contract your calf to push yourself up to your starting position. Continue visualizing and repeat your reps.

Moving from a stretch to a contraction in a smooth, controlled motion allows for greater calf muscle utilization and maximizes the effectiveness of the exercise. An explosive and jerky motion would create momentum and cause your entire body to overcompensate.

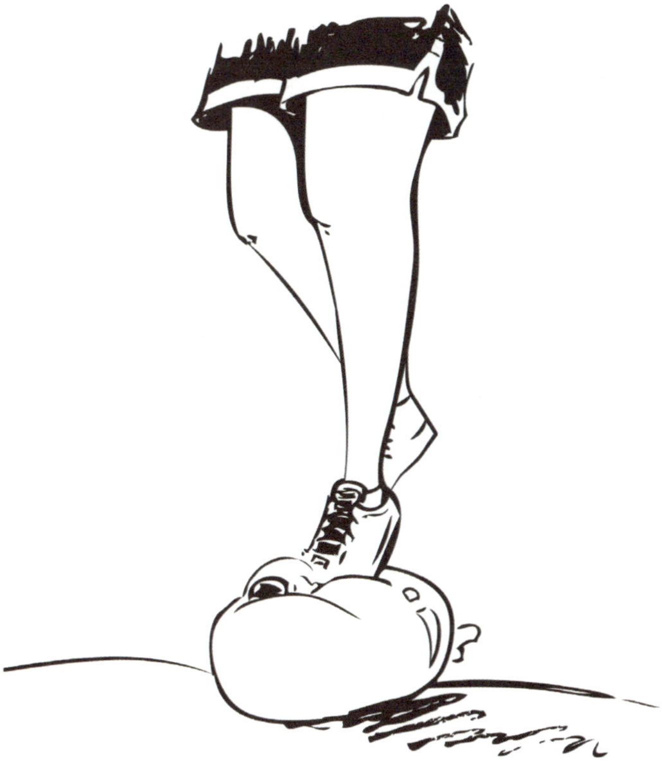

Questions and Answers

How do I position my foot for single calf raises?

Place your foot on the edge of the calf stand. The ball of your foot should stay on the edge of the stand while the heel of your foot hangs off the edge. If you notice your foot slipping off the stand then adjust your footing. Be sure you are not using momentum to push youself up. This forces the calves to do the work and keeps your toes from overcompensating.

Why do I need to maintain a neutral lower back position when I'm training my calves?

The neutral lower back position is proper posture. It relieves the pressure in your lower back, helps to prevent overcompensation, and forces your calves to do most of the work. For that reason, pull your hips back, lean slightly forward, and squeeze your abs to push your lower back into a neutral position.

The Secrets to Success!

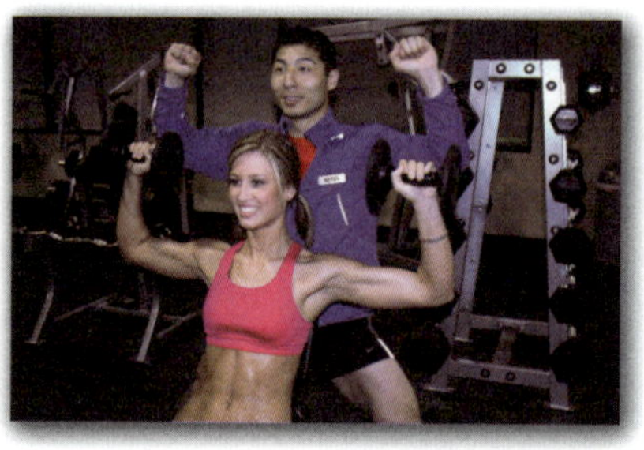

From Your Personal Trainer, Kevin Orr

Balancing your meals with a specific ratio of PFCs is definitely a big step and provides another big learning curve. Since you know what proteins, fats, and carbohydrates are, you can simply look at your nutrition facts to calculate exactly what you are eating. Yes, it is a little more time consuming to learn, but it is imperative you know how many PFCs you are eating so you can fine tune the balance of your meals. This fine tuning will give you another leap in energy and performance. Your body's hormones do not perform at their maximum based on a point system or simply in moderating the amounts of foods you eat. The proper balance of proteins, fats, and carbohydrates synergize with each other to accelerate body fat loss and help you meet your fitness goals. Balance is the secret!

Kevin is truly one of a kind: focused, disciplined, and has a great amount of compassion. The first six months with him were like magic. I lost 30 pounds and through his system became in great shape. He understands fitness completely and I respect him completely.

- Mort Kelsey

I cannot emphasize enough just how grateful I am to Kevin for his training program and philosophy. It was only a few months, but I gained the most results from those few months of training than I did in a lifetime of high level athletics and team sports. Recently, I was selected for a law enforcement position working as an enforcement agent. My mental preparation for training and police academy starts with the fitness lessons he taught me. Step one, two, and three: Nutrition, nutrition, nutrition! Being a lifetime athlete, my belief about nutrition was that as long as I worked out, I could eat whatever I wanted. That proved to be a myth if I wanted to tone and have more energy. I also believed I was strong enough to begin my workouts at a much higher standard and level than the non-athlete. I was wrong on both accounts. Kevin showed me that nutrition was the foundation of feeling good and healthy and maintaining the results I was working for in the gym. He helped me to get stronger and maximize the results necessary for a career in law enforcement.

- Michelle Ackerman

Example Weight & Cardio Routine

Continue to choose a workout routine based on your level of fitness and your schedule before progressing to Week Eight. Write it down in your schedule, page 249. If none of the example routines work for you, configure a routine that fits your needs, and write it down. Planning ahead will help you set yourself up for success.

Weight Routine 1

Sunday	Monday	Tuesday	Wednesday	Thursday	Friday	Saturday
	Arms: 4x15 Abs: 4x20		Legs: 3x20 Chest/Back/ Shoulders 4x15		Arms: 4x15 Abs: 4x20	

Weight Routine 2

Sunday	Monday	Tuesday	Wednesday	Thursday	Friday	Saturday
		Arms: 4x15 Abs: 4x20	Legs 3x20	Chest/Back/ Shoulders 4x15		Arms: 4x15 Abs: 4x20

Weight Routine 3

Sunday	Monday	Tuesday	Wednesday	Thursday	Friday	Saturday
	Legs 3x20	Chest/Back/ Shoulders 4x15	Arms: 4x15 Abs: 4x20	Legs 4x20		

Continue to choose routine 1, 2, or 3 to begin your weekly cardio routine, or rearrange your cardio training to best fit you.

Cardio Routine 1

Sunday	Monday	Tuesday	Wednesday	Thursday	Friday	Saturday
	EFX: 15 Stairs: 15		EFX: 15 Stairs: 15		EFX: 15 Stairs: 15	

Cardio Routine 2

Sunday	Monday	Tuesday	Wednesday	Thursday	Friday	Saturday
		EFX: 15 Stairs: 15	EFX: 15 Stairs: 15	EFX: 15 Stairs: 15		EFX: 15 Stairs: 15

Cardio Routine 3

Sunday	Monday	Tuesday	Wednesday	Thursday	Friday	Saturday
	EFX: 15 Stairs: 15	EFX: 15 Stairs: 15	EFX: 15 Stairs: 15	EFX: 15 Stairs: 15	EFX: 15 Stairs: 15	

Example Schedule

On your schedule, page 249, continue to write down which cardio machines along with the duration you plan to complete this week.

	Sunday	Monday	Tuesday	Wednesday	Thursday	Friday	Saturday	
Week 5 Weight: Body fat: Cardio: Duration:		218 30% Chest/Back Shoulders: 4x15 Cycle: 15 Stepper: 15	Arms: 4x15 Abs: 4x20 Cycle: 15 Stepper: 15	Legs: 4x20 Cycle: 15 Stepper: 15	Chest/Back Shoulders: 4x15 Cycle: 15 Stepper: 15	Legs: 4x20 Cycle: 15 Stepper: 15	Chest/Back Shoulders: 4x15 Cycle: Stepper:	Why Sick! Solution Make it up another day when feeling better
Week 6 Weight: Body fat: Weights: Sets: Cardio: Duration:		216 Arms: 4x15 Abs: 4x20 Stairs: 15 Cycle: 15	Legs: 4x20 Stairs: 15 Cycle: 15	Chest/Back Shoulders: 4x15 Stairs: 15 Cycle: 15	Arms: 4x15 Abs: 4x20 Stairs: 15 Cycle: 15	Stairs: 15 Cycle: 15		Why Solution Perfect week!
Week 7 Weight: Body fat: Weights: Sets: Cardio: Duration:		214 29% Legs: 4x20 EFX: 15 Stairs: 15	Chest/Back Shoulders: 4x15 EFX: 15 Stairs: 15	Arms: 4x15 Abs: 4x20 EFX: 15 Stairs: 15	Legs: 4x20 EFX: 15 Stairs: 15	EFX: 15 Stairs: 15		

Before moving on...

Did you follow through with your plan? If not, cross out what you did not complete on your schedule and write in what you did complete before moving on to the next week.

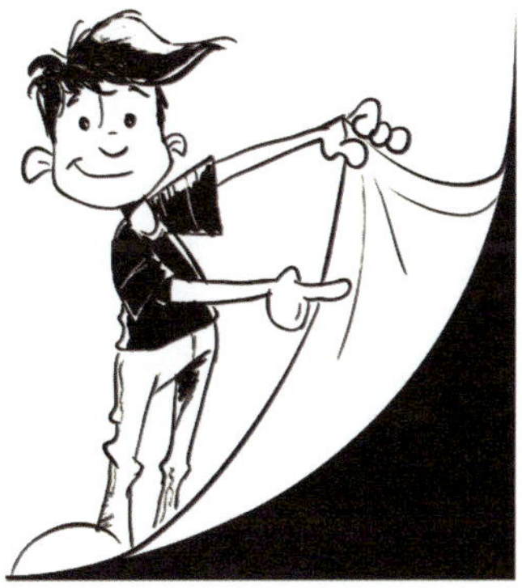

Week 7

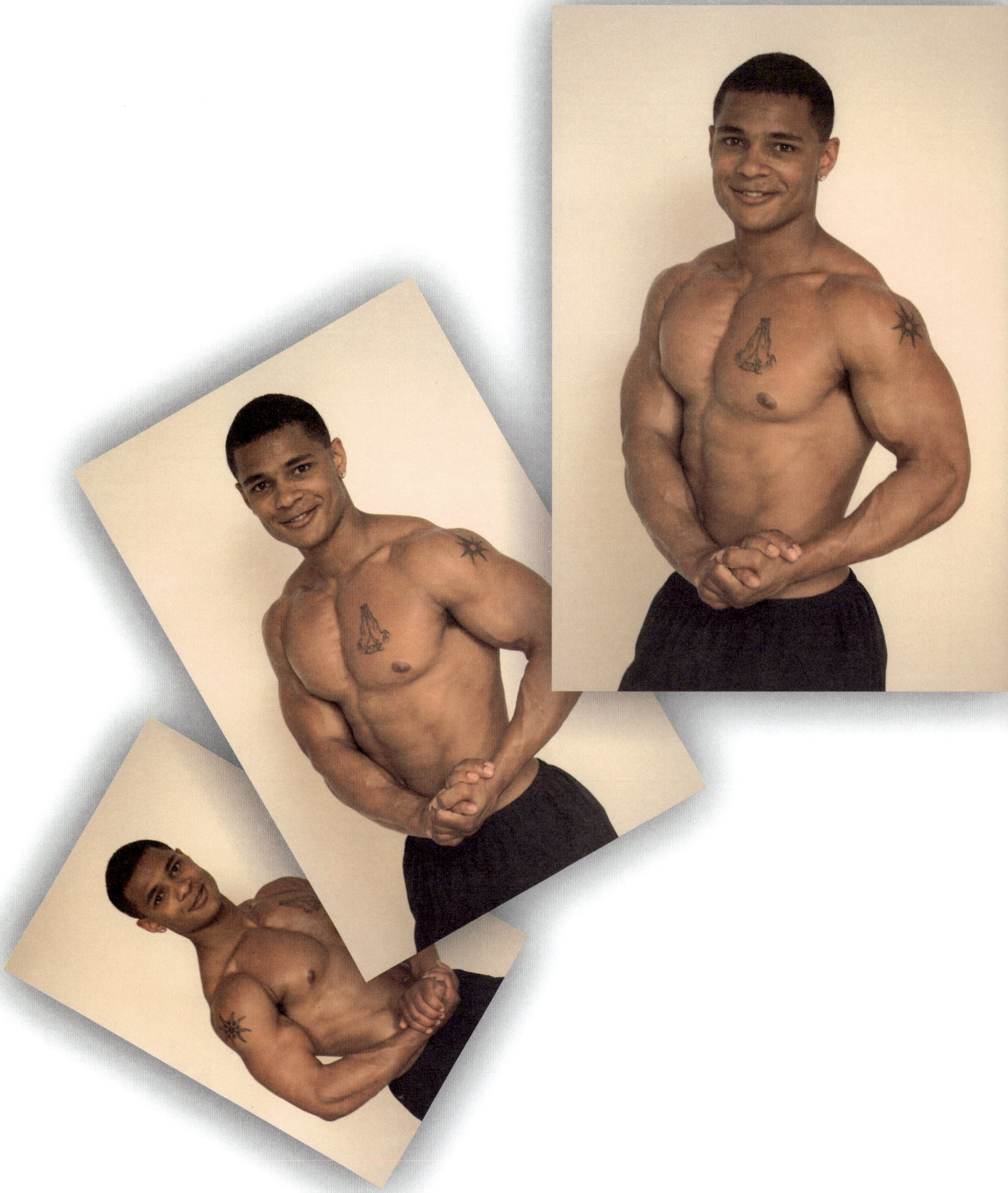

Week 8

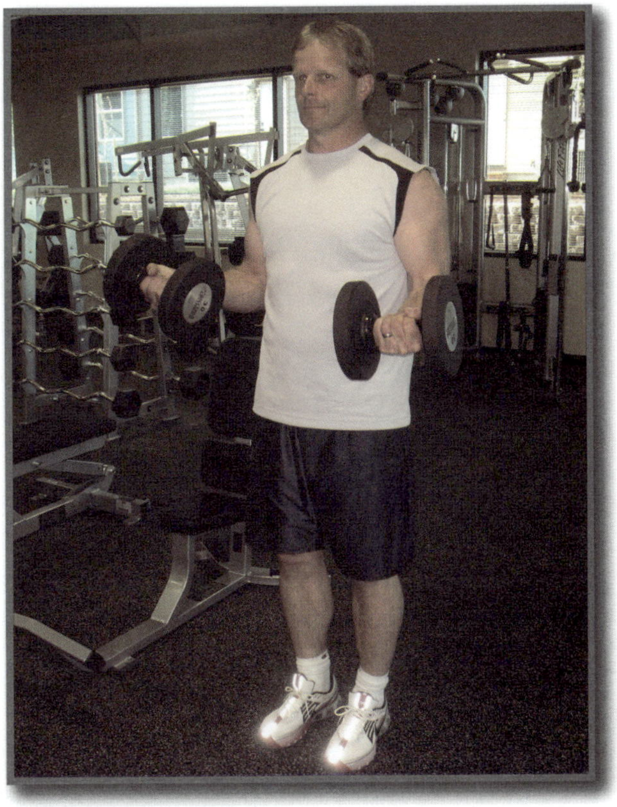

I am a 46-year-old construction superintendent. My wife introduced me to Kevin in the fall of 2006. After meeting and beginning to work out with Kevin, it became apparent that he was an expert in nutrition and exercise. After four months, I had reached my weight loss goal and was feeling 100% better than I had since I was in my 20s. I cannot say enough about the structured workouts and nutrition plans that Kevin taught us

-Tim Kofstad

Goal:

Plan meals and prepare your foods ahead of time.

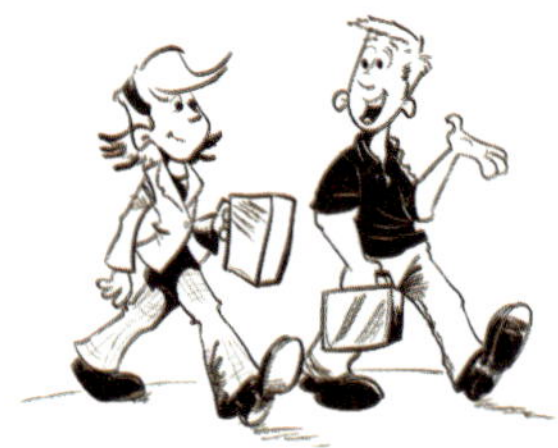

Why?

Have you ever heard the phrase, "failing to plan is planning to fail"? When it comes to your nutrition, this is very true. Planning is essential to your success. To stay on track with your goals, you need to have the right foods, in the right amounts, at the right times. Making a meal plan and following through sets you up to succeed. Having planned and prepared meals ready and on hand will ensure that you have the good food you need at the time you need it. Otherwise, you will find yourself eating whatever is available when you get hungry. You know how it works: You are in your car without a healthy snack handy, suddenly feeling like you are starving and you see your favorite fast food restaurant. Next thing you know, you are in the drive-thru making a choice you know you will regret. A similar scenario happens at the office: You are hungry. You don't have your snack with you. There are donuts in the break room... If you don't have good food ready and available at work, in your car, whereever you are, the chances of eating something unhealthy when you're feeling hungry is quite high. This is where your meal plan comes in. Having a plan and preparing your meals in advance brings you one step closer to achieving your goals because it helps you avoid pitfalls and sets you up to succeed. All you have to do is follow your plan. It's that simple.

How?

Get organized! Create a meal plan at the beginning of each week using your recommended foods chart and your PFC ratios. Put together meals and snacks using the foods you like. Keep it simple. Choose meals that are easy to prepare and convenient to take with you. Write down exactly what you are going to eat and post it where you can see it.

Make a grocery list and go shopping.

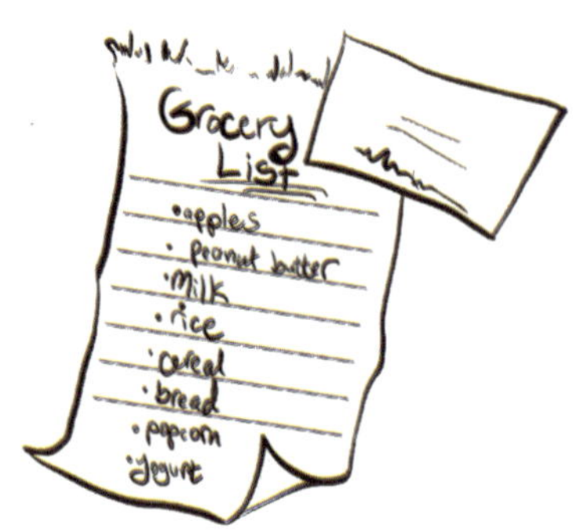

- Create a master grocery list on your computer or go to page 250. Include a column for the Proteins, Fats, Carbohydrates, & Miscellaneous Items (Cooking spray, seasonings, toppings, condiments, plastic bags, etc.)

- Print your list. Circle the food items you need for this week's meal plan.

- Go shopping once a week. Only buy the circled items on your list. Having too much food in the fridge may tempt you to eat more, so stick to your list.

Make sure you have small containers and plastic bags on hand for taking food to work. If not, add them to your list.

Cook once, eat several times. Maximize your meal prep time by cooking most of the foods you will need for meals and snacks for the next three or four days, at one time.

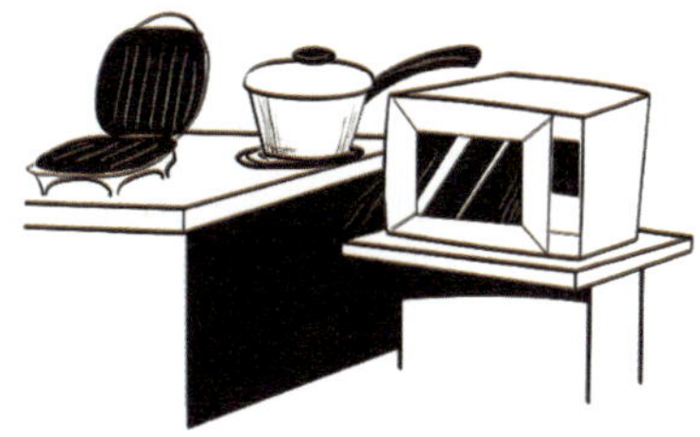

Meats:
- Cook your chicken, turkey, ham, or any other meats. Cut them into your specific serving size.
- Store them in portable containers so you can "grab and go."

Whole grains and complex carbohydrates:
- Cook your whole grain pastas, brown rice, or sweet potatoes.
- Measure into your specific serving size.
- Store each individual serving in its own container, so it is ready to "grab and go."

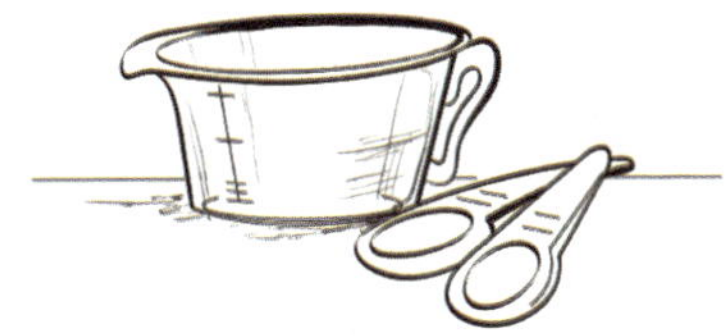

Fruits and vegetables:
- Cook vegetables or cut up fresh vegetables. Buy fresh fruits that are "serving size" whenever possible.
- Cut and slice your fruits and vegetables into your specific serving size.
- Store each individual serving in its own container so it is ready to "grab and go."
- Although fresh is best, keep canned and frozen vegetables on hand to use when fresh isn't available.
- Try to avoid canned fruit. These are typically high in added sugars and don't have near the amount of nutrients as fresh fruit does.

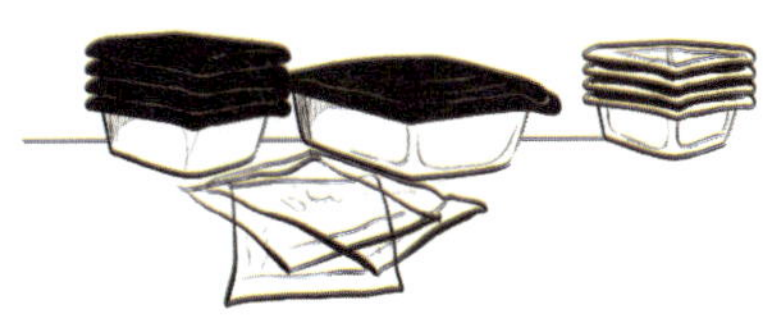

Prepare your lunch ahead of time. A sandwich and a piece of fruit are the most popular items in a sack lunch. You can also think beyond bread. How about chicken or turkey wraps? What about ham and swiss on a whole wheat English muffin? These foods are easy to prepare and eat. These combos are also easy to balance your PFCs.

Week 8

PFC Combos:

Proteins:
- Chicken, turkey, low-fat ham, canned tuna, egg whites, etc.

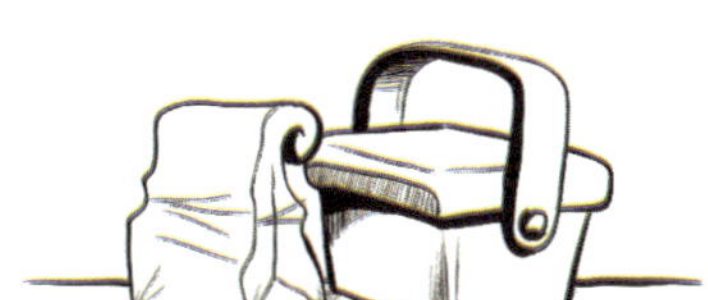

Fats:
- 100% natural peanut butter, nuts, cheese, avocado, egg yolk, olives.

Carbohydrates:
- 100% whole wheat bread, 100% whole wheat tortillas, spinach tortillas, 100% whole wheat English muffin.
- Vegetables such as tomatoes, lettuce, onions, alfalfa or broccoli sprouts, pickles, peppers, onions.

Healthy Condiments:

- Relish, mustard (yellow or Dijon), salsa, ketchup, horseradish, low-fat, low-sugar, and low-sodium sauces and dressings, etc.

Salads are also a great "grab and go" lunch. Greens, proteins, and extras can easily travel in ziplock bags. Add your low fat-or low-calorie dressing to the bag right before eating and shake. Voilà!

Prepare your snacks ahead of time. Keep your snacks simple and predictable. Here are a few examples:

- String cheese and an apple
- String cheese and whole wheat crackers or pretzels
- Yogurt
- Portable fruits and vegetables with sliced turkey or nuts
- Whole wheat crackers and tuna

Have all ingredients for breakfasts and dinners on hand so those meals, as designed in your weekly meal plan, can be put together with ease.

Whatever you do, follow your plan!

Questions and Answers

Preparing my meals sounds like a lot of work! Why do I need to have a plan?

We all know that at times life can get a little hectic. With all the events and stresses of daily life, your nutrition plan can get lost in the shuffle. Let's go over a scenario: You're running late for work, the kids aren't ready for school, and the baby is crying! You speed to the office, phones are ringing off the hook, and your boss has stacked a pile of paperwork on your desk that has a noon deadline. Around 10:00 a.m., your stomach is growling and you haven't had a bite to eat. You don't have anything prepared and healthy foods are hard to find around the office. Tired and frustrated, you end up getting coffee and a muffin from the lobby and hurry back to your desk. You work through your lunch break and around 2:00 p.m., you find yourself starving and searching for whatever is available. You rummage through the break room and come out with a Costco-sized tub of trail mix, a handful of chocolates, and a donut left over from yesterday's meeting. By the end of the day you are exhausted. It is 5:00 p.m. and you're on your way home. Your mind is racing, you're stuck in traffic, and your cell phone rings. In all the chaos, you totally forgot about your daughter's 6 pm basketball game. You wind up making a quick detour to the closest fast food restaurant. The next thing you know, you are in the drive-thru making a choice you know you will regret. After the game, you head home, open the fridge only to find the kids have eaten you out of house and home. You sigh, thinking to yourself, "so much for my nutrition plan," and throw a frozen pizza in the oven. What a day! You can say that again! Fortunately, days like this can be avoided with proper planning. As you can see, creating a fool-proof plan is vital to your success.

I don't have time to cut my vegetables!

Buy them already cut up. Most grocery stores have a variety of pre-cut, pre-packaged vegetables in the produce section. However, they can be more expensive than whole vegetables. Still no time for fresh veggies? That's OK. Frozen veggies are almost as healthy. If you pull out your frozen veggies the night before, they will be thawed out and ready to eat the next day. Warm them up and you are set to go. Canned veggies are quick and easy, too, but unfortunately not as nutritious. Pop the top and they are ready to eat. Although, stick to low GI canned vegetables.

I still have difficulty eating the proper amount of fruits and vegetables!

Keep your fruits and vegetables at eye-level and easily accessible in your refrigerator or in a bowl on your counter. Try some of the following tips:

- Buy low GI seasonal fruits and vegetables **that you like.**
- Buy them "serving size."
- Keep them washed and ready to eat. This will help you eat them more often.
- Don't really like vegetables? Dip them in the low fat or low calorie dressing of your choice.
- Don't like them raw? Try steaming, roasting, or grilling vegetables.
- Experiment with seasonings: A drizzle of olive oil and a sprinkle of dried cilantro, basil, garlic, paprika, cayenne pepper, or rosemary can jazz up any vegetable.
- Sneak them into other dishes. Add chopped vegetables to your scrambled eggs or tuck very thin slices between the meat and cheese on your sandwich. They count as part of the servings you need and you will hardly even notice them!

Are there any methods for keeping my sliced fruits looking fresh and not turning brown?

The best method is to cut your fruits as close to serving time as possible. But, if that's not an option, you can sprinkle your sliced fruits with some lemon, orange, or pineapple juice to keep them from turning brown.

Can I refreeze my big bag of chicken breasts that I didn't have time to cook?

Though safe to eat after refreezing, meat and poultry that has been thawed and then refrozen may lose quality. The texture may be rubbery when cooked. It is best to refreeze after cooking.

I'm bored with the same foods all the time. Is there a solution?

Eating healthy doesn't have to be boring. Some people find it easier to keep it simple and eat the same meals for awhile, but others like more variety. Try using different herbs and spices for an added kick to your meals. Experiment with garlic or onion powders, herbs, lemon or lime juices, soy sauce or Worcestershire sauce, or a variety of different seasonings, to add some excitement to your meals. The brand, Mrs. Dash® makes excellent no-salt seasoning. A personal favorite is the chicken blend. Continue to experiment a little bit. You may discover a new flavor that really appeals to your taste buds. MILLIONS of delicious, simple, healthy recipes can be found on-line. More ideas on overcoming food boredom follow in the next chapter.

What are some of the best methods for cooking meats, brown rice, and vegetables?

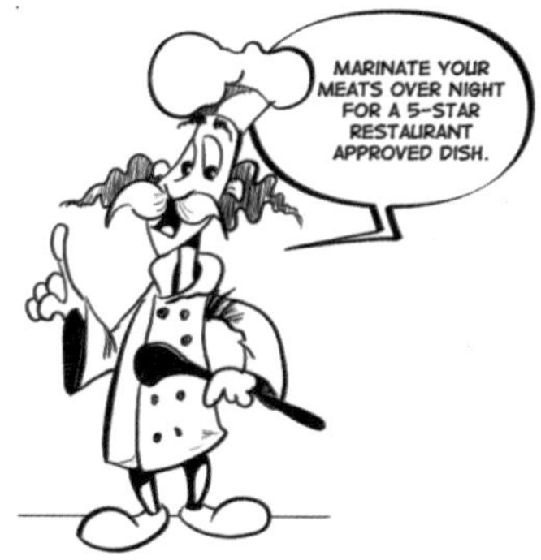
MARINATE YOUR MEATS OVER NIGHT FOR A 5-STAR RESTAURANT APPROVED DISH.

Meats:

- *George Foreman Grill* your meats. It's easy to use. Just set the temperature and timer. It's also known to "knock out the fat."
- Crock pot your meats. Toss meat in at night, turn the pot on low, and in the morning you're ready to go!
- Bar-B-Que is quick, easy, and tasty. You can work wonders with foods on the BBQ and there is very little clean up.

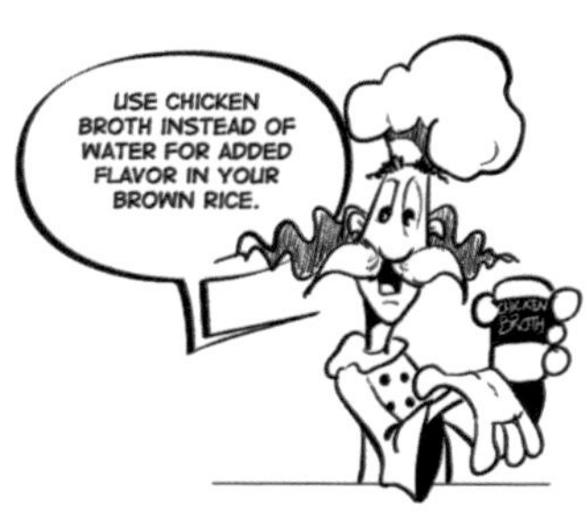
USE CHICKEN BROTH INSTEAD OF WATER FOR ADDED FLAVOR IN YOUR BROWN RICE.

Brown rice:

- Brown or wild rice can be made on the stovetop or in a rice cooker.

Vegetables:

- Yams can be baked, boiled, BBQ'd, or even microwaved.

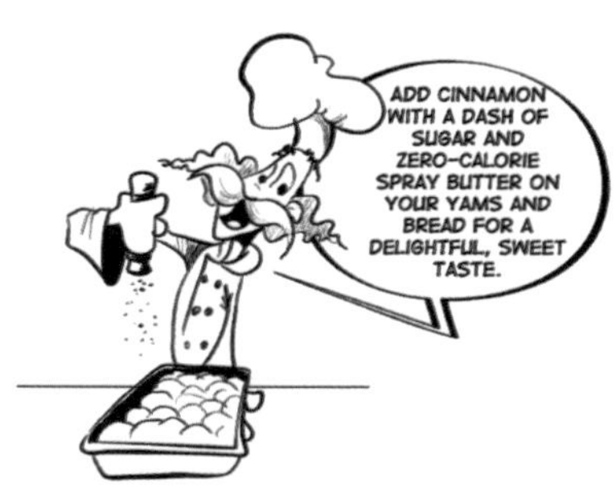
ADD CINNAMON WITH A DASH OF SUGAR AND ZERO-CALORIE SPRAY BUTTER ON YOUR YAMS AND BREAD FOR A DELIGHTFUL, SWEET TASTE.

- *George Foreman Grill* your veggies, too. It's easy to cook, leave alone, clean up, and gives a great grilling flavor.

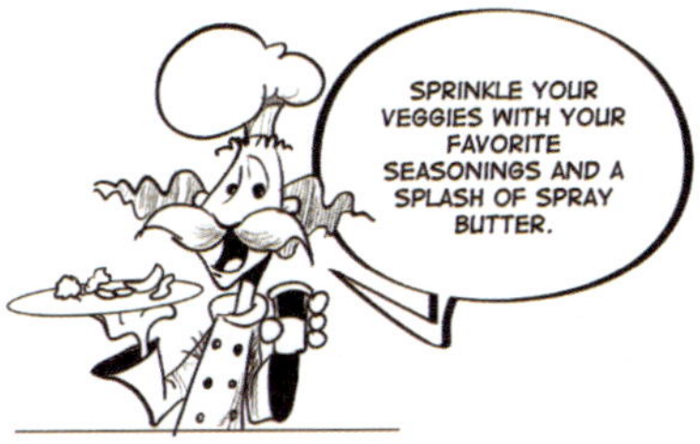
SPRINKLE YOUR VEGGIES WITH YOUR FAVORITE SEASONINGS AND A SPLASH OF SPRAY BUTTER.

- Steam in a steamer basket on your stove top.
- Microwave with a small amount of liquid.
- Roast – Most vegetables can be roasted in the oven at high heat (400 to 425 degrees) for a relatively short amount of time. Try laying asparagus on a cookie sheet. Spray with olive oil and sprinkle with chopped garlic or garlic salt. Roast for 10 minutes. Delicious!

What are the best methods of storing foods for on-the-go meal planning?

There are several ways to store prepared food items:

- Cook a fairly large quantity of the foods you will be eating and store them together. For example, you can cook several chicken breasts and store them in your refrigerator in a gallon-size Ziploc® freezer bag. These bags are great for storing fresh, as well as prepared fruits and vegetables.

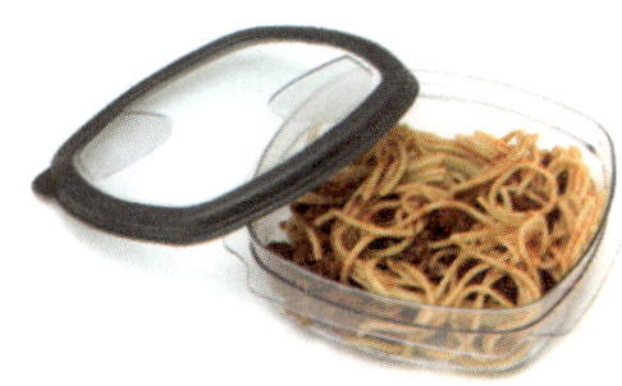

- A big pot of cooked brown rice or whole grain pasta can be stored in a large plastic container.
- When it's time to eat, you simply pull out a piece of chicken, scoop out a serving of rice, measure out your veggies, and heat them in the microwave. You instantly have a healthy, home-made meal.

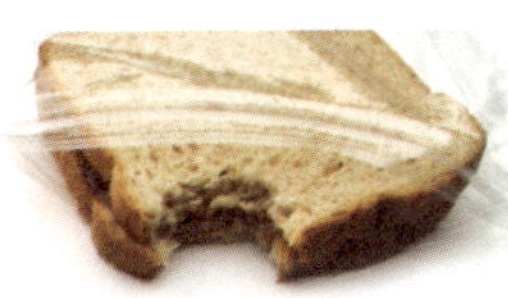

- Placing individual servings in individual Tupperware®-type containers is another way to be "grab-and-go" ready at all times. Besides, these are more environmentally friendly.

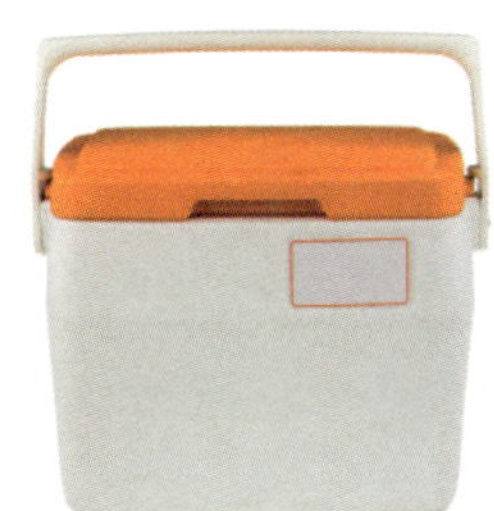

- Zip-type baggies are another alternative. They are great for the on-the-go lifestyle. You can get all different sizes, they are inexpensive, and if you lose or break one, it's not a big deal. Just do not resuse them.
- You may also want to purchase a small cooler to store and carry your food for the day.

Having nutritious meals ready and waiting will keep you on track when life gets hectic or you're on the go.

How long is it okay to store my prepared food items in my refrigerator?

The shelf life of food varies and will depend upon the food itself, the manufacturing process, packaging, temperature, and humidity. To ensure quality, practice FIFO (First-In-First-Out). Place newly prepared and/or purchased food items behind existing food items. Your prepared foods should be stored in clean, shallow containers with a cover. Don't forget to label and date all the big batches of food you prepare at one time.

Cooked Meats can be stored in the refrigerator for up to four days. Fresh meat such as ground beef, veal, and lamb can be stored in the freezer for up to four months. Poultry can be stored in the freezer for up to 12 months. Fish can be stored for up to six months, while ham can be stored for up to two months. Whole eggs, egg whites, and processed packaged meats do not freeze well.

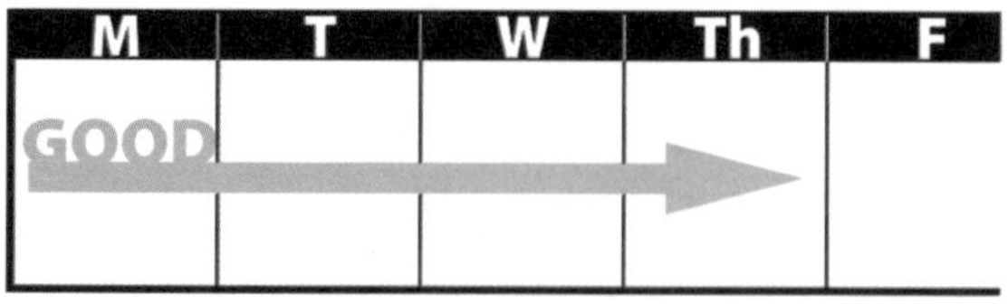

Cooked brown rice can be stored, when tightly covered, in the refrigerator for up to seven days, or in the freezer for six months. Brown rice has a shorter shelf life than white rice due to the natural oil in its bran layer.

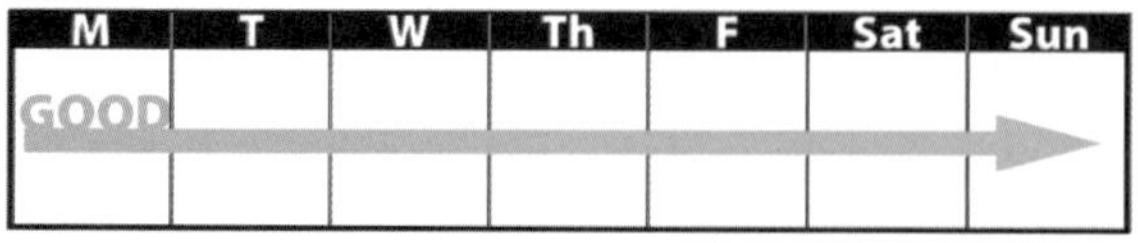

100% whole wheat bread can be stored at room temperature for up to a week and twice as long when stored in the refrigerator. If stored in the freezer, it can last up to three months.

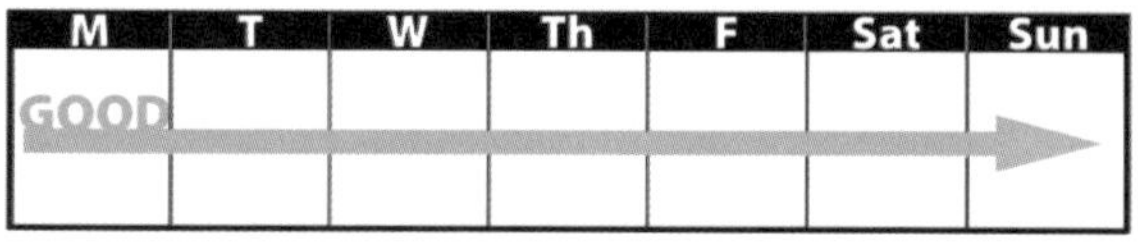

Fresh vegetables can be stored up to five days in the refrigerator. Canned vegetables are good for up to one year while frozen vegetables are good for up to eight months. **Note:** Sweet potatoes, onions, squash, and eggplants should be stored in a cool, well-ventilated place and tomatoes should be stored at room temperature to maintain their quality and nutritional value.

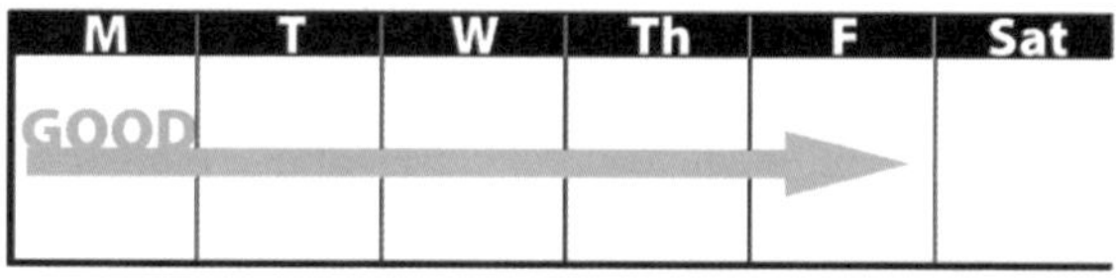

Fresh fruit varies from two days to one month. Apples are good for up to seven days at room temperature and can last up to one month in the refrigerator. Ripe strawberries, melons, peaches, and grapes can be stored in the refrigerator for up to five days.

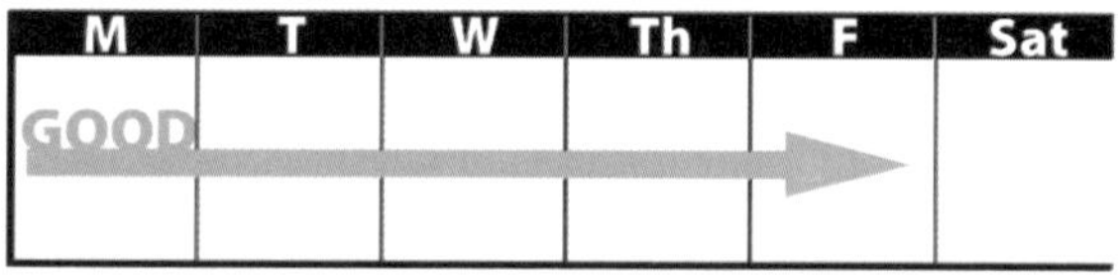

When is the best time to shop and cook?

Shopping and cooking can be time consuming. Try shopping on a day when you don't work or when you have a light schedule. Remember, don't shop when you are hungry! You will buy more food than you planned. Stick to your list. The same goes for cooking. Your day off, or the day of the week you have the most time available for cooking, is the best day to set aside for this task. If you don't have time to cook and prepare several days worth of meals at one time, just prepare meals for one day at a time, but do it the night before so they are ready for you when you wake up. The most important part of meal planning and preparing is creating a system that works best for you and helps you stick to your meal plan for the week.

I lost 16 pounds in one month by following Kevin's simple plan. He advised me to eat every three hours and avoid carbohydrates for my last meal of the day. His 30-minute cardio routine and nutrition plan was a perfect guide for me. His training has given me more energy and clarity every day! Thanks Kevin!

- Otoniel Rosales

He helped me put the focus back onto me, my person. My life wasn't just about working and getting ahead. Taking time for my body was critical to living a happy, fulfilling life. Kevin's positive attitude, his patience, as well as his honest concern and care for his clients, are invaluable. They are what make him so effective. Kevin's help has changed weight training from an awful thing to something that's even enjoyable. I no longer go into the weight room embarrassed, not wanting anyone to see me workout for fear it's obvious I don't know what I'm doing. Now, I know what to do. It's almost unbelievable to me that I can go into the gym with confidence!

- Patricia Hale

Nutrition Log

Date:__________	Sun Mon Tues Wed Thurs Fri Sat	
	Food	**PFC**
Meal 1	*Food & Amount*	*P F C*
Time:_____		
Meal 2		
Time:_____		
Meal 3		
Time:_____		
Meal 4		
Time:_____		
Meal 5		
Time:_____		
Meal 6		
Time:_____		

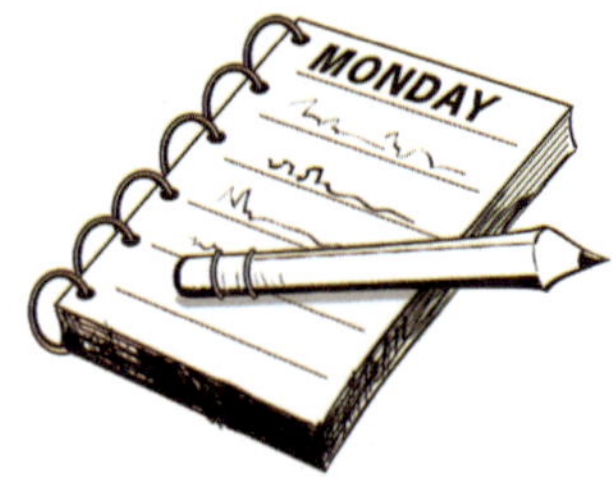

Checklist

Achieved:

- ✓ Consume meal or snack every 3 hours
- ✓ Water every 3 hours
- ✓ Sleep optimal hours
- ✓ Intake multivitamin
- ✓ Weights and cardio
- ✓ Consume PFCs every meal or snack
- ✓ Foods low on the GI
- ✓ PFC ratio balance
- ✓ **Planned meals**

Avoided:

- ✓ Sugars
- ✓ White flour
- ✓ Processed foods

Key Points

Week 1
- Eat a small meal or snack once every three hours – five to six meals per day.
- Drink at least 1 cup (8 ounces) of water per meal and at least one cup before, during, and after your workouts.
- Keep a nutrition log.
- Sleep is vital!
- Take a daily multivitamin.

Week 2
- Avoid bad sugars.

Week 3
- Avoid white flour and white rice.

Week 4
- Avoid processed foods.

Week 5
- Balance your meals and snacks with a combination of proteins, fats, and carbohydrates.

Week 6
- Eat foods that are low on the Glycemic Index.

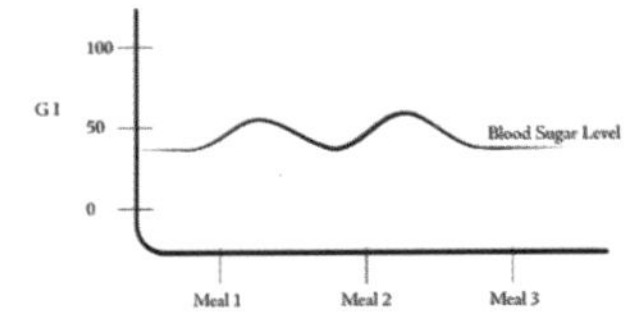

Week 7
- Balance your meals and snacks with a specific ratio of proteins, fats, and carbohydrates.

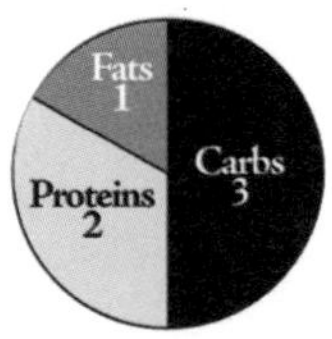

Week 8
- **Plan and prepare your foods for meals and snacks ahead of time.**
- **Keep your prepared food selection simple.**
- **Continue to record everything you're eating and drinking in your nutrition log daily.**

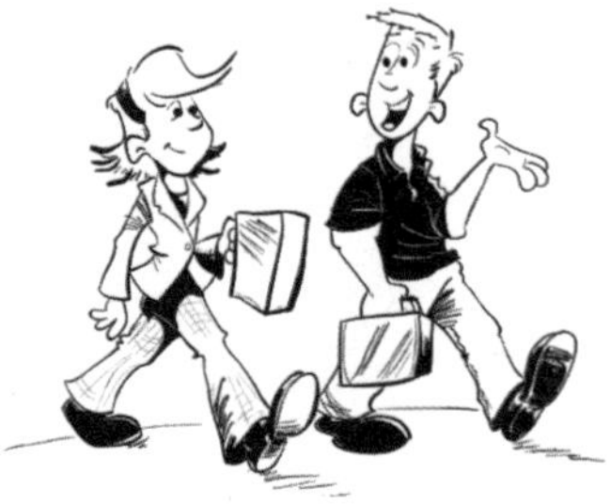

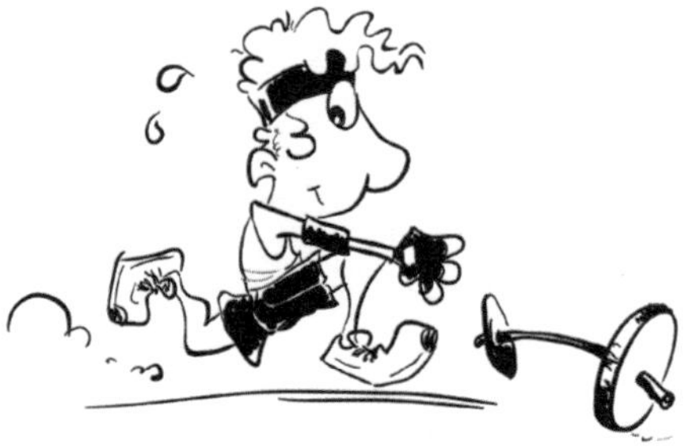

Chest

Goal:

Complete four sets of 15 reps on the **cable chest press**.

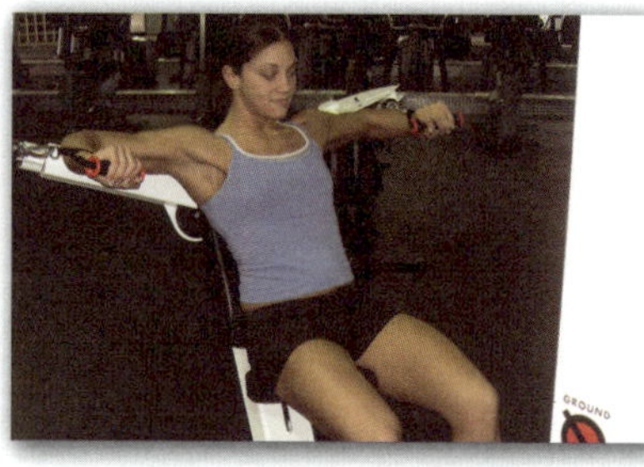

Primary
Chest

Stabilizers
Shoulders
Triceps
Forearms
Core

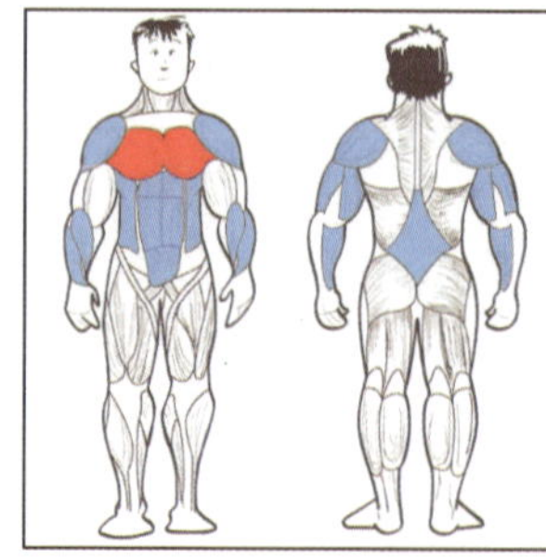

Why?

The cable chest press is a machine exercise targeting your chest. The muscle stabilizers include your shoulders, triceps and forearms, as well as the rest of your core. The seated cable chest press combines the elements of a dumbbell exercise with a machine exercise by simulating the dumbbell bench press in a seated position. Like dumbbells, cables activate all of the little stabilizers throughout your entire body in order to perform the motion of the chest press.

How?

Step 1 - Sit with your legs bent in a 90-degree angle, feet flat on the floor, pointed forward. Grab the handles.

Step 2 - Squeeze your abs to push your lower back flat against the bench.

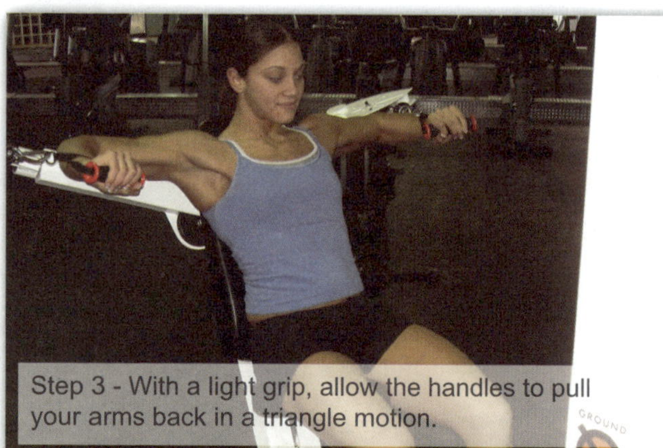

Step 3 - With a light grip, allow the handles to pull your arms back in a triangle motion.

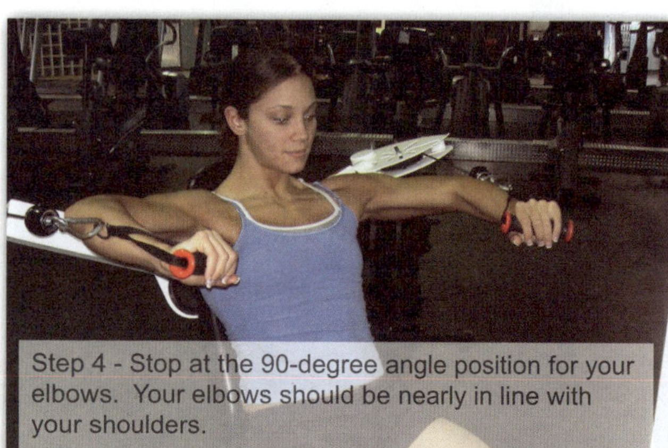

Step 4 - Stop at the 90-degree angle position for your elbows. Your elbows should be nearly in line with your shoulders.

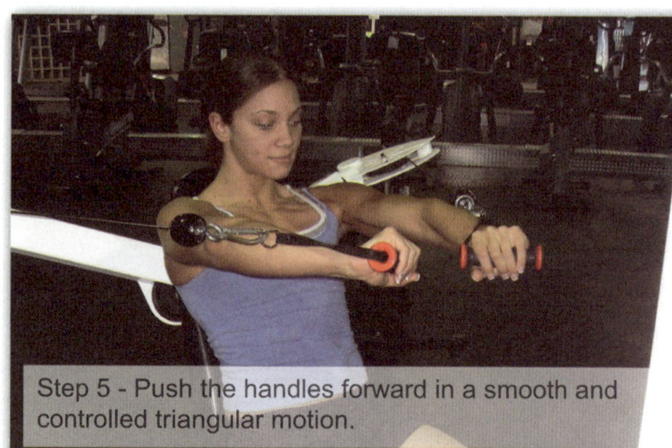

Step 5 - Push the handles forward in a smooth and controlled triangular motion.

Your goal is to complete four sets of 15 (4 x 15).

Range of Motion Techniques

To Maximize Muscle Tension and Minimize Overcompensation

Dos | **Don'ts**

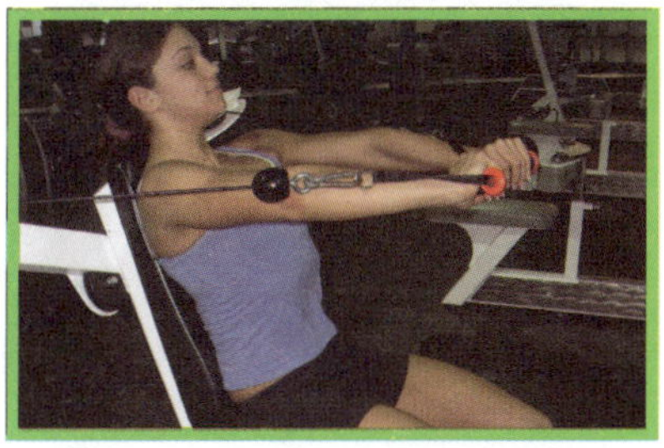
Squeeze Your Chest While Keeping Elbows Bent

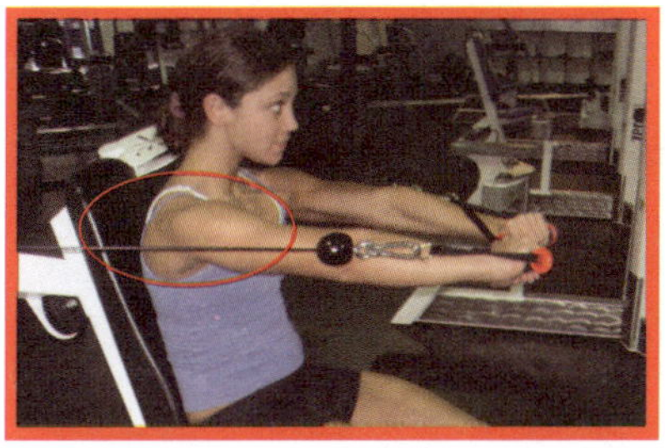
Avoid Leaning Forward

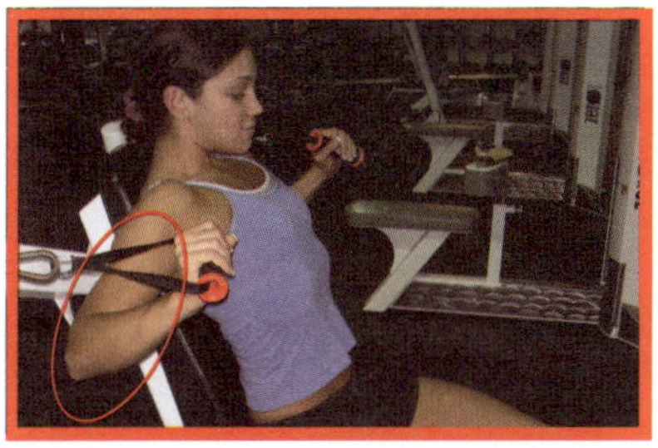
Avoid Elbows Too Low and Too Far Back

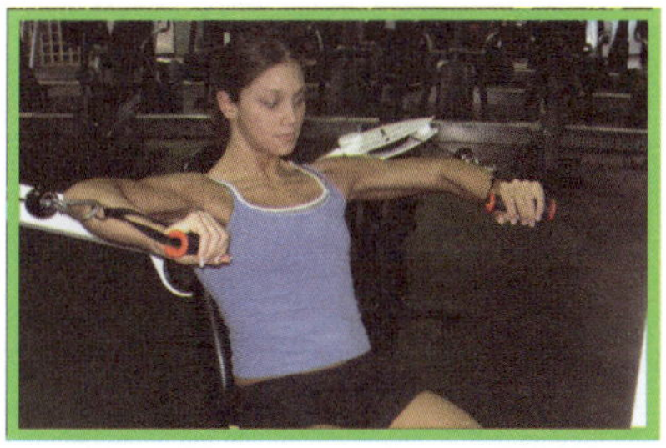
Feel Light Stretch in Chest While Elbows are in line with Shoulders

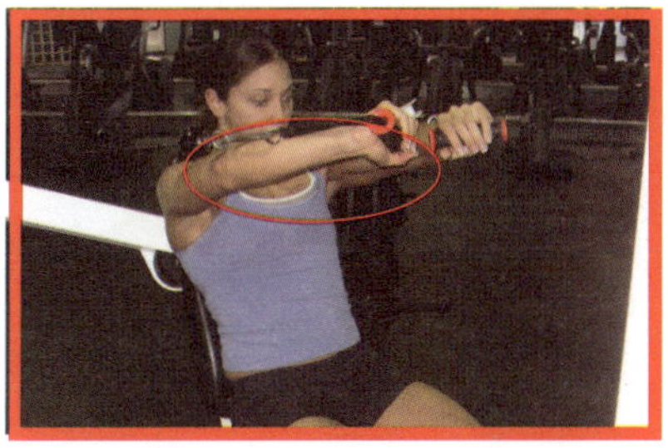
Avoid Pushing Too High

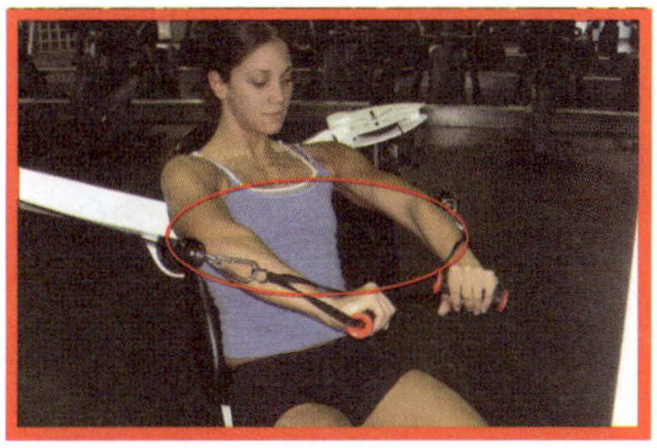
Avoid Pushing Too Low

Visualize

"Semicircle and Cable Effect"

Sit against the back support with a cable in each hand. At your starting position, resist the weight with your chest as the cables pull your arms back toward you. Focus on feeling a stretch in your chest before pushing forward. Squeeze and flex your chest muscles to push the cables forward in a semicircular motion. Imagine that you are contracting your chest so much that your hands are about to touch.

Visualize cables attached to your hands. Allow the cables to guide you through a smooth and controlled semicircular motion. At the starting position, the cables pull your arms forward and together completing a semicircle. Just before your hands touch at the center of the semicircle, allow the cables to pull your arms back to repeat. Continue contracting your chest, and repeat your visualization throughout the entire range of motion.

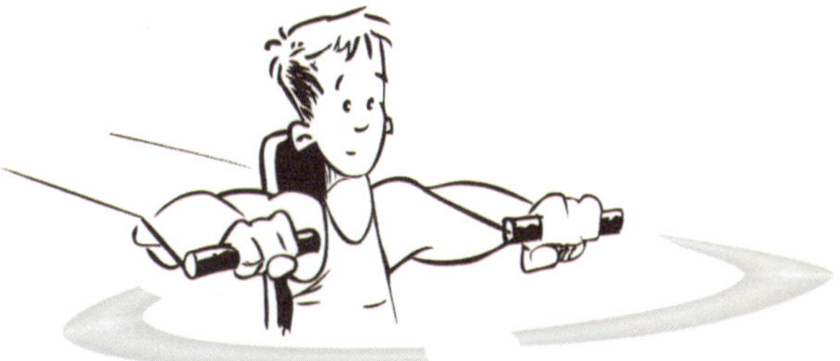

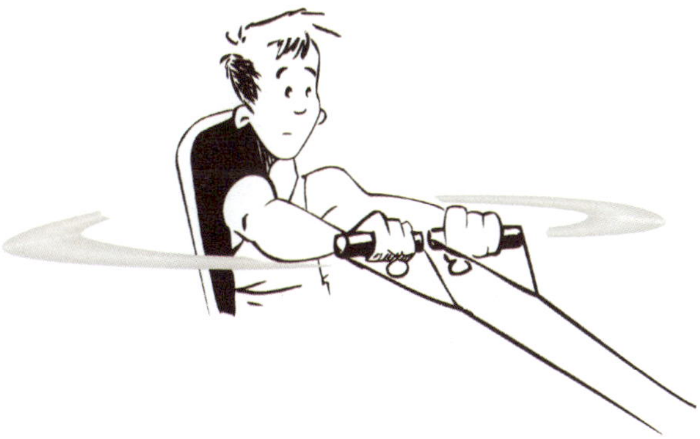

Week 8

Questions and Answers

Is it still important to keep my lower back flat?

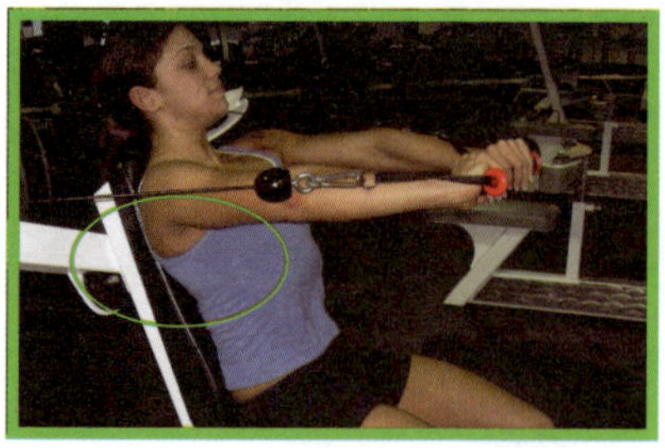

You bet! Keeping your lower back flat is always important. When your back is in a neutral position, it relieves the pressure in your lower back. By reducing the tension in your lower back, you will increase the tension in your chest leading to a more effective workout. Hold your abs in tightly to flatten the arch in your lower back and push it flat against the bench.

I feel my shoulders! Am I doing something wrong?

Your shoulders are a stabilizer in this exercise. It is normal to feel your stabilizers burn, especially if this is a new exercise, and you might not yet be conditioned enough. As you get stronger, you will be able to work your chest without feeling your shoulders. Be sure to keep the handles aligned with your chest. This will allow you to use more of your chest and less of your shoulders.

How fast should I perform my reps?

Your tempo should continue to stay at two seconds back and two seconds forward. Remember, your form is most important, so use a smooth, controlled motion. Just like dumbbells, both sides of your body are having to work independently. This means you should expect to have less stability than you do when performing the bench press. As your stabilizers strengthen, it will be easier to stabilize yourself throughout the motion.

How do I practice visualization when I can't even control my form?

Visualization requires mental focus, concentration, and practice. At this point, you might not be able to feel your chest muscles contract and reach the "pump" effect. That is OK. Continue working out, and you will get stronger. The more muscle you have, the easier it is to feel the muscles contract. Remember, visualization allows you to strengthen your targeted muscles, so continue to practice, and it will come together.

Can I pause in this exercise?

Yes. If you need to pause, you should pause at your starting position. Pausing is an effective way to gain control of your motion. If you are fatigued and need to take a break, pausing can serve as a short break before ultimately fatiguing. Pausing for one to two seconds before trying to continue with another rep may assist you in reaching your optimal goal of reps.

How do I get into my starting position without it hurting my shoulders?

To avoid injuring your shoulders and lower back use the following steps:

1. Stand up and lean against the back pad.
2. Grab the handles and pull them forward into your starting position.
3. Slide down the back pad into a seated position. Now you're ready to perform your set.

Why do I need to perform a triangle motion?

A triangular motion allows you to maximize the tension and contraction of your chest muscles. Pushing the handles straight forward and backward is much easier to complete and much less effective. Why? This motion allows your shoulders to overcompensate for your chest. If you want to get the most effective chest workout, you'll want your handles to travel in the triangular motion.

Back

Goal:

Complete four sets of 15 reps on the **independent lat pulldown.**

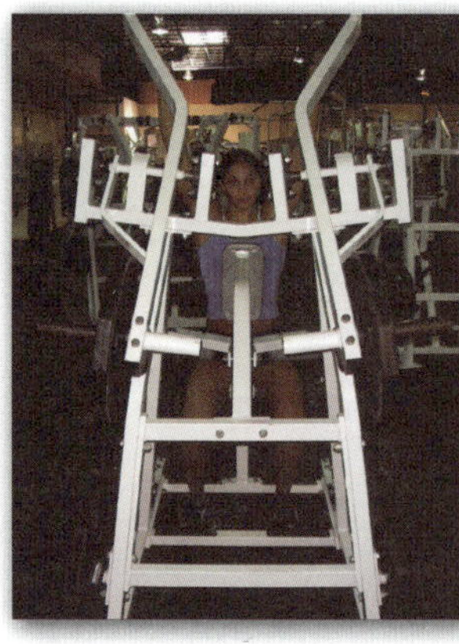

Primary
Lats

Stabilizers
Shoulders
Biceps
Forearms
Core

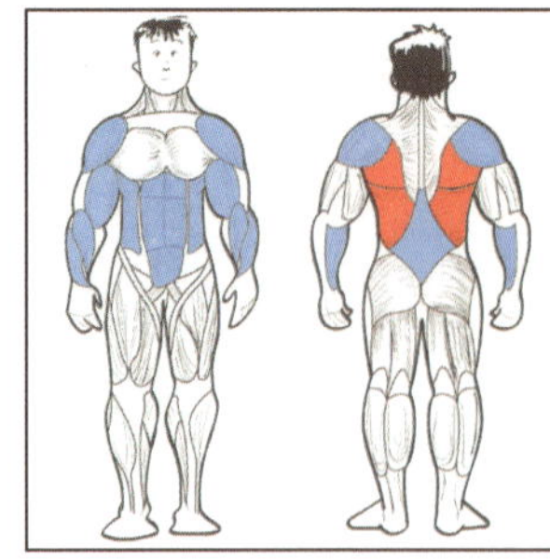

Why?

The independent lat pulldown is a machine exercise targeting your lats. The muscle stabilizers include your shoulders, traps, biceps, and forearms, as well as the rest of your core. The independent lat pulldown combines the elements of a dumbbell exercise with a machine exercise. Like dumbbells, more stabilizers are required to be activated in order to complete the exercise. The independent lat pulldown adds variety to your training and variety helps to prevent your body from adapting to any one machine.

How?

Step 1 - Grab the bar at a 90-degree angle grip and sit down.

Step 2 - Squeeze your abs to push your lower back into a neutral position.

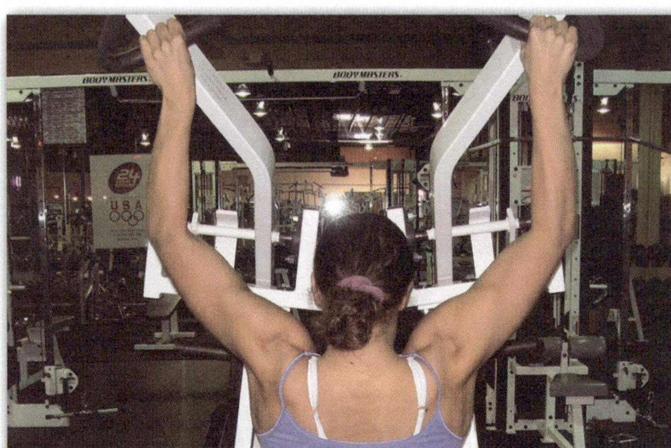

Step 3 - Begin with a light grip with your elbows unlocked and slightly flared out.

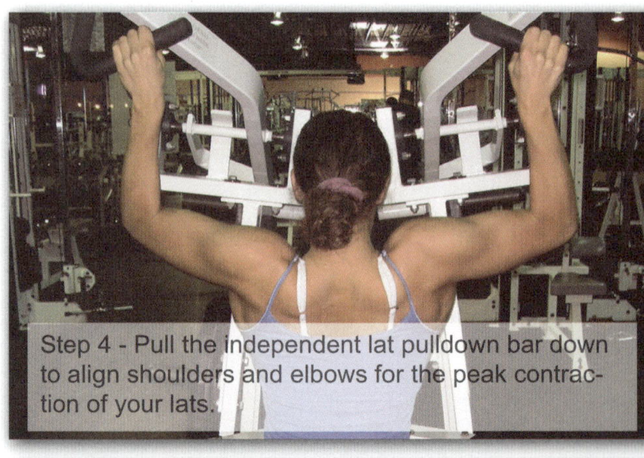

Step 4 - Pull the independent lat pulldown bar down to align shoulders and elbows for the peak contraction of your lats.

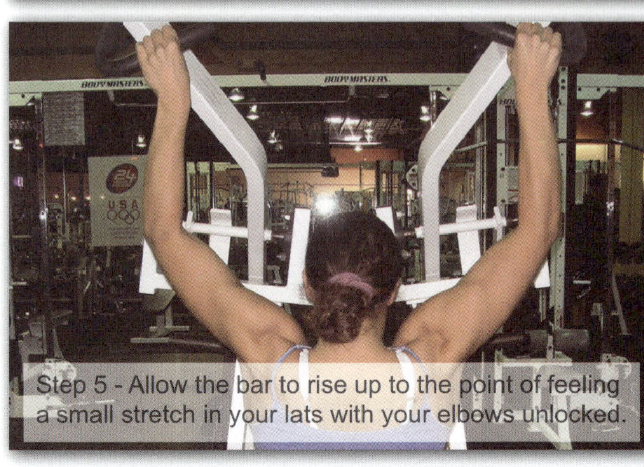

Step 5 - Allow the bar to rise up to the point of feeling a small stretch in your lats with your elbows unlocked.

Step 6 - Repeat using a smooth, controlled motion to maximize the tension in your lats.

Your goal is to complete four sets of 15 (4 x 15).

Range of Motion Techniques

To Maximize Muscle Tension and Minimize Overcompensation

Dos | **Don'ts**

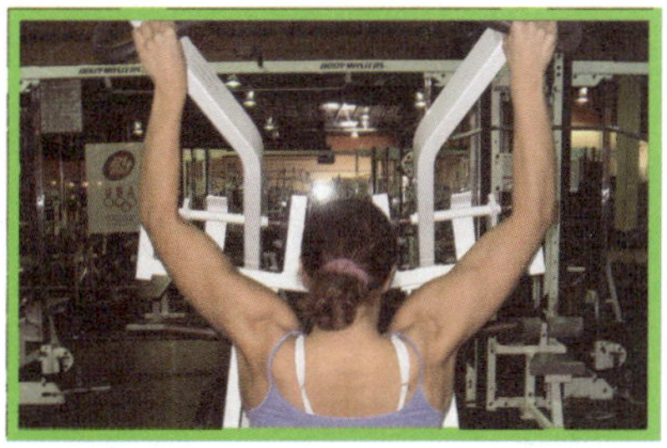

Stretch Lats While Keeping Elbows Bent

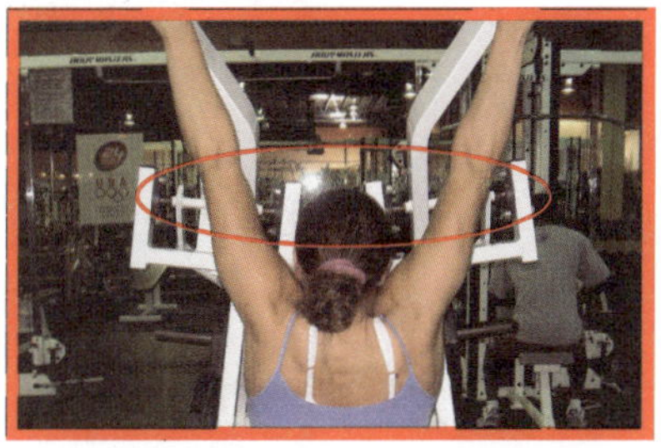

Avoid Locking Out Elbows

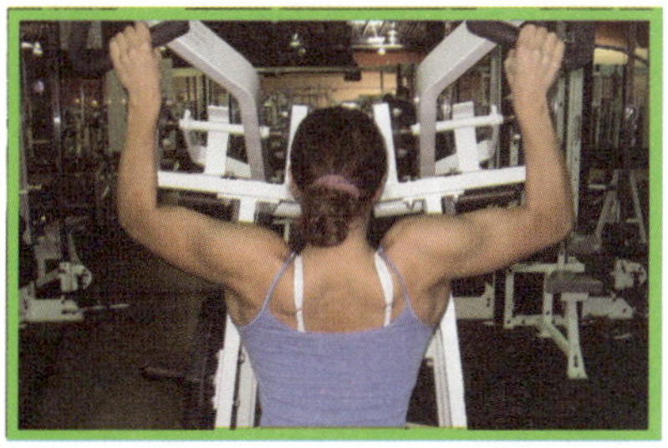

Elbows Flared Out and Slightly Parallel with Shoulders

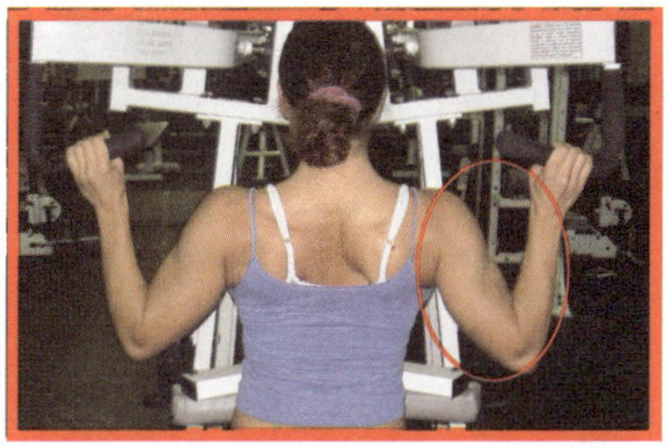

Avoid Pulling Elbows Beyond Shoulders

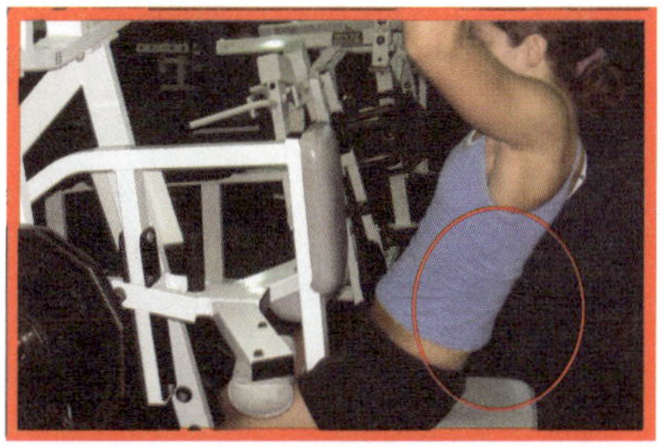

Avoid Leaning Back Too Far

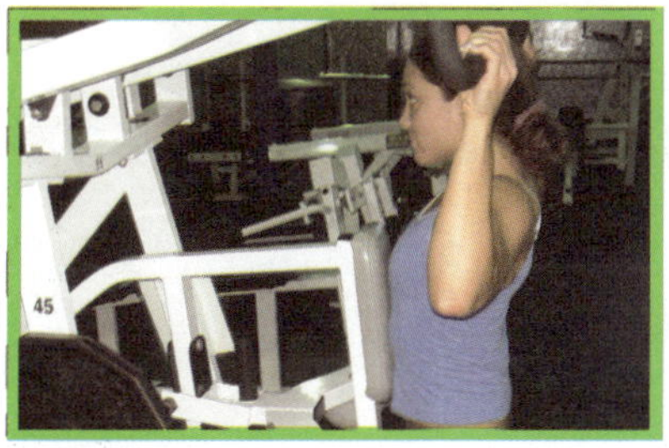

Maximize Lat Tension When Elbows are Aligned With Shoulders

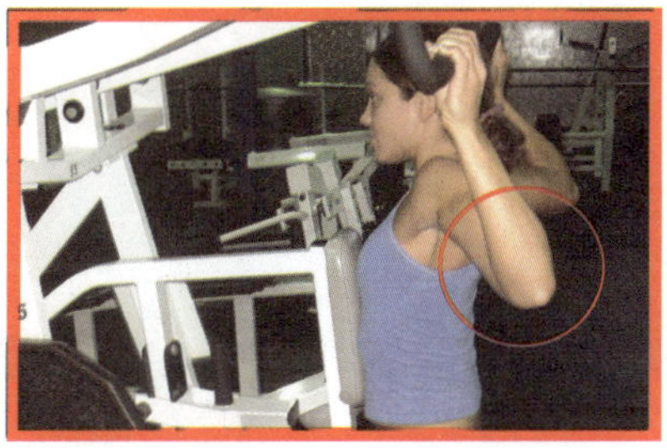

Avoid Pulling Elbows Too Far Back

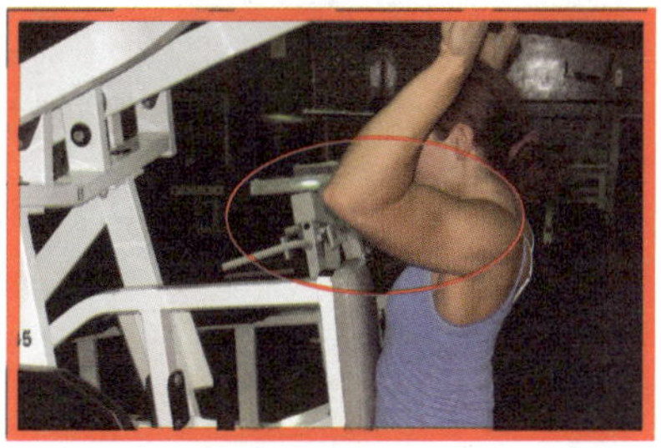

Avoid Pulling Elbows Too Far Forward

Visualize

"Flare, Stretch, and Cable Effect"

Visualize flaring your lats out at your starting position, making your upper back feel as wide as possible. Your elbows are slightly forward and your upper back is rounded. Keeping your lats flared, pull down to your peak lat contraction. Resist the weight as you allow the independent bars to raise up. Focus on feeling the stretch in your lats at the top of your starting position. Continue to visualize your lats flaring outward, and stay within the proper range of motion. Repeat the visualization for every rep.

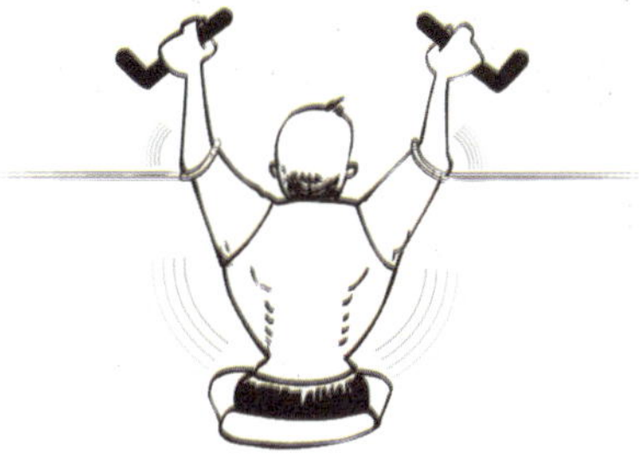

You can also try another technique: Visualize cables attached to your elbows. They are pulling and stretching your arms apart. This forces your shoulders to relax and allows you to keep your lats flared.

Shoulders

Goal:

Complete four sets of 15 reps of the **dumbbell lateral raises**.

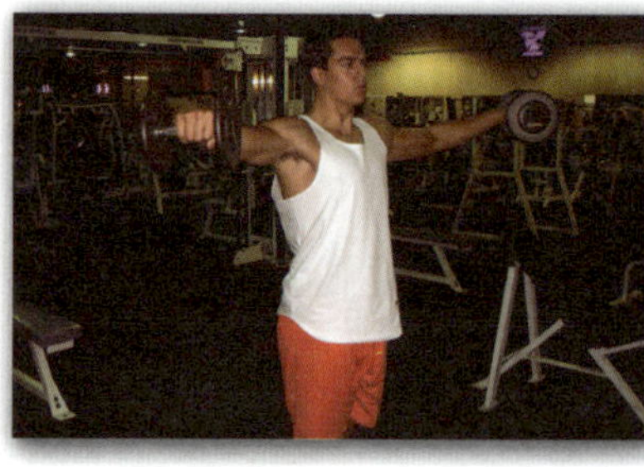

Primary
Shoulders

Stabilizers
Biceps
Forearms
Core

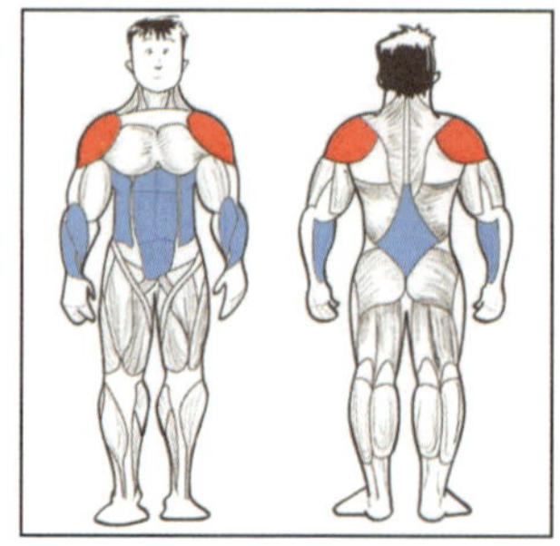

Why?

The dumbbell lateral raise is a free weight exercise targeting your shoulders. The muscle stabilizers include your biceps and forearms, as well as the rest of your core. Dumbbell exercises are a great way to add training variety and increase the strength of your stabilizers. Dumbbell lateral raises work your shoulder muscles from a different angle than the vertical motion of the dumbbell shoulder press.

How?

Step 1 - Stand with your feet shoulder-width apart, one dumbbell in each hand.

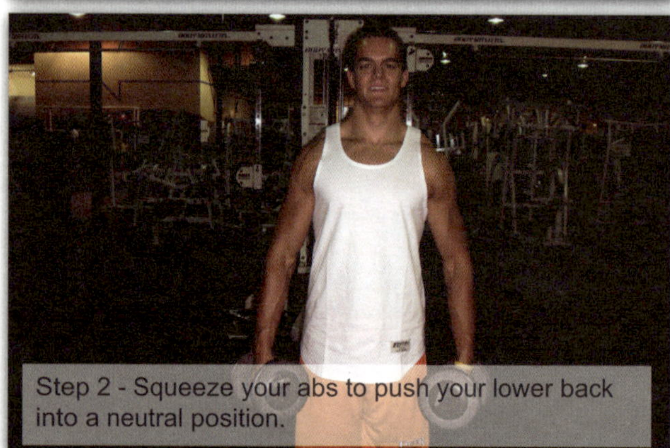

Step 2 - Squeeze your abs to push your lower back into a neutral position.

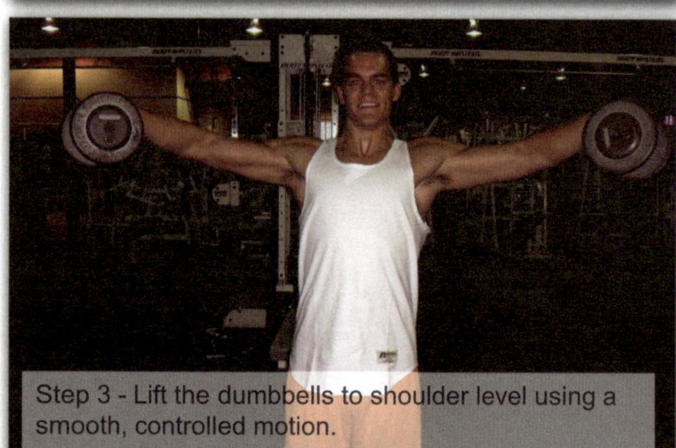

Step 3 - Lift the dumbbells to shoulder level using a smooth, controlled motion.

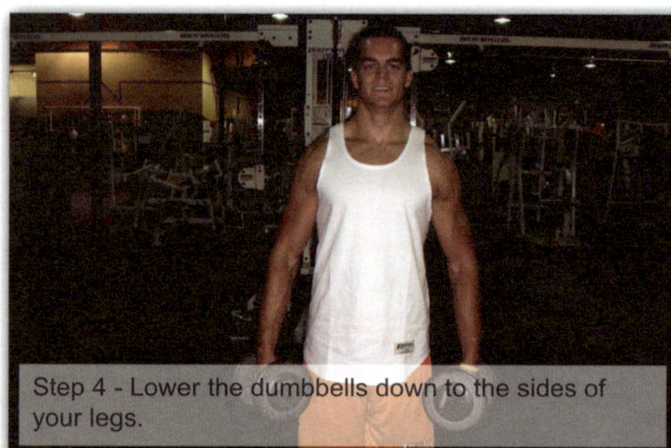

Step 4 - Lower the dumbbells down to the sides of your legs.

Step 5 - Repeat.

Your goal is to complete four sets of 15 (4 x 15).

Range of Motion Techniques

To Maximize Muscle Tension and Minimize Overcompensation

Dos

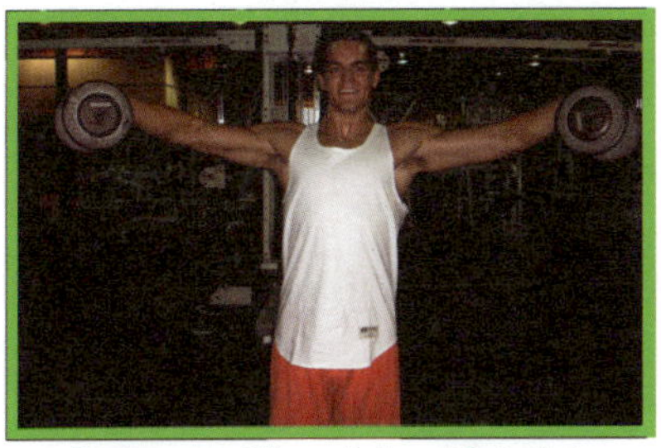

Raise to Shoulder Height

Don'ts

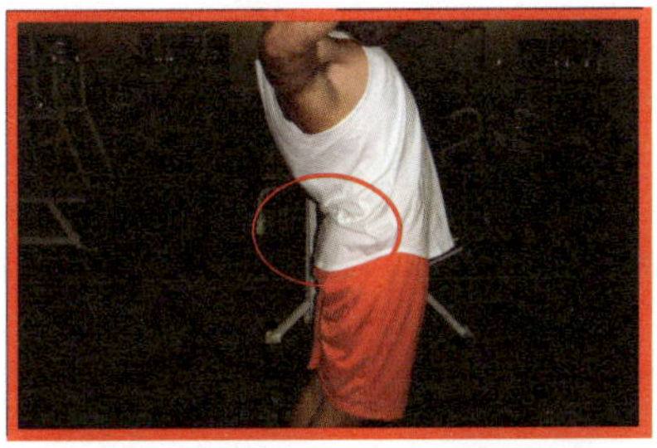

Avoid Arching Lower Back

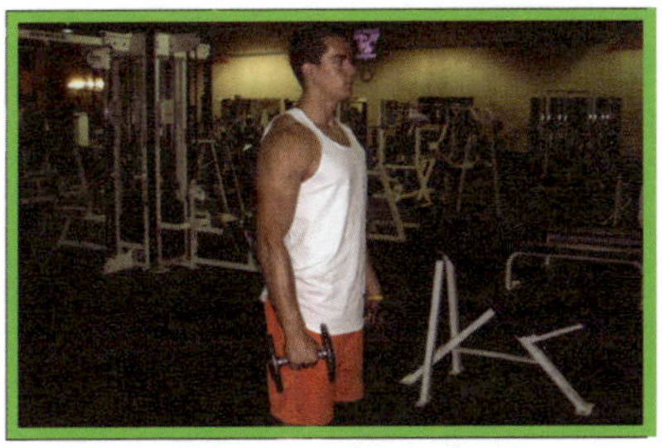

Keep Elbows Slightly Bent

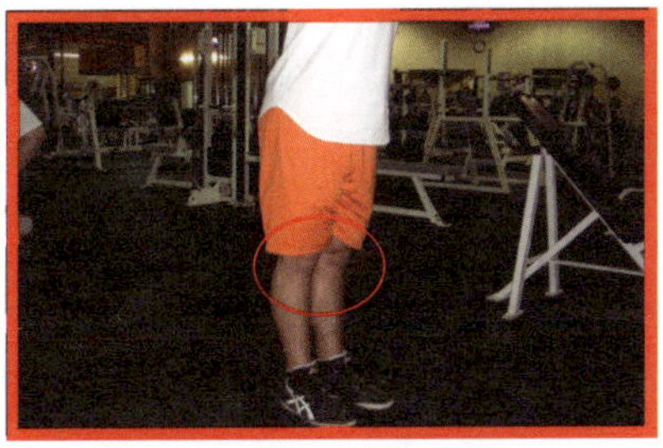

Avoid Locking Out Knees

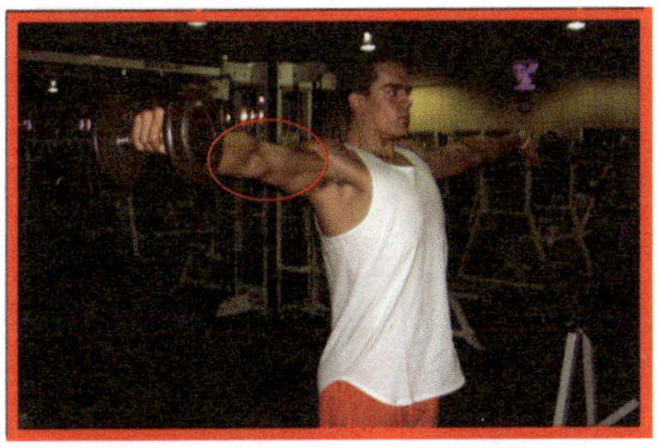

Avoid Locking Out Elbows

Visualize

"Semicircle and Cable Effect"

While performing lateral raises, visualize cables attached to your dumbbells pulling them up towards the ceiling in a semicircular motion. At the same time, imagine another set of cables attached to your dumbbells that are pulling and stretching your dumbbells out to your sides.

Your goal is to visualize every rep and to stay within the proper range of motion. When performed correctly, this visualization minimizes the use of your shoulder joints, biceps, forearms, and wrists.

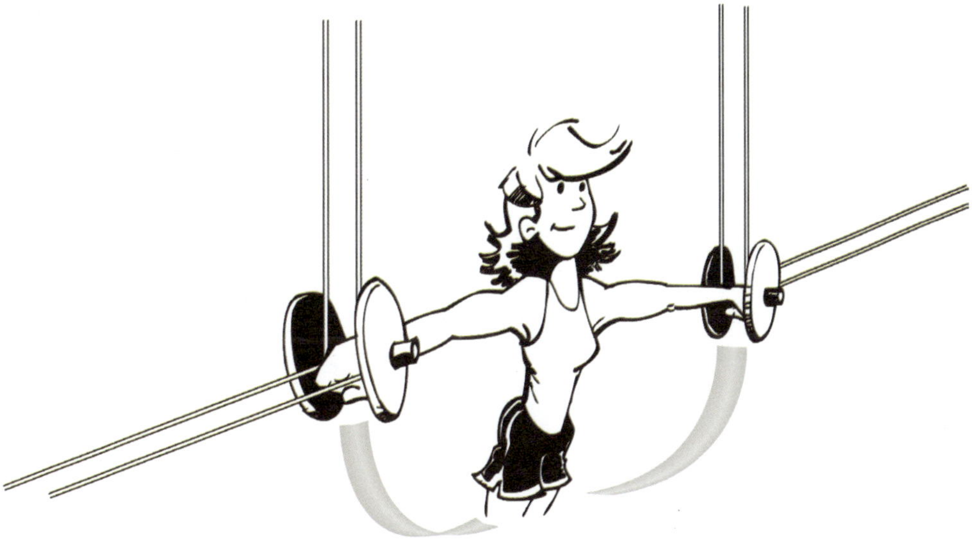

Questions and Answers

Can I keep my arms in a 90-degree angle instead of extending out?

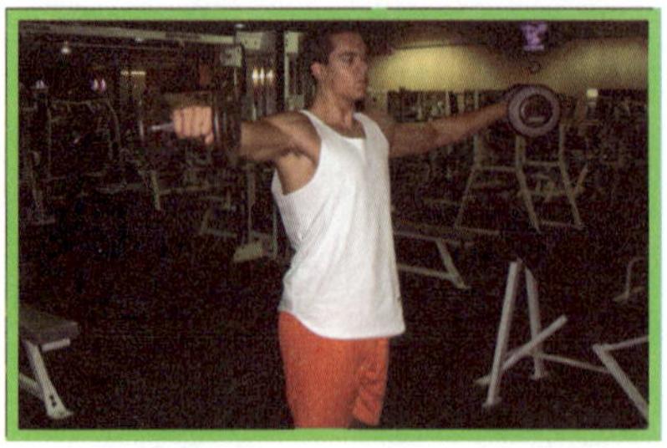

Keeping your arms extended out while traveling in a semi-circular motion allows you to maximize the tension and contraction of your shoulders. Keeping your arms bent at a 90-degree angle allows your biceps and forearms to overcompensate for your shoulders. Your goal is to work your shoulders without the assistance of your stabilizer. If you want the most effective shoulder workout, you will want your dumbbells extended.

Can I weight train with the two exercises I've learned and perform four sets each?

Weight training with two different exercises and four sets each on the same muscle group is not the most ideal weight training routine for foundation training. Foundation training conditions your body to progress toward your next goal. Once you have a solid foundation, you can focus on body fat loss, strength, or endurance. Without a solid foundation, you are at a much higher risk of injury.

I have been exercising for 20+ years. Running was my main exercise. I could never lose weight. I thought about all the hours I put in running and an occasional step class - what's up with that? So, I signed up with Kevin at a local gym and in two-and-a-half months, I lost 12 lbs. His education about the whole body was the key. I had the cardio down but Kevin added weights to my workout. He also added an eating schedule that had me eating more frequently throughout the day. Kevin also had me write down everything I ate and at what time I ate it. Kevin is so inspirational that he makes you want to succeed in getting fit.

- Susie Falter

The Secrets to Success!

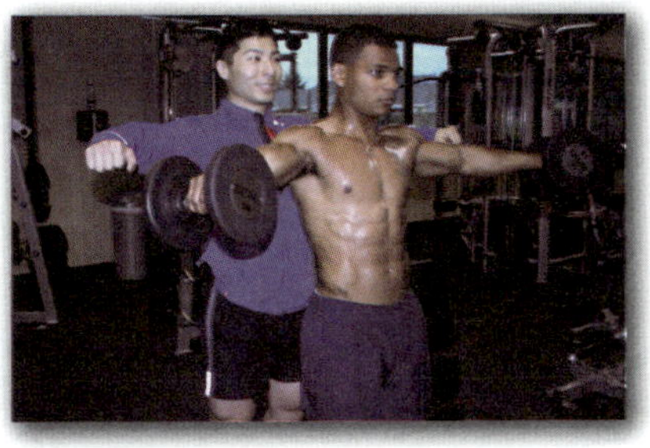

From Your Personal Trainer, Kevin Orr

I believe success is a state of mind. I also believe achieving that success comes from planning ahead. Fail to plan, plan to fail.

You have learned so much about how to work around the obstacles of life. Your commitment to maintaining a workout schedule and a nutrition plan has already grounded you in a healthy, positive lifestyle. But there is always that one meal or event that can throw you a curve ball. If you don't plan ahead, it's very likely you will spend a day living on fast food, no water, and no workout. Of course, this doesn't sound too bad for just one day, meal, or event. However, once you let yourself go a little bit, you may find it's harder to get back into your positive lifestyle routine. So, make sure you do everything you can to plan your meals, snacks, and workouts ahead of time. Planning ahead is the secret!

Example Weight & Cardio Routine

Continue to choose a workout routine based on your level of fitness and your schedule before progressing to Week 9. Write it down in your schedule, on page 249. If none of the example routines work for you, configure a routine that fits your needs, and write it down. Planning ahead will help you set yourself up for success.

Weight Routine 1

Sunday	Monday	Tuesday	Wednesday	Thursday	Friday	Saturday
	Chest/Back/ Shoulders 4x15		Legs: 4x20 Arms: 4x15 Abs: 4x20		Chest/Back/ Shoulders 4x15	

Weight Routine 2

Sunday	Monday	Tuesday	Wednesday	Thursday	Friday	Saturday
		Chest/Back/ Shoulders 4x15	Arms: 4x15 Abs: 4x20	Legs 4x20		Chest/Back/ Shoulders 4x15

Weight Routine 3

Sunday	Monday	Tuesday	Wednesday	Thursday	Friday	Saturday
	Chest/Back/ Shoulders 4x15	Arms: 4x15 Abs: 4x20	Legs 4x20	Chest/Back/ Shoulders 4x15		

Continue to choose routine 1, 2, or 3 to begin your weekly cardio routine, or rearrange your cardio training to best fit you.

Cardio Routine 1

Sunday	Monday	Tuesday	Wednesday	Thursday	Friday	Saturday
	Tread:R 15 EFX: 15		Tread:R 15 EFX: 15		Tread:R 15 EFX: 15	

Cardio Routine 2

Sunday	Monday	Tuesday	Wednesday	Thursday	Friday	Saturday
		Tread:R 15 EFX: 15	Tread:R 15 EFX: 15	Tread:R 15 EFX: 15		Tread:R 15 EFX: 15

Cardio Routine 3

Sunday	Monday	Tuesday	Wednesday	Thursday	Friday	Saturday
	Tread:R 15 EFX: 15	Tread:R 15 EFX: 15	Tread:R 15 EFX: 15	Tread:R 15 EFX: 15	Tread:R 15 EFX: 15	

Example Schedule

On your schedule, page 249, continue to write down which cardio machines along with the duration you plan to complete this week.

	Sunday	Monday	Tuesday	Wednesday	Thursday	Friday	Saturday	
Week 5 Weight: Body fat: Cardio: Duration:		218 30% Chest/Back Shoulders: 4x15 Cycle: 15 Stepper: 15	Arms: 4x15 Abs: 4x20 Cycle: 15 Stepper: 15	Legs: 4x20 Cycle: 15 Stepper: 15	Chest/Back Shoulders: 4x15 Cycle: 15 Stepper: 15	Legs: 4x20 Cycle: 15 Stepper: 15	Chest/Back Shoulders: 4x15 Cycle: Stepper:	Why Sick! Solution Make it up another day when feeling better
Week 6 Weight: Body fat: Weights: Sets: Cardio: Duration:		216 Arms: 4x15 Abs: 4x20 Stairs: 15 Cycle: 15	Legs: 4x20 Stairs: 15 Cycle: 15	Chest/Back Shoulders: 4x15 Stairs: 15 Cycle: 15	Arms: 4x15 Abs: 4x20 Stairs: 15 Cycle: 15	Stairs: 15 Cycle: 15		Why Solution Perfect week!
Week 7 Weight: Body fat: Weights: Sets: Cardio: Duration:		214 29% Legs: 4x20 EFX: 15 Stairs: 15	Chest/Back Shoulders: 4x15 EFX: 15 Stairs: 15	Arms: 4x15 Abs: 4x20 EFX: 15 Stairs: 15	Legs: 4x20 EFX: 15 Stairs: 15	EFX: 15 Stairs: 15		Why Class Exam Solution Shift workouts one day
Week 8 Weight: Body fat: Weights: Sets: Cardio: Duration:		211 Chest/Back Shoulders: 4x15 Tread:R 15 EFX: 15	Arms: 4x15 Abs: 4x20 Tread:R 15 EFX: 15	Legs: 4x20 Tread:R 15 EFX: 15	Chest/Back Shoulders: 4x15 Tread:R 15 EFX: 15	Tread:R 15 EFX: 15		

Before moving on...

Did you follow through with your plan? If not, cross out what you did not complete on your schedule and write in what you did complete before moving on to the next week.

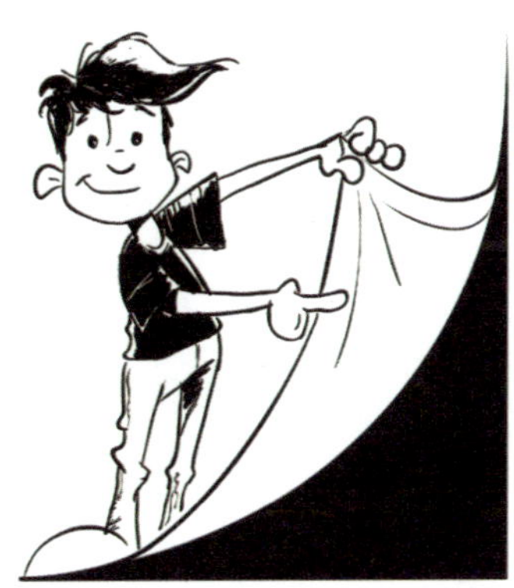

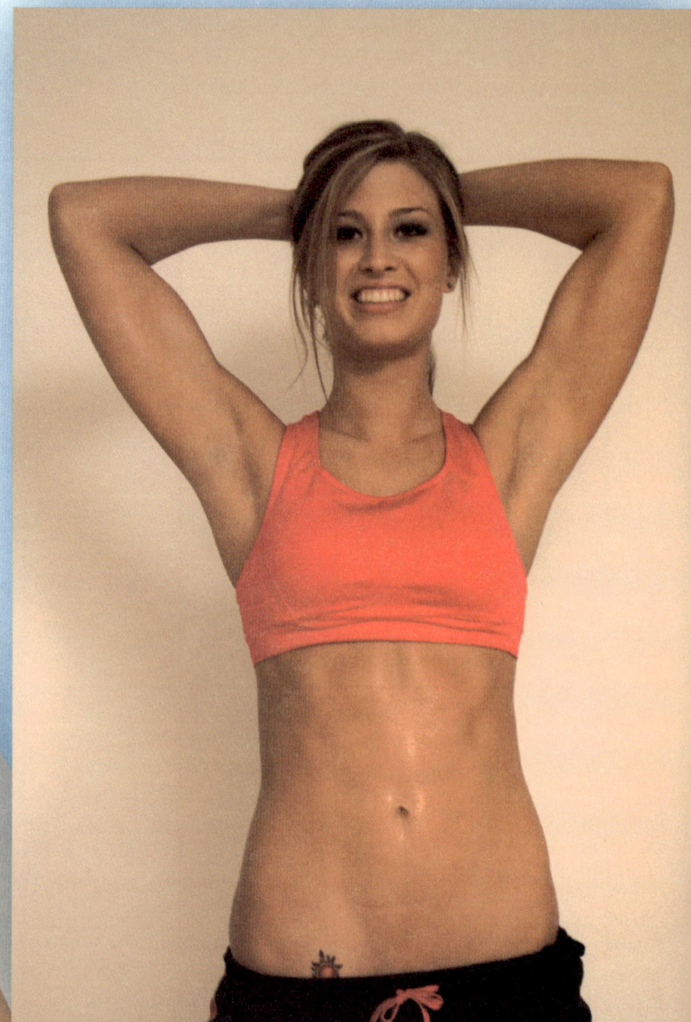
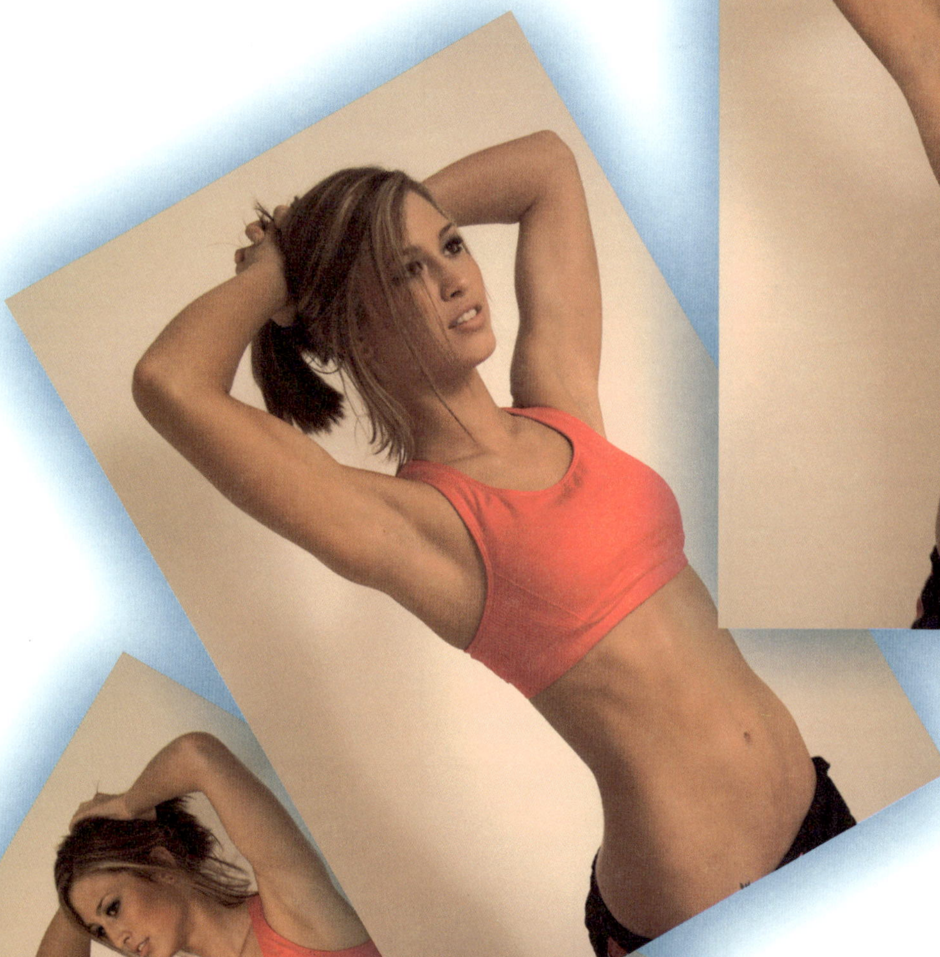
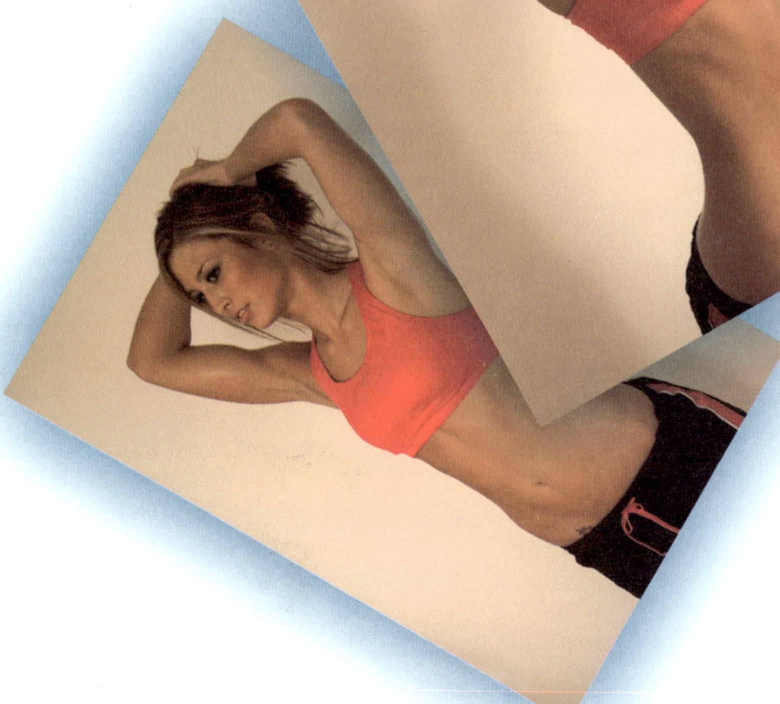

Week 9

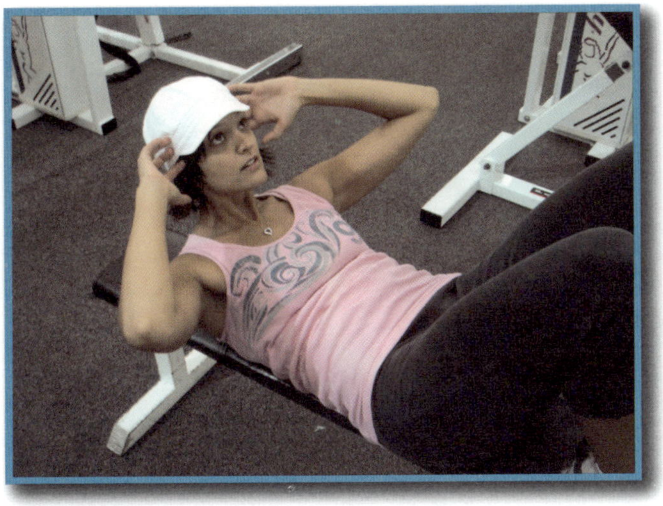

I believe that with proper instruction and lots of motivation everyone can look and feel the way they want. The combination of exercise, nutrition, accountability, and setting goals give you what you need to succeed. All of these things combined will give you the education you need to maintain a healthy lifestyle. I thank Kevin Orr's method for teaching me what I know today. Because of him, I am happier and healthier, and I know how to maintain my new look.

- Heather Cowell

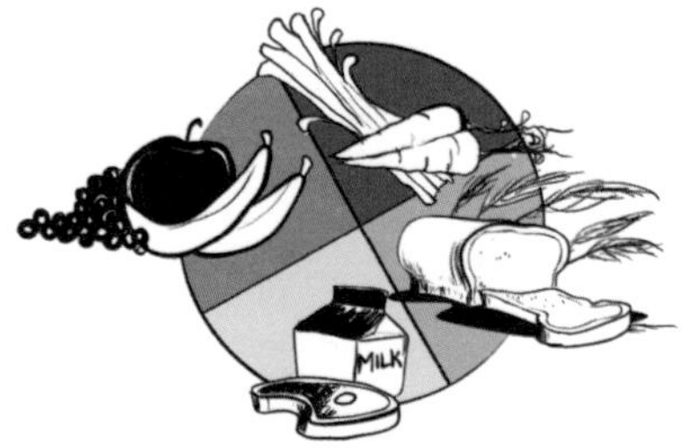

Goal:

Eat a variety of healthy foods.

Why?

Including a variety of foods in your meal plans is the key to ensuring you are eating all the nutrients that your body requires to be healthy and strong. While eating the same foods every day makes meal planning a breeze, for most people, it will eventually lead to boredom. And that can lead to making food choices you will later regret. To keep that from happening and to keep you on track for meeting your goals, you need to shake up your menu by adding variety. Mix things up and have fun with your ingredients! There is a big caution here: revitalizing your meals can also wake up your desire to overeat. As we proceed with expanding your food choices, portion control is a must!

How?

Eat a wide variety of meats, fruits, vegetables, whole grains, legumes, herbs, and spices. New colors, flavors, and textures in new combinations make meal times exciting and get you past the boredom slump.

Here's a list of basic healthy options:

Protein*		**Fat**	**Carbohydrates**		
Meats	**Poultry**	**Oils**	**100% Whole Grain, etc.**	**Fruits**	**Vegetables**
Lean Beef	Chicken Breast	Canola Oil	Brown Rice	Apples	Asparagus
Lean Ham	Ground Turkey	Flax Oil	Cream of Wheat	Apricots	Bell Pepper
Lean Pork	Turkey Breast	Olive Oil	Oatmeal	Bananas	Broccoli
Round Steak	Turkey Sausage	Sunflower Oil	Popcorn	Blackberries	Cauliflower
Top Sirloin			Wild Rice	Blueberries	Carrots
			Whole Wheat Bagel	Cantaloupe	Celery
Fish	**Dairy**	**Nuts**	Whole Wheat Bread	Cherries	Corn
Catfish	Cottage Cheese	Almonds	Whole Wheat Buns	Grapefruit	Cucumber
Cod	Eggs	Peanuts	Whole Wheat Crackers	Grapes	Eggplant
Clams	Egg Substitutes	Walnuts	Whole Wheat English Muffins	Guava	Green Beans
Crab	Egg Whites		Whole Wheat Pasta	Honeydew	Legumes
Haddock			Whole Wheat Pita		Lettuce

continued on next page

*Most protein food items contain fat.

Protein		Fat	Carbohydrates		
Fish	**Dairy**	**Nut Butters**	**100% Whole Grain, etc.**	**Fruits**	**Vegetables**
Halibut	Milk	Almond	Whole Wheat Rolls	Kiwi	Peas
Lobster	String Cheese	Cashew	Whole Wheat Tortilla	Mangoes	Potato
Tilapia	Yogurt	100% Natural PB		Oranges	Pumpkin
Trout				Papaya	Spinach
Tuna		**Seeds**		Peaches	Squash
Salmon		Avocados		Pears	Sweet Potatoes
Scallops		Flax Seeds		Pineapple	Tomatoes
Shell Fish		Olives		Pomegranate	Yams
Shrimp		Sunflower Seeds		Raspberries	Zucchini
White Fish				Strawberries	
				Watermelon	

Which foods do you like? Which foods would you like to try? Which foods are you *willing* to try? Start mixing and matching! Try some of the following healthy enhancements for new flavors and colors:

Breakfast

- Add sliced banana and strawberries to your cottage cheese to take the "blah" out of this power protein.
- Sliced banana, blueberries, peaches, or nectarine stirred into oatmeal adds color, texture, and taste appeal.
- Diced ham, low fat mozzarella cheese, and pineapple turn dull scrambled eggs into a tropical surprise. For added zing, add minced jalapeños.
- Fold chopped onions, mushrooms, olives, red and green peppers into your egg white omelet. Sprinkle with cayenne pepper and fresh cilantro. Enjoy with a side fruit salad.

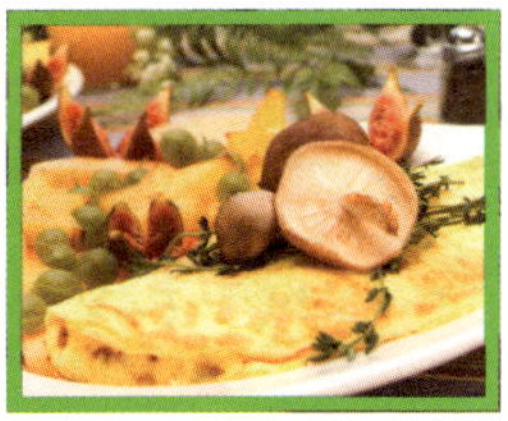

Lunch

- Perk up your chicken salad or whole wheat pasta with green, red, and orange pepper strips, broccoli florets, carrot or cucumber slices, they will add crunch and color.
- In small amounts (1-2 tablespoons), these ingredients can enliven your salad. (Remember to count them in with your PFCs):
  - Crumbled cheese (blue, feta, goat)
  - Dried fruit (cranberries, blueberries, apricots, cherries)
  - Pomegranate seeds
  - Chopped nuts, pine nuts, sunflower seeds, sliced almonds

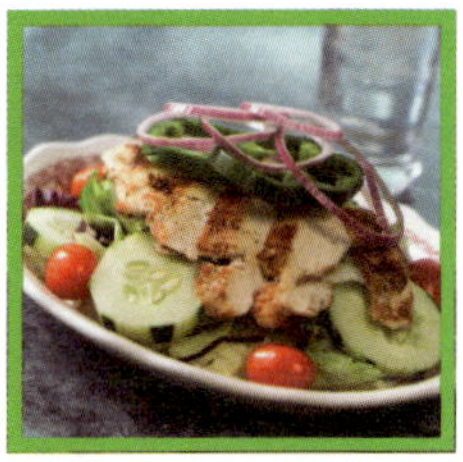

- Sliced kiwi fruit, red grapes, and blueberries added to your tossed green salads provide a little sweetness. Chopped nuts add crunch. Red onions add zip.
- Oranges, grapefruit, or nectarine slices transform any turkey salad.

...continued

- Some chopped tomatoes, onions, jalapeños, and Dijon ensure a new experience for your chicken sandwich.

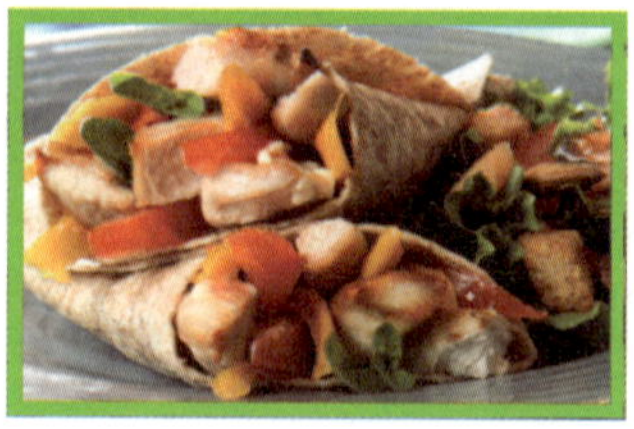

- Small amounts of thinly sliced fruits, such as apples or mangos, can turn a ho-hum sandwich into a gourmet delight.
- Apple chunks, pineapples, mangos, red grapes, or kiwi slices perk up chicken, ham, or tuna salads. Add red onion for some heat.
- Wrap any of those combos in a spinach or whole wheat tortilla and the boring sandwich is history!

<u>Snacks</u>

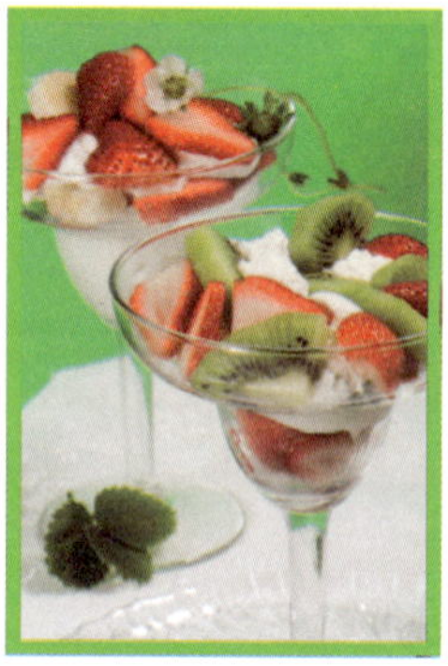

- Try eating kiwi fruit from its own container. Simply cut it in half and scoop out each half with a spoon. Good for you and EASY! You can also try this with personal sized cantaloupe and watermelon. No bowl needed! Remember to add some protein to this snack.
- Create a zesty dip for your chicken strips: salsa made with tomatoes, mangoes, avocados, minced onions, cilantro, lemon or lime juice, and chili peppers.
- Fruit salad on the go? Sliced banana, blueberries, peaches and grapes topped with low-fat vanilla yogurt. Yum!

<u>Dinner</u>

- Grill everything! Pineapple, peaches, zucchini, cucumber, tomatoes, onions, or mushrooms are easy to grill and make a delicious combination for chicken or fish.

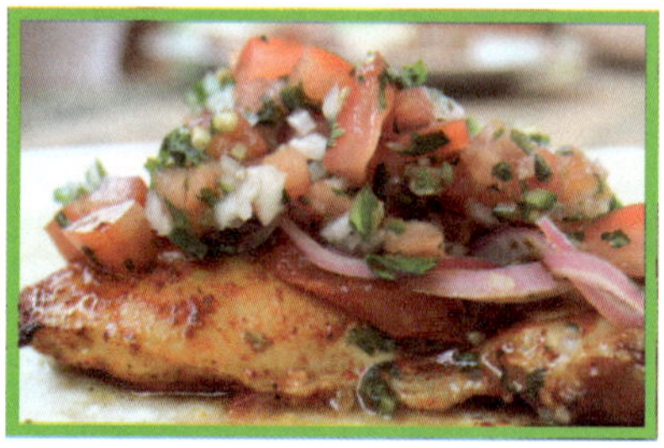

- Make shish kabobs. Alternate chunks of meat, zucchini, pepper, onion, pineapple, tomato. Baste with low calorie raspberry vinaigrette.
- Spice up your salmon. Spray a salmon fillet with olive oil. Sprinkle with dried dill, Beau Monde or celery salt, and cracked black pepper. Grill, bake, or microwave.
- “Fry” up some skinless chicken breasts. Spray chicken breasts with olive oil. Sprinkle with garlic salt, cayenne pepper, dried cilantro and dried parsley. Spray a pan with olive oil. Cook the chicken for 7 minutes a side. Cover the pan and let the chicken set for 5 minutes. (Basil and rosemary is another great combo for perking up that same old chicken.)

Time to review your nutrition log.

1. Cross out a few food items that can be replaced with another healthy food item and add the new variation.

2. Keep your "variety choice" food selections simple.

3. Continue to record everything you eat and drink in your nutrition log daily.

For Example:

Time	Food and Amount	Substitute
7:00 AM	WW toast, Adam's® PB, ½ cup cottage cheese	**Blueberries, strawberries, chopped nuts**, ½ cup cottage cheese
10:00 AM	WW crackers, white cheese, lean meats: turkey, chicken, tuna	**100% WW tortilla, avocado slice, turkey slice, mozzarella cheese, fresh cilantro**
12:30 PM	WW sandwich	**Yam, chicken with salsa**
3:00 PM	Apple, string cheese	**Kiwi**, string cheese
6:00 PM	Workout	Workout
8:00 PM	WW pasta, chick-en	**Fruit & veg-etable salad**, chicken

WW = 100% whole wheat

Week 9

Questions and Answers

Why is it so important to have a variety of fruits and vegetables?

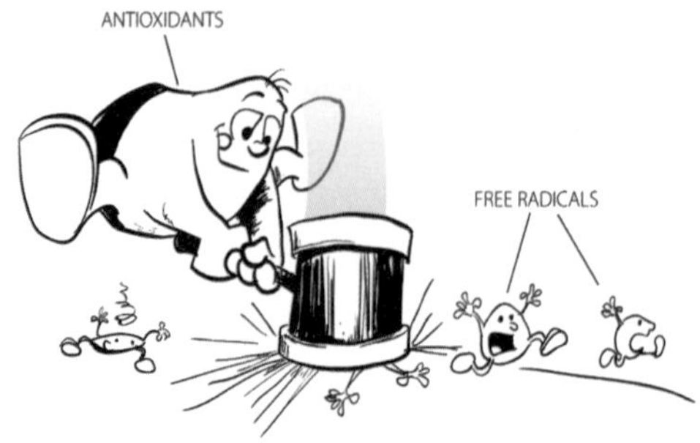

Two words: Fiber and antioxidants. Phytonutrients (or phytochemicals) are antioxidants, enzymes that block free radicals (forms of pollution and carcinogens in foods) from damaging cells. They have been shown to boost the immune system and lower the risk of a variety of cancers and chronic diseases including stroke, diabetes, cardiovascular disease and hypertension. One of these nutritional warriors is Beta-carotene (a carotenoid and flavonoid), which gives fruits and vegetables their bright colors. Beta-carotene is present when you see orange. It gives carrots, sweet potatoes, cantaloupe, and oranges their bright, orange color. This color is associated with reducing the risk of lung cancer. Flavonoids are in the skin, so it's important to avoid peeling most fruits and vegetables. They assist in eliminating mutagens and carcinogens, which decrease the risks of several types of cancers.

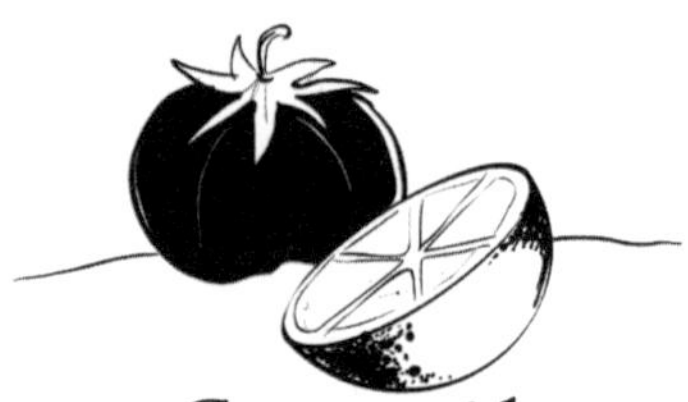

Carotenoids

Another carotenoid is alpha-carotene, which can be found in orange-and red-colored fruits and vegetables such as carrots, squash, kiwi, spinach, and mangos. These colors have been shown to decrease the risks of heart disease and several forms of cancers. Red tomatoes, watermelon, and pink grapefruit are associated with reducing the risk of several types of cancer, such as prostate cancer. Bright yellow, orange, dark green leafy vegetables include alpha-carotene, which has been shown to decrease the risks of heart disease and various forms of cancer. Many other carotenoids such as lutein, lycopene, and zeaxanthin are in fruits and vegetables. They pack an antioxidant punch that affects the health of your skin, bones, vision, and immune system. Generally, the brighter and darker your fruits and vegetables, the more antioxidants they will have and the more nutrient-dense they will be.

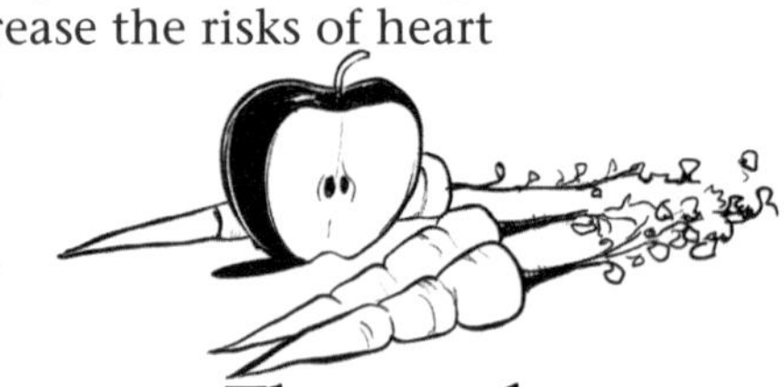

Flavonoids

If you continue to eat the same fruits and vegetables every day, you may be missing out on many nutrients that can have a huge impact on your health and longevity. All fruits and vegetables contain fiber which is essential for proper digestion. If you eat the same ones all the time, you may be missing those that have more fiber and better taste. When you add variety, you can ensure that you are getting all the powerful nutrients you need.

I am getting tired of whole wheat. Are there alternatives?

The whole grains in your meals are probably coming in the form of oatmeal, 100% whole grain breads, and cereals. Why not try different whole grains such as barley, amaranth, rye, buckwheat, and others? These are just as nutritious as whole wheat, and help you keep food boredom at bay.

Why do I feel the need to eat more when I add variety?

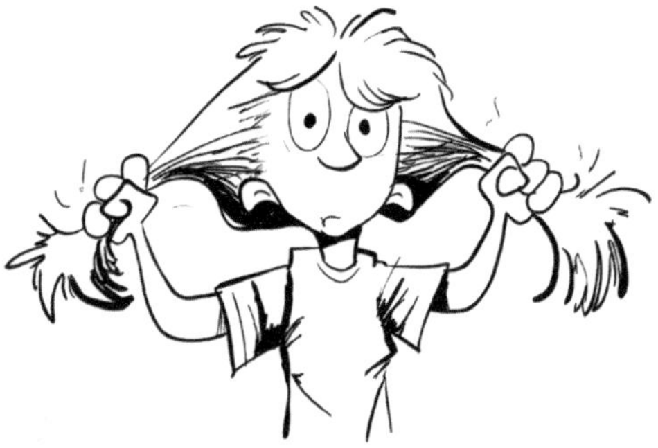

Address one challenge to develop a healthier lifestyle and up pops another. However, this new challenge is your opportunity to solidify your new lifestyle change. Feeling the need to eat more when you're increasing food variety is a typical response when you've been focused on your weight and hunger control. Introducing new foods excites several of your sensory receptors such as taste and smell. Your brain and body react in ways that can reignite your old emotions related to food and eating. Those emotions include appetite, anger, fear, anxiety, depression, and pleasure. They can also surface food-related memories. This emotional connection can increase your emotional urge to eat more. Eating the same food day after day normally leads to less overeating. On the other hand, the more variety and choices you have, the more it can excite your emotional hunger, which can make it harder to control your food intake. By being aware of this, you can pay attention to body signals when you're adding variety. As always, moderation is the key! Eat slowly. Savor your meals. Practice portion control. Soon, eating healthy and eating well will be a painless part of your new healthy lifestyle.

Do I still need to follow my PFC ratios when I'm adding a little more variety?

Yes, your PFC ratios are vital in continuing to balance your blood sugar for optimal energy and metabolism. Adding variety is simply a method to avoid boredom with your nutrition plan.

What should I drink?

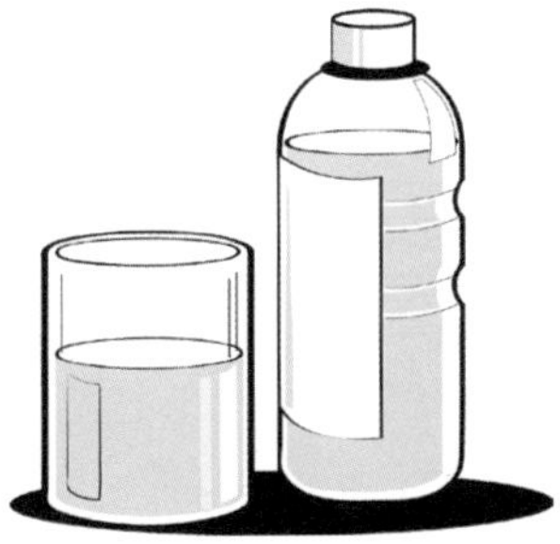

Water should always be your beverage of choice. Fruit drinks are high in sugar and very high glycemic. Crystal Light® is OK in moderation. Again, for some people, it could create a sweet tooth. Taste something sweet and you may crave more sweet. Be very careful and know your limit.

Every day there is new nutritional information in the news! How can I really know what I SHOULD be eating?

The amount of information that you receive about the health benefits of certain foods is vast, and we are being overloaded with information as the press jumps on nutrition stories – often times prematurely. Good, solid, scientific information that is more than a headline in the newspaper should factor into your nutritional decisions. Avoid changing your eating habits based on headlines in the news. The recommendations I have given you have solid research support.

Nutrition Log

Date:___________	Sun Mon Tues Wed Thurs Fri Sat			
	Food	**PFC**		
Meal 1	*Food & Amount*	*P*	*F*	*C*
Time:_____				
Meal 2				
Time:_____				
Meal 3				
Time:_____				
Meal 4				
Time:_____				
Meal 5				
Time:_____				
Meal 6				
Time:_____				

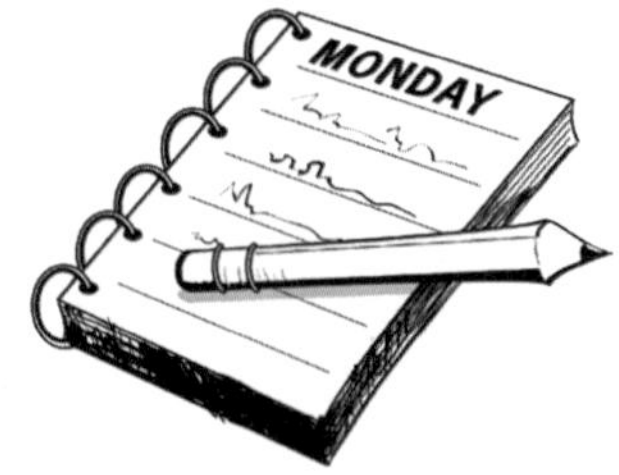

Checklist

Achieved:

- ✓ Consume meal or snack every 3 hours
- ✓ Water every 3 hours
- ✓ Sleep optimal hours
- ✓ Intake multivitamin
- ✓ Weights and cardio
- ✓ Consume PFCs every meal or snack
- ✓ Foods low on the GI
- ✓ PFC ratio balance
- ✓ Planned meals
- ✓ **Add nutritional variety**

Avoided:

- ✓ Sugars
- ✓ White flour
- ✓ Processed foods

Key Points

Week 1
- Eat a small meal or snack once every three hours – five to six meals per day.
- Drink at least 1 cup (8 ounces) of water per meal and at least one cup before, during, and after your workouts.
- Keep a nutrition log.
- Sleep is vital!
- Take a daily multivitamin.

Week 2
- Avoid bad sugars.

Week 3
- Avoid white flour and white rice.

Week 4
- Avoid processed foods.

Week 5
- Balance your meals and snacks with a combination of proteins, fats, and carbohydrates.

Week 6
- Eat foods that are low on the Glycemic Index.

Week 7
- Balance your meals and snacks with a specific ratio of proteins, fats, and carbohydrates.

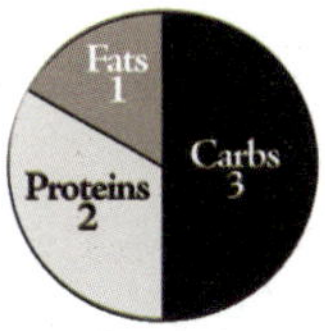

Week 8
- Plan and prepare your foods for meals and snacks ahead of time.
- Keep your prepared food selection simple.
- Continue to record everything you're eating and drinking in your nutrition log daily.

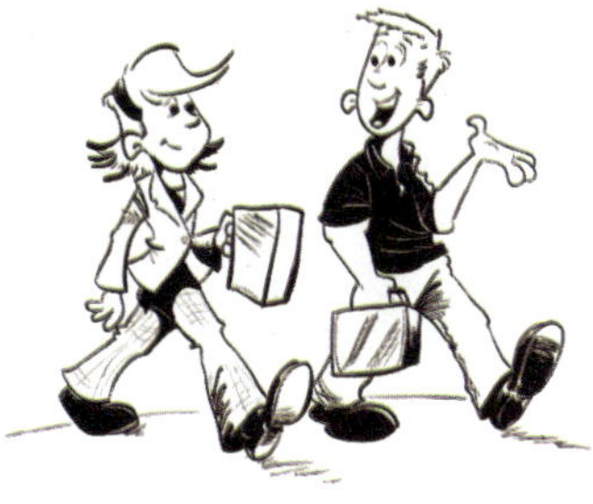

Week 9
- **Adding a variety of foods to your meal plans** is the key to ensuring that you're eating the wide variety of nutrients that your body requires to keep your body healthy and strong.

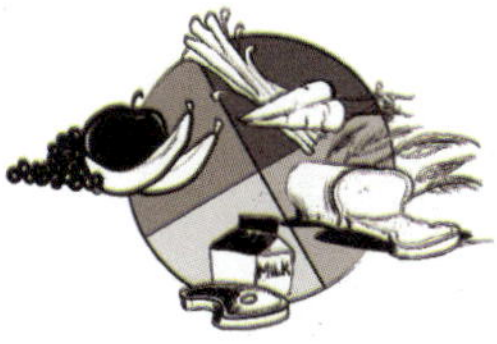

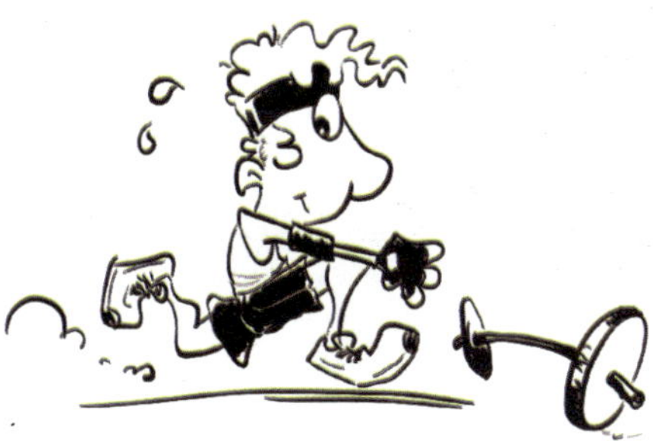

Biceps

Goal:

Complete four sets of 15 reps of the **straight bar biceps curl**.

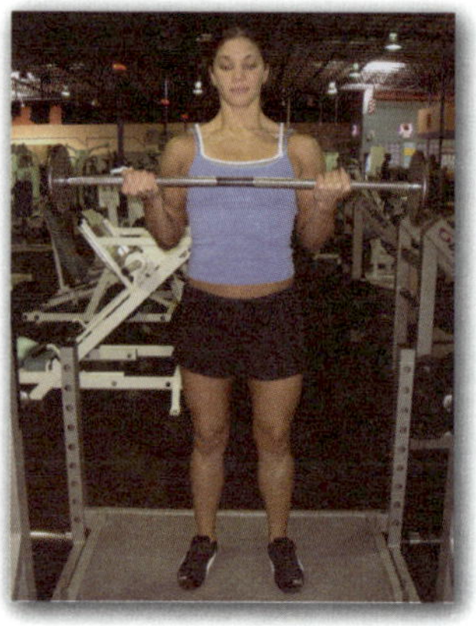

Primary
Biceps

Stabilizers
Shoulders
Forearms
Core

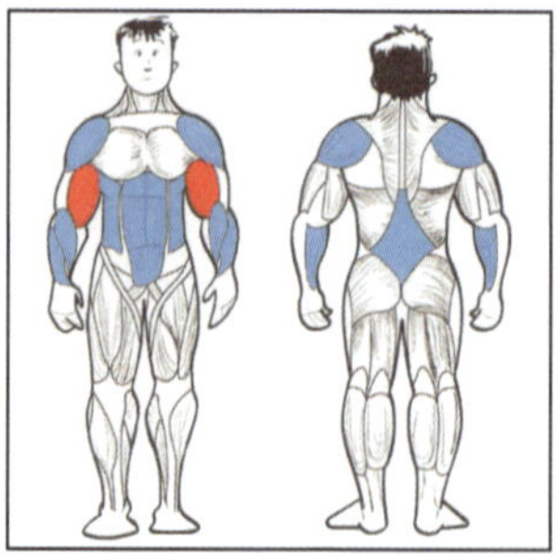

Why?

The straight bar biceps curl is a compound exercise targeting your biceps. The muscle stabilizers include your shoulders and forearms, as well as the rest of your core.

How?

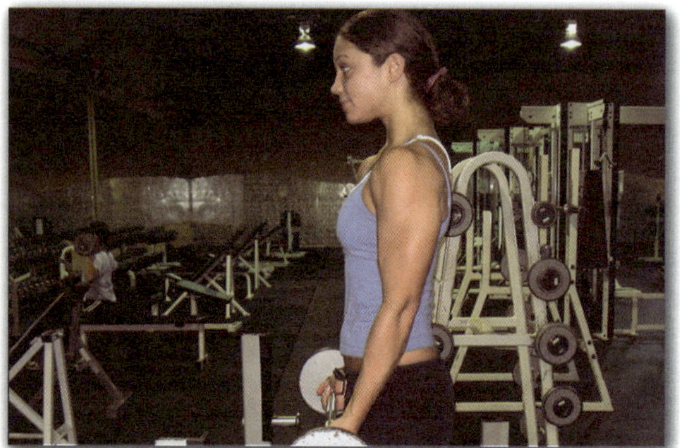

Step 1 - Begin with your feet shoulder-width apart. Hold the straight bar with your palms facing forward.

Step 2 - Squeeze your abs to push your lower back into a neutral position.

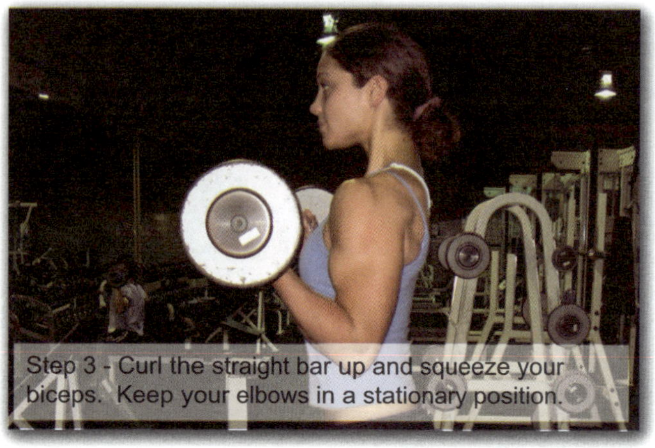

Step 3 - Curl the straight bar up and squeeze your biceps. Keep your elbows in a stationary position.

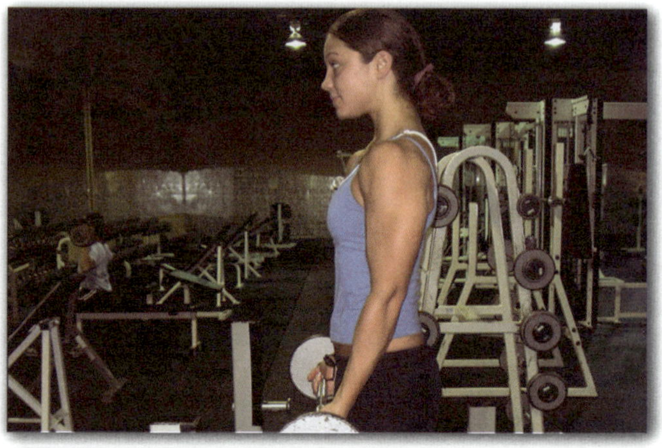

Step 4 - Lower the straight bar back to your starting position using a smooth and controlled motion. Repeat.

Your goal is to complete four sets of 15 (4 x 15).

Range of Motion Techniques
To Maximize Muscle Tension and Minimize Overcompensation

Dos	Don'ts
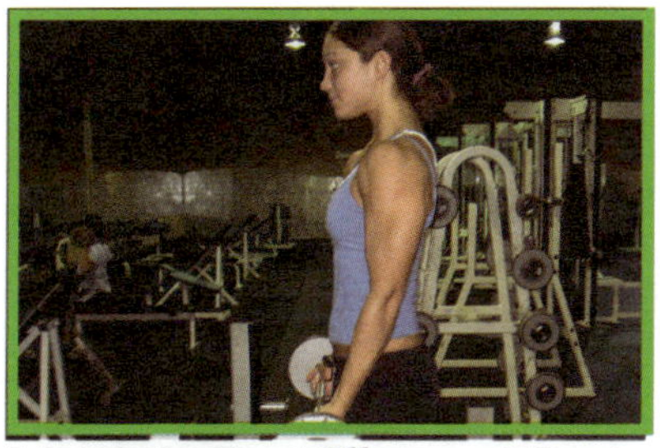 Maintain Bent Elbows at Starting Position	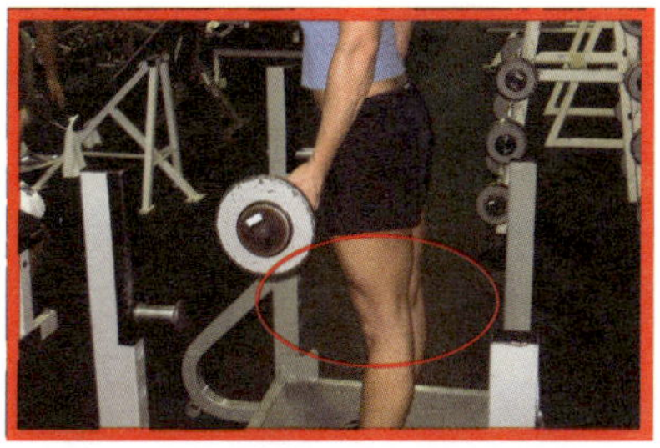 Avoid Locking Out Knees
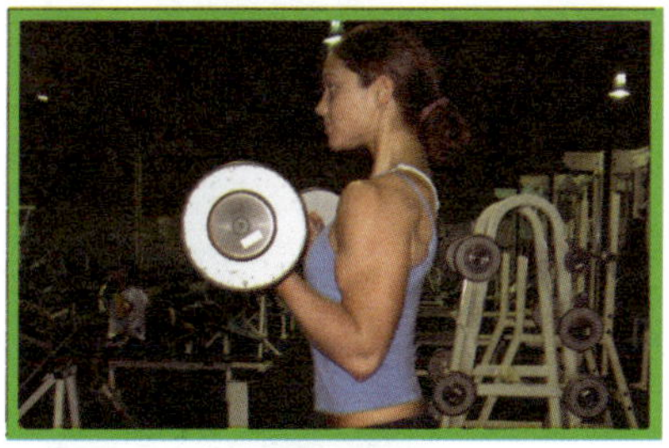 Squeeze Biceps to Peak Contraction	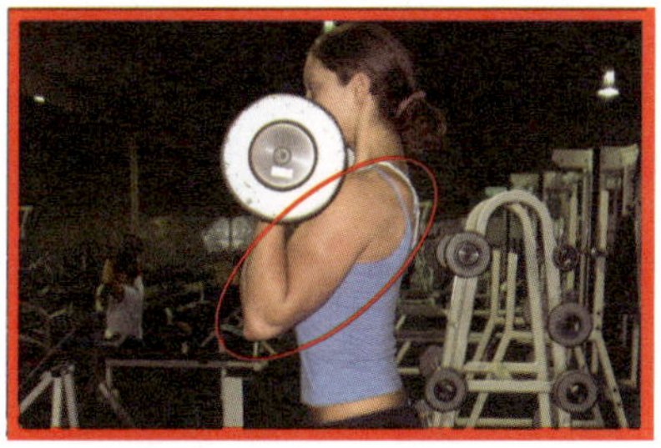 Avoid Exceeding Peak Contraction
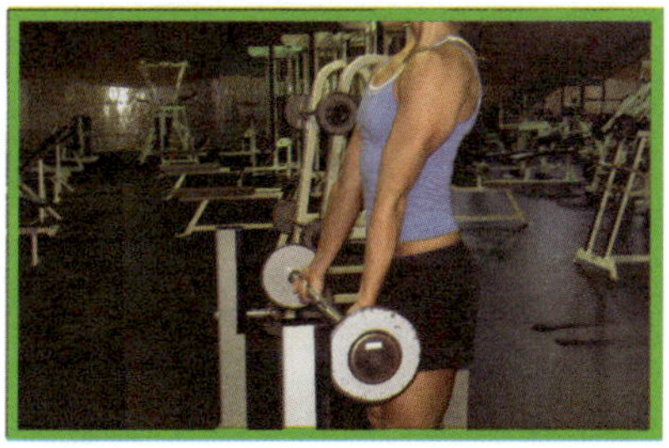 Lower to Resist and Lock Out Elbows to Stretch Biceps	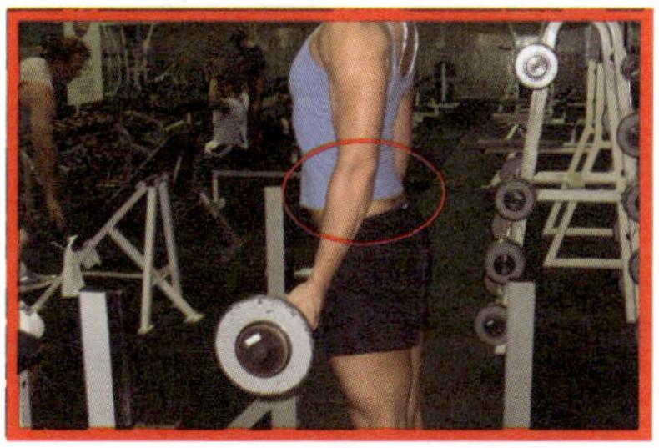 Avoid Maintaining Bent Elbows When Biceps Need to Stretch for Optimum Biceps Tension

Visualize

"Ball, Stretch, Semicircle Effect"

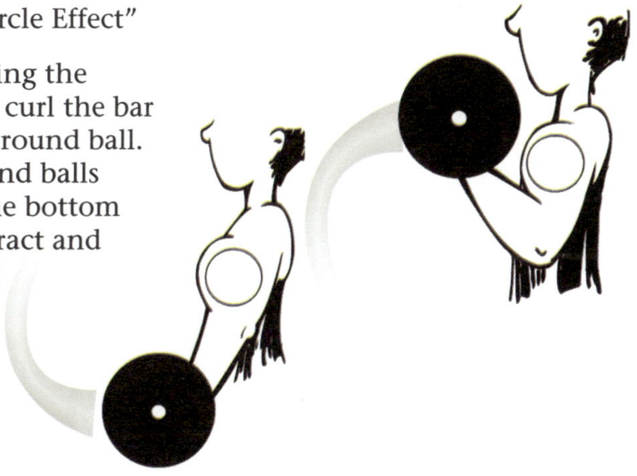

While performing standing straight bar curls, visualize curling the straight bar up and down in a semicircular motion. As you curl the bar up, flex your biceps and imagine curling them into a tight, round ball. As you lower the bar, resist the weight and imagine the round balls stretching. Focus on feeling the stretch in your biceps at the bottom of your range of motion. As you curl the bar back up, contract and squeeze your biceps back into the biggest balls you can curl them into.

Repeat and continue to visualize with each rep. Visualizing allows you to maximize the tension in your biceps, while reducing tension in your lower back, forearm, and wrists.

Questions and Answers

What's the purpose of feeling a stretch in my biceps?

Feeling a stretch in your biceps ensures that your biceps are resisting, not your shoulders, forearms, or any other stabilizers.

Why am I feeling tension in my elbows when lowering my straight bar to lock out?

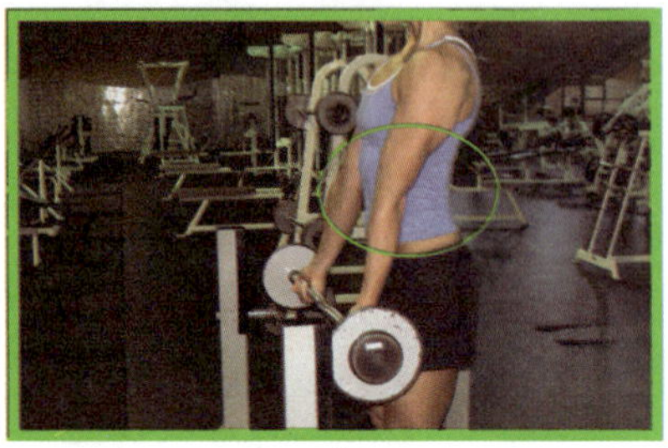

If you are feeling tension in your elbows when coming down to lock-out, your elbow position may be too far back. Be sure to maintain an elbow position that's slightly in front of your body. Otherwise, the pressure will be in your elbows, not your biceps.

How do I know when I've reached my peak contraction for biceps?

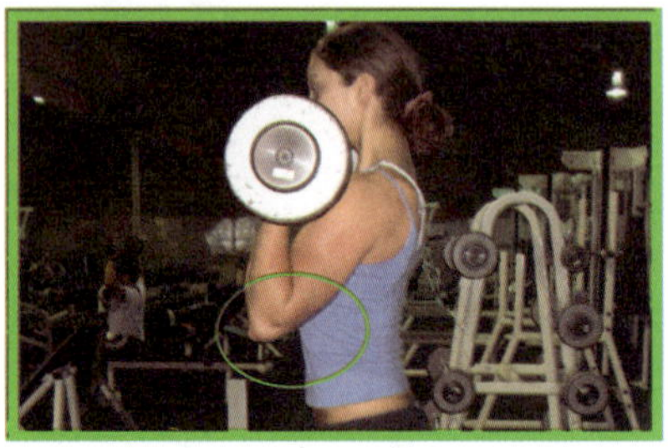

Keep your elbows slightly forward and in a stationary position while curling the straight bar up. The moment your elbows begin to move forward, you have reached your peak contraction. If you allow your elbows to go forward, your shoulders and lower back will begin to overcompensate.

I have been working out for over 20 years and have always been in reasonably good shape. However, I never quite saw the results I had hoped for considering all the effort I'd put forth. After a short while on Kevin's program, I finally achieved the success and saw the results I have been striving for all these years. If you're in good shape and want to achieve great shape, then this program can get you there in record time. My hat is off to Kevin for supplying me with this very livable program that has moved me beyond a 20-year plateau.
-Dolly Fisher Bales

Triceps

Goal:

Complete four sets of 15 reps on the **preacher triceps extension**.

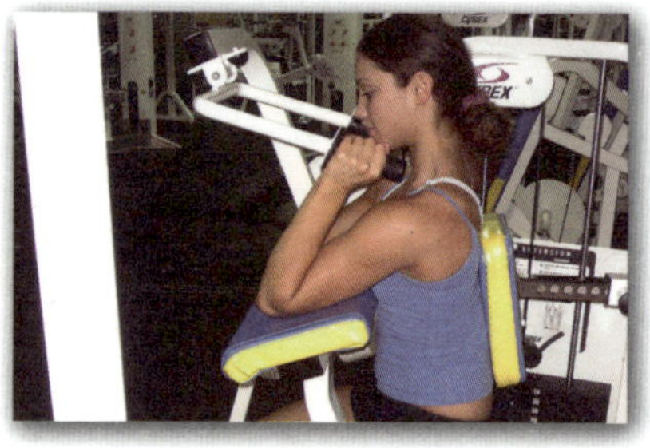

Primary
Triceps

Stabilizers
Shoulders
Forearms
Core

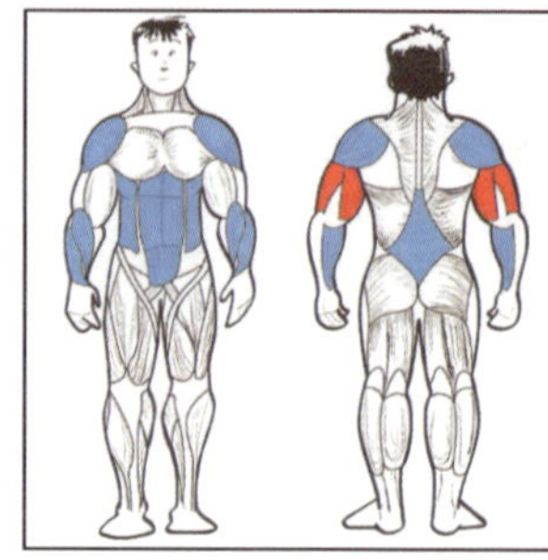

Why?

The preacher extension is a machine exercise targeting your triceps. The muscle stabilizers include your shoulder and forearms, as well as the rest of your core. This machine is very effective in reducing overcompensation and relieving joint pressure, especially in your elbows and wrists. It is similar to the preacher biceps curl. The preacher pad acts as a stabilizer causing your elbows to become the lever. Your triceps muscle must work hard to extend the weight forward to your peak contraction.

How?

Step 1 - Before sitting down, adjust the seat and back support to fit you comfortably.

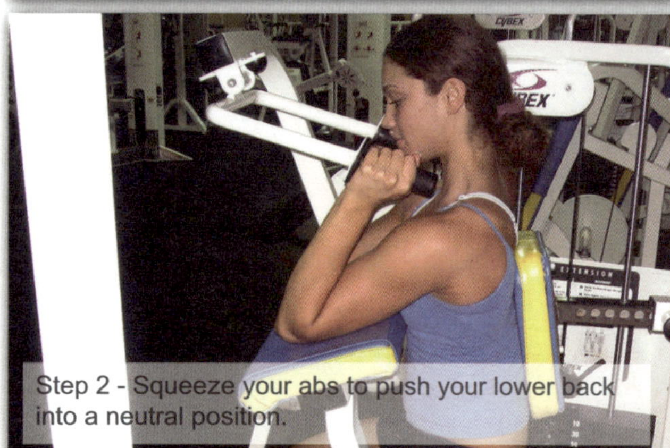

Step 2 - Squeeze your abs to push your lower back into a neutral position.

Step 3 - Align your elbows with your shoulders. Lightly grip the bar and keep your elbows unlocked.

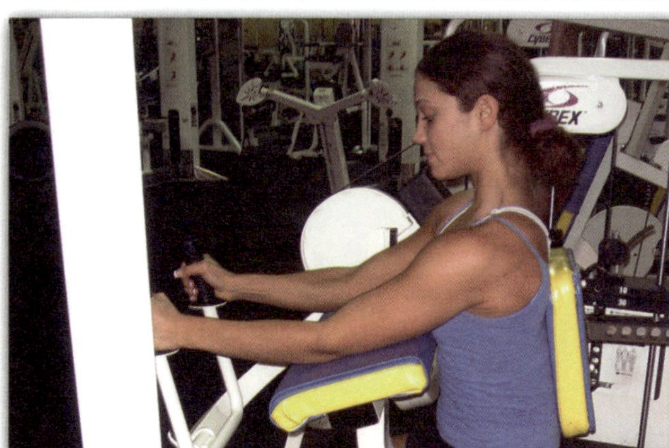

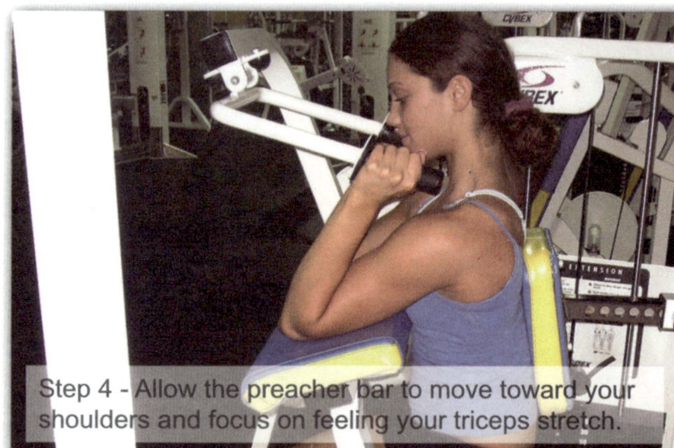

Step 4 - Allow the preacher bar to move toward your shoulders and focus on feeling your triceps stretch.

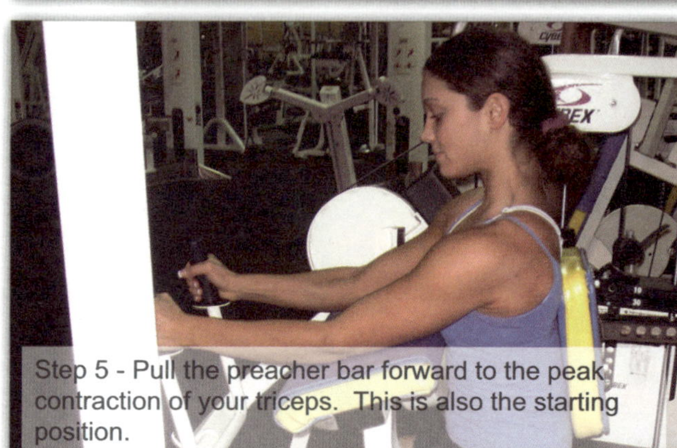

Step 5 - Pull the preacher bar forward to the peak contraction of your triceps. This is also the starting position.

Step 6 - Repeat with a smooth, controlled motion to maximize the tension in your triceps.

Your goal is to complete four sets of 15 (4 x 15).

Range of Motion Techniques

To Maximize Muscle Tension and Minimize Overcompensation

Dos

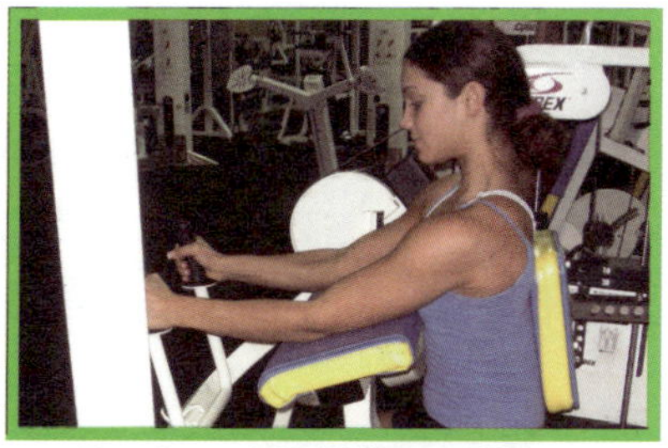

Begin with Elbows Bent

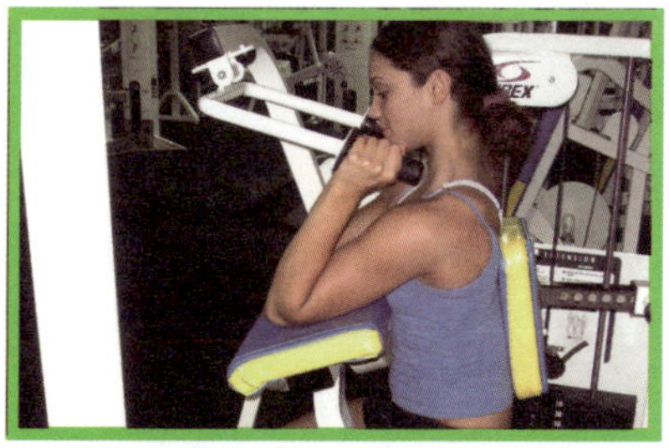

Stretch to Resist and Feel Stretch in Triceps

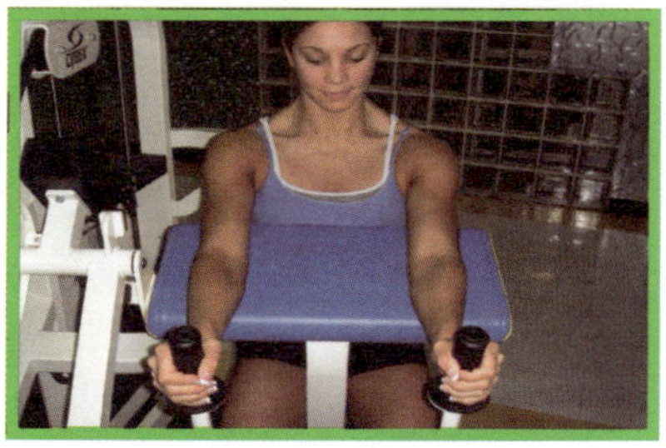

Maximize Triceps Tension When Shoulders, Elbows, and Wrists are Aligned

Don'ts

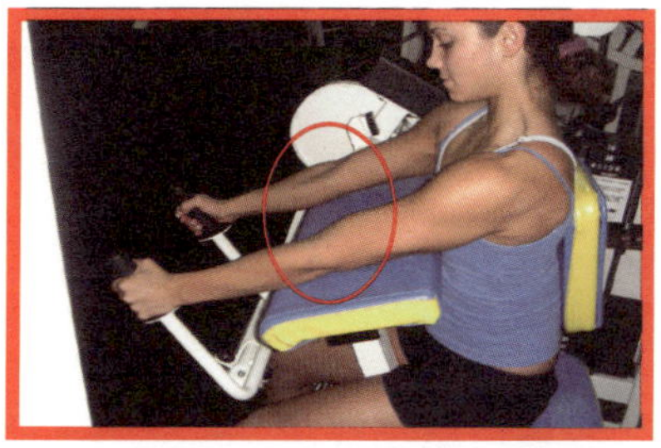

Avoid Locking Out Elbows

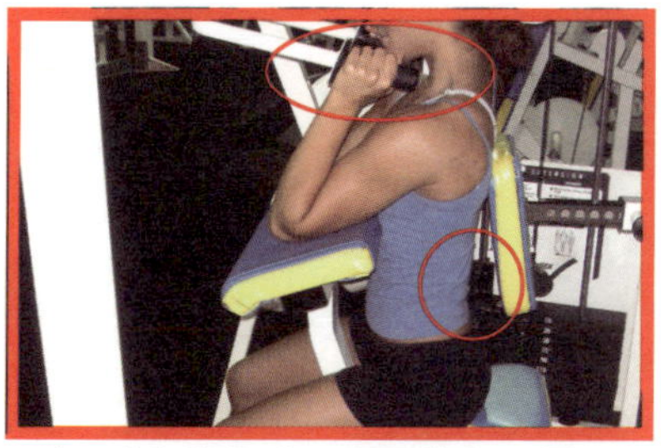

Avoid Coming Back too Far and Arching

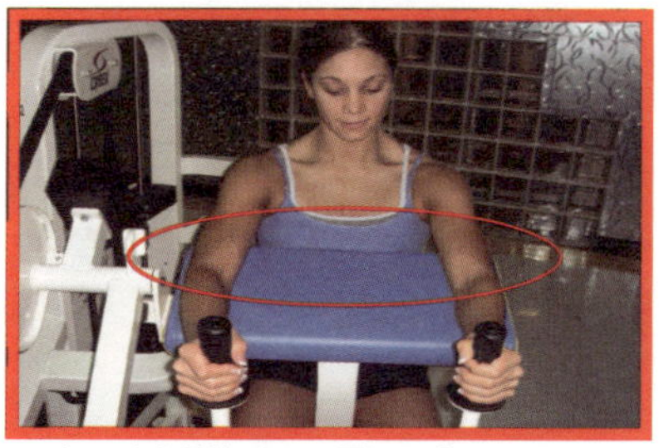

Avoid Elbows Too Apart or Too Close Together

Visualize

"Cable and Rubber Band Effect"

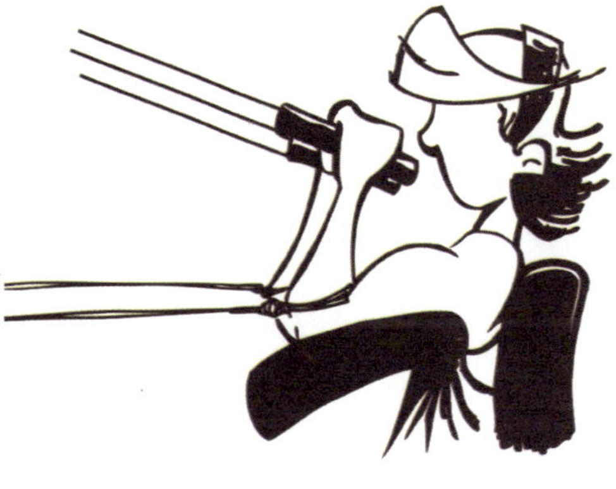

While performing preacher triceps extension, visualize cables attached to your elbows pulling them forward. Press your back against the back support. Imagine your triceps are a rubber band. As you resist the preacher bar coming towards you, the rubber band lengthens and tightens. When pushing the bar forward, the rubber band shortens and you feel tension in your triceps.

This allows you to squeeze and flex your triceps. The tension in your triceps tightens the rubber band, which pulls the preacher bar to your peak contraction.

Repeat the visualization with each rep. This maximizes the tension in your triceps and helps to reduce overcompensation from your shoulders, forearms, and wrists.

Questions and Answers

What if I feel my elbows?

Elbow pain is commonly felt in this motion. Try the following:

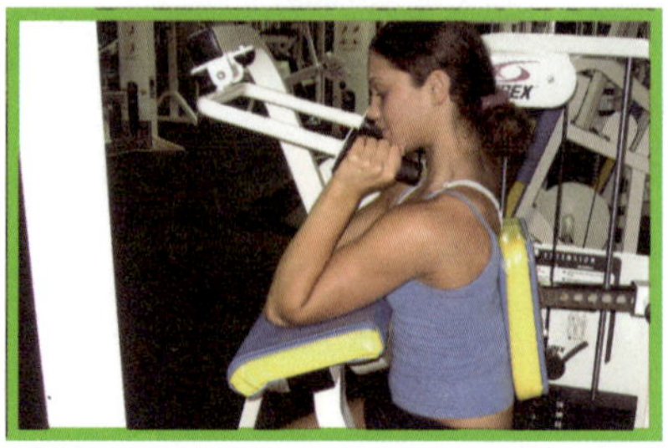

1. Avoid allowing the preacher bar to come too close to your shoulders.
2. Maintain a light hand grip.
3. Avoid pushing the preacher bar forward. Instead, visualize contracting your triceps to pull the preacher bar forward.
4. Lastly, visualize!

What if I feel my wrists?

Lightly grip the bar and wrap your thumbs around the bar to secure your wrists. Wrist stability helps to keep the wrists strong. Gripping too tightly increases wrist joint tension and forearm overcompensation. Overcompensation leads to injuries, and injuries are obstacles that get in the way when you're trying to reach your goal.

What if my lower back won't stay flat?

Keeping your lower back flat against the back support is very important! It relieves the pressure in your lower back, reducing overcompensation, forcing your triceps to do the work. Don't forget to squeeze your abs. Squeezing your abs helps to flatten the arch in your lower back.

Why do I need to feel a stretch in my triceps every rep?

Feeling a stretch in your triceps ensures your triceps are doing the work and no other muscle groups are overcompensating.

The training sessions that Kevin led me through were a very important part of my new approach to a healthier lifestyle. He taught me how to visualize the goal of what a particular exercise was intended to achieve. I noticed at that time that there were, in some cases, very subtle differences in how I had previously done a particular exercise and how Kevin had demonstrated the proper way to perform the exercise. Yet, even these small differences made a tremendous difference in how I felt after working out this way.

- Dave Tremain

I came to be a client of Kevin's due to knee problems I was having. Kevin taught me not only how to eat right but, how to read my body. We then started working out and this is where I got the most out of being a client. Kevin worked me hard and taught me how to push myself to places I had never been. All of these things I have maintained to this day. I'm 39 years old and play soccer five times a week. Because of what Kevin taught me, I feel like I'm 25. Thank you, Kevin, you changed my life!

- Tim Adamsen

Abs

Goal:

Complete four sets of 20 reps on the **incline reverse crunches**.

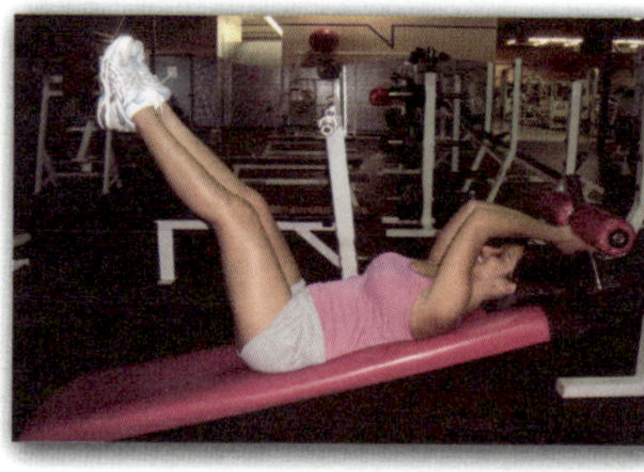

Primary
Abs

Stabilizers
Lower Back
Hip Flexors
Quads
Neck

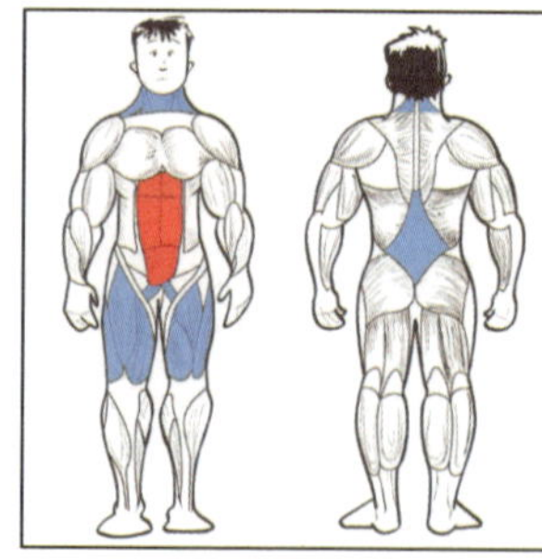

Why?

Incline reverse crunches target the entire region of your abs. The muscle stabilizers include your quads, hip flexors, neck, and lower back. The incline increases the intensity of the exercise and reinforces your core strength.

How?

Step 1 - Lay flat on your back on an incline bench.

Step 2 - Squeeze your abs to push your lower back into a neutral position against the bench.

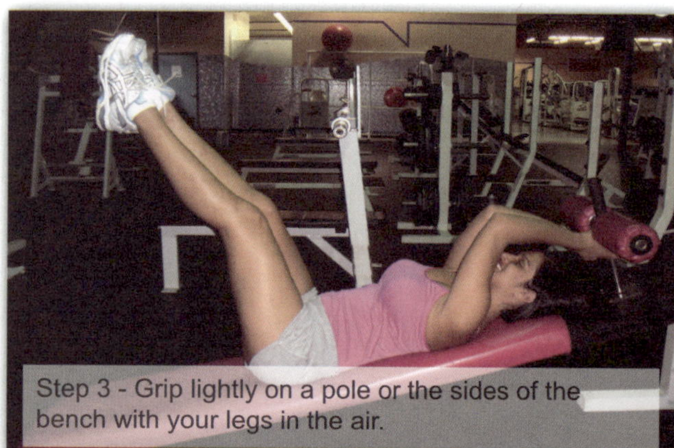

Step 3 - Grip lightly on a pole or the sides of the bench with your legs in the air.

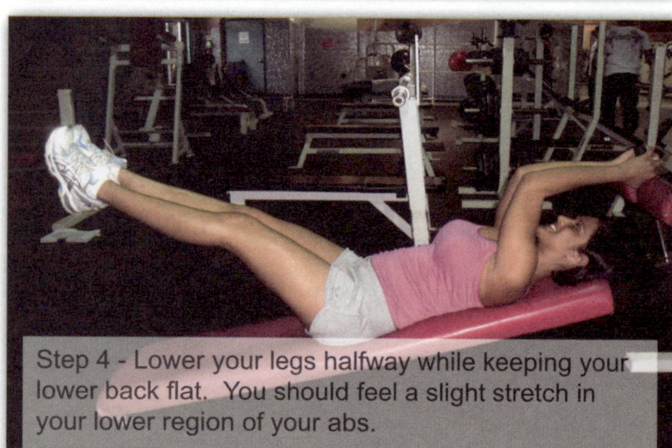

Step 4 - Lower your legs halfway while keeping your lower back flat. You should feel a slight stretch in your lower region of your abs.

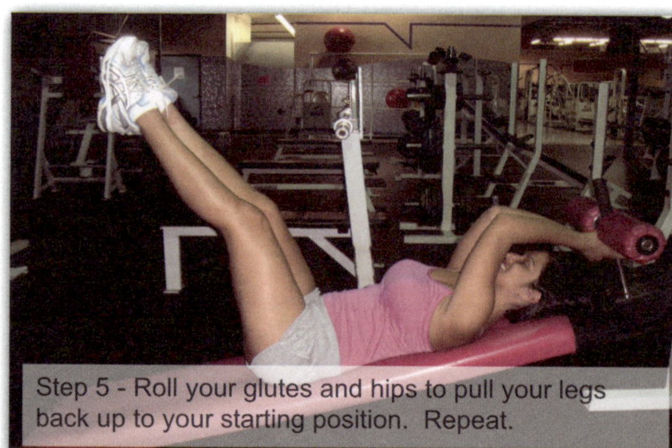

Step 5 - Roll your glutes and hips to pull your legs back up to your starting position. Repeat.

Your goal is to complete four sets of 20 (4 x 20).

Range of Motion Techniques

To Maximize Muscle Tension and Minimize Overcompensation

Dos

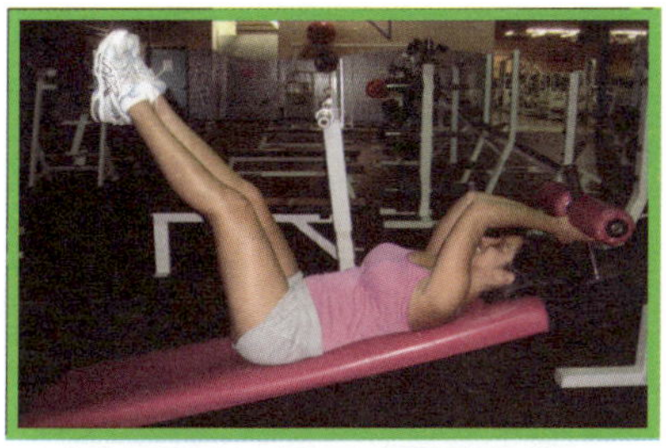

Maximize Tension in Abs When Contracting

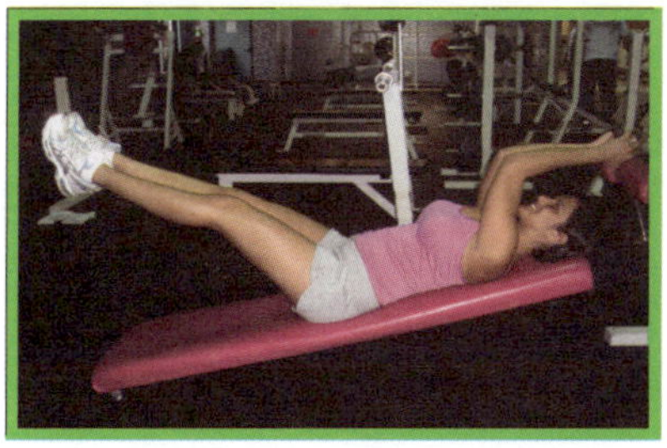

Maximize Tension in Abs When Resisting and Stretching

Don'ts

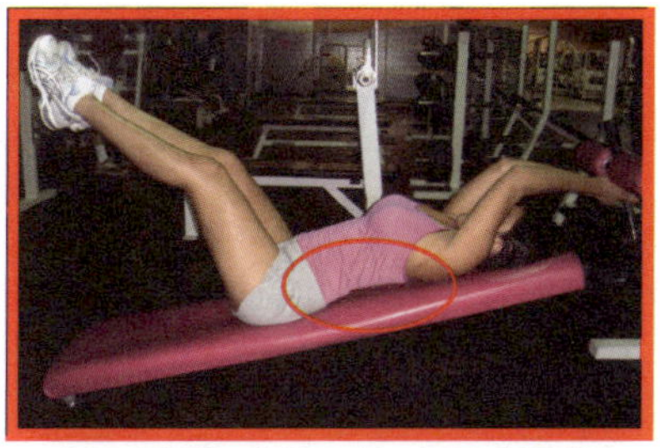

Avoid Arching Lower back

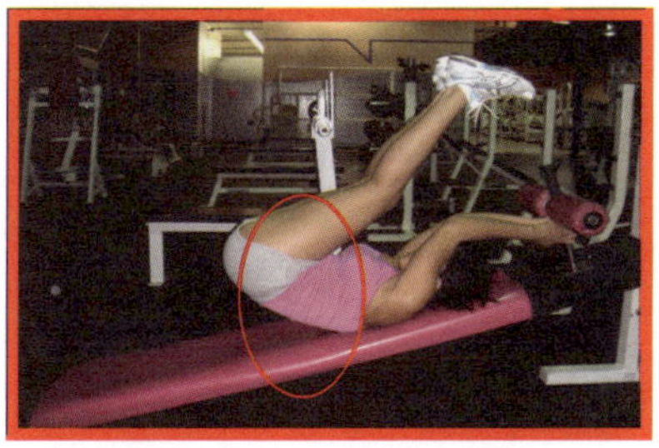

Avoid Curling Beyond Peak Contraction

Visualize

"Rubber Band Effect"

As you lower and raise your legs, squeeze your abs, and visualize your abs as a rubber band. As you lower your legs, the rubber band lengthens. You are squeezing your abs so much that the rubber band tightens, pulling your legs back up to your peak contraction.

Continue to visualize the rubber band. This will help to maintain the tension and squeeze of your abs. Repeat. Visualizing, while staying within the proper range of motion, will maximize your ab workout.

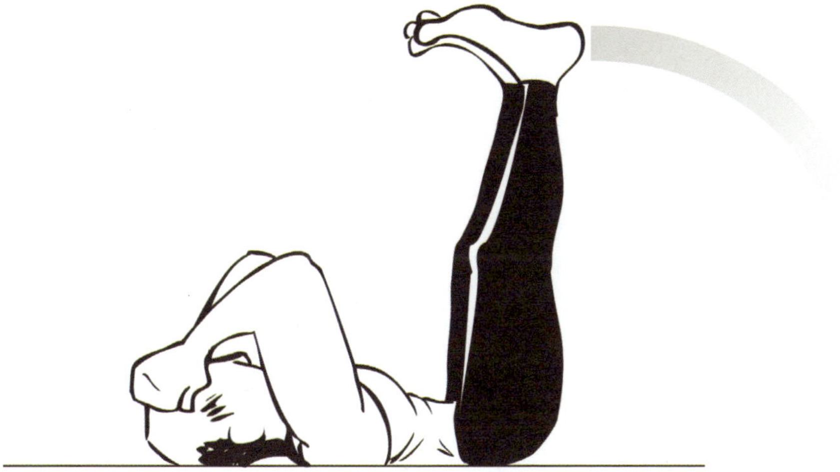

Questions and Answers

What should I do if I feel burning in my lower back?

If you are experiencing a light burning sensation in your lower back, that is great! Your muscles are fatigued! Muscle fatigue leads to strengthening and conditioning. However, if you're feeling pain in your lower back while performing crunches, you may be arching too much. Focus on squeezing your abs to push your lower back into a neutral position against the bench. This relieves the pressure in your lower back and forces your abs to do the muscle work.

Why do I need to feel a stretch in my abs?

Feeling a stretch in the lower region of your abs ensures that your abs are resisting. This reduces overcompensation and allows your abs to do the work.

Can I lower my legs further than halfway?

Yes. Lower your legs as far as possible. As long as you can maintain a flat lower back position, it is OK to lower your legs farther for a deeper, more intense stretch. However, if your lower back arches, you've lost form. Lower your legs until your lower back is about to arch and then raise them up. This maximizes the resistance, strength, and tension in your abs. Just be sure to avoid using your lower back, hip flexors, or quads. If you can feel them, you are overcompensating!

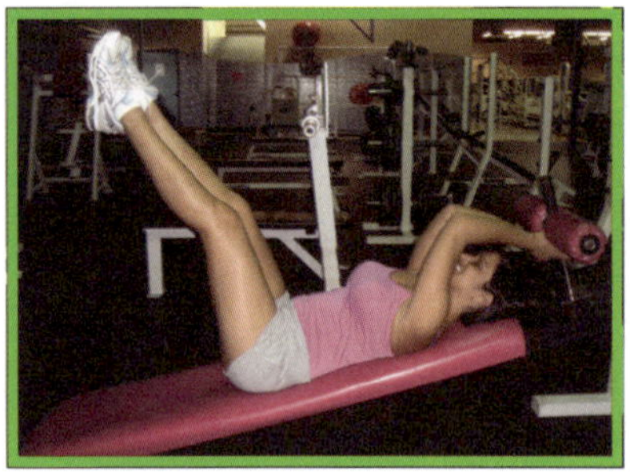

Starting Position

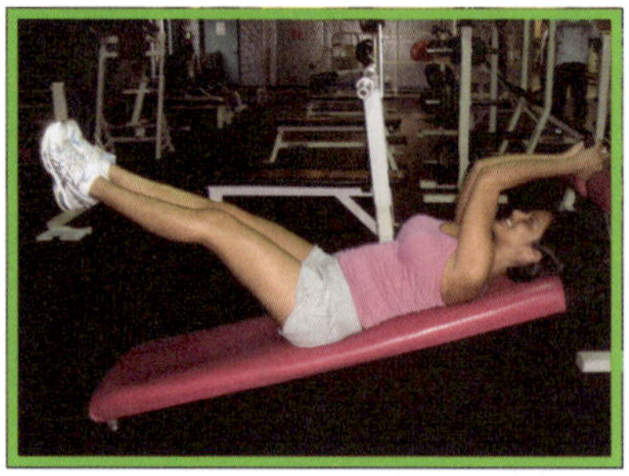

Lower Your Legs

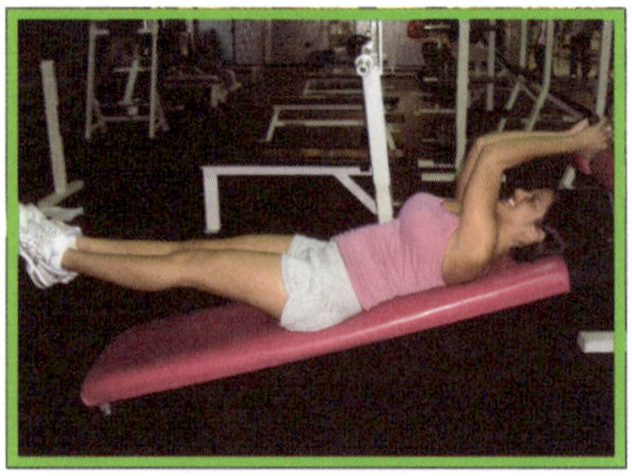

Minimize Arch in Your Lower Back

What if I feel my legs more than my abs?

Feeling your legs is caused by overcompensation. Basically, your abs are fatigued and cannot continue. The moment you feel your legs, you are done with that set. If you continue to overcompensate, your legs, the stabilizers, will be fatigued and you will train less of your abs.

How fast should I perform my reps?

Your tempo should be two seconds down and two seconds up.

The Secrets to Success!

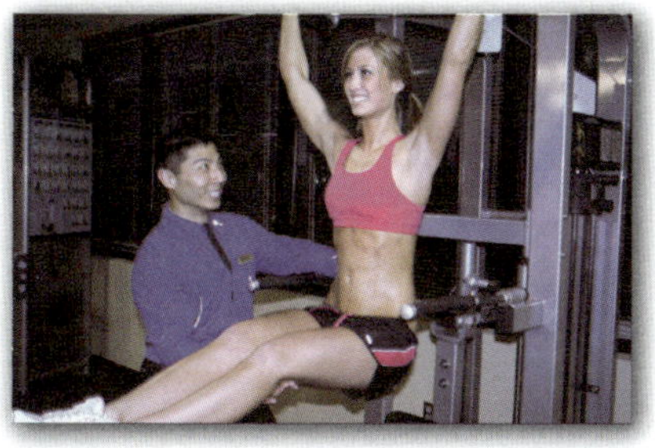

From Your Personal Trainer, Kevin Orr

Are you tired of eating the same foods over and over again? Here are some positive reasons for staying consistent with the same foods every day:

- It allows you to plan ahead and be more time-efficient.
- It is easy to prepare the same foods every day.
- It takes the focus off food.
- It makes it easy to control your appetite.
- It helps control cravings.
- You are unlikely to overeat.
- You don't have to think about what you're going to eat.
- It makes meal preparation easy!

Eating the same foods every day might lead to the accidental "cheat" day or meal. The moment you taste something very sweet or crunchy, you set yourself up to crave more at another time. Variety does add a little spice and zip to your life but you don't need variety every day. If it helps you stay on track, purposely spice it up a little on the weekend or a specific day of the week. As long as you stay aware of your portions, servings, and PFC ratios, you'll have no problems in staying the course. Purposeful variety is the secret!

Example Weight & Cardio Routine

Continue to choose a workout routine based on your level of fitness and your schedule before progressing to Week Ten. Write it down in your schedule, page 249. If none of the example routines work for you, configure a routine that fits your needs, and write it down. Planning ahead will help you set yourself up for success.

Weight Routine 1

Sunday	Monday	Tuesday	Wednesday	Thursday	Friday	Saturday
	Arms: 4x15 Abs: 4x20		Legs: 4x20 Chest/Back/ Shoulders 4x15		Arms: 4x15 Abs: 4x20	

Weight Routine 2

Sunday	Monday	Tuesday	Wednesday	Thursday	Friday	Saturday
		Arms: 4x15 Abs: 4x20	Legs 4x20	Chest/Back/ Shoulders 4x15		Arms: 4x15 Abs: 4x20

Weight Routine 3

Sunday	Monday	Tuesday	Wednesday	Thursday	Friday	Saturday
	Arms: 4x15 Abs: 4x20	Legs 4x20	Chest/Back/ Shoulders 4x15	Arms: 4x15 Abs: 4x20		

Continue to choose routine 1, 2, or 3 to begin your weekly cardio routine, or rearrange your cardio training to best fit you.

Cardio Routine 1

Sunday	Monday	Tuesday	Wednesday	Thursday	Friday	Saturday
	Stairs: 15 Tread:R 15		Stairs: 15 Tread:R 15		Stairs: 15 Tread:R 15	

Cardio Routine 2

Sunday	Monday	Tuesday	Wednesday	Thursday	Friday	Saturday
		Stairs: 15 Tread:R 15	Stairs: 15 Tread:R 15	Stairs: 15 Tread:R 15		Stairs: 15 Tread:R 15

Cardio Routine 3

Sunday	Monday	Tuesday	Wednesday	Thursday	Friday	Saturday
	Stairs: 15 Tread:R 15	Stairs: 15 Tread:R 15	Stairs: 15 Tread:R 15	Stairs: 15 Tread:R 15	Stairs: 15 Tread:R 15	

Example Schedule

On your schedule, page 249, continue to write down which cardio machines along with the duration you plan to complete this week.

	Sunday	Monday	Tuesday	Wednesday	Thursday	Friday	Saturday	
Week 5 Weight: Body fat: Cardio: Duration:		218 30% Chest/Back Shoulders: 4x15 Cycle: 15 Stepper: 15	Arms: 4x15 Abs: 4x20 Cycle: 15 Stepper: 15	Legs: 4x20 Cycle: 15 Stepper: 15	Chest/Back Shoulders: 4x15 Cycle: 15 Stepper: 15	Legs: 4x20 Cycle: 15 Stepper: 15	Chest/Back Shoulders: 4x15 Cycle: Stepper:	Why Sick! Solution Make it up another day when feeling better
Week 6 Weight: Body fat: Weights: Sets: Cardio: Duration:		216 Arms: 4x15 Abs: 4x20 Stairs: 15 Cycle: 15	Legs: 4x20 Stairs: 15 Cycle: 15	Chest/Back Shoulders: 4x15 Stairs: 15 Cycle: 15	Arms: 4x15 Abs: 4x20 Stairs: 15 Cycle: 15	Stairs: 15 Cycle: 15		Why Solution Perfect week!
Week 7 Weight: Body fat: Weights: Sets: Cardio: Duration:		214 29% Legs: 4x20 EFX: 15 Stairs: 15	Chest/Back Shoulders: 4x15 EFX: 15 Stairs: 15	Arms: 4x15 Abs: 4x20 EFX: 15 Stairs: 15	Legs: 4x20 EFX: 15 Stairs: 15	EFX: 15 Stairs: 15		Why Class Exam Solution Shift workouts one day
Week 8 Weight: Body fat: Weights: Sets: Cardio: Duration:		211 Chest/Back Shoulders: 4x15 Tread:R 15 EFX: 15	Arms: 4x15 Abs: 4x20 Tread:R 15 EFX: 15	Legs: 4x20 Tread:R 15 EFX: 15	Chest/Back Shoulders: 4x15 Tread:R 15 EFX: 15	Tread:R 15 EFX: 15		Why Family get together Solution Make up missed workout
Week 9 Weight: Body fat: Weights: Sets: Cardio: Duration:		209 27% Arms: 4x15 Abs: 4x20 Stepper: 15 Tread:R 15	Legs: 4x20 Stepper: 15 Tread:R 15	Chest/Back Shoulders: 4x15 Stepper: 15 Tread:R 15	Arms: 4x15 Abs: 4x20 Stepper: 15 Tread:R 15	Stepper: 15 Tread:R 15		

Before moving on...

Did you follow through with your plan? If not, cross out what you did not complete on your schedule and write in what you did complete before moving on to the next week.

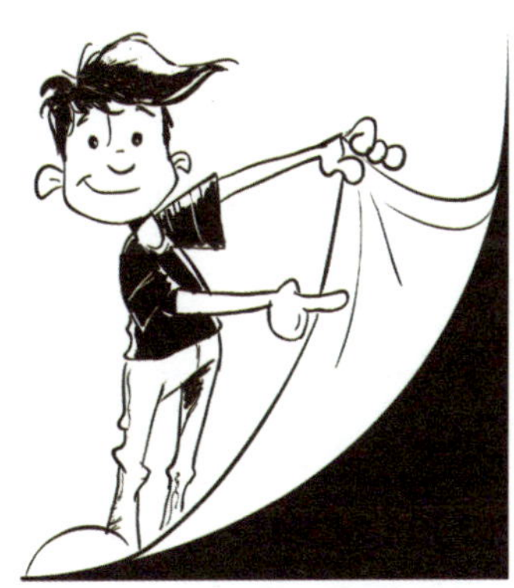

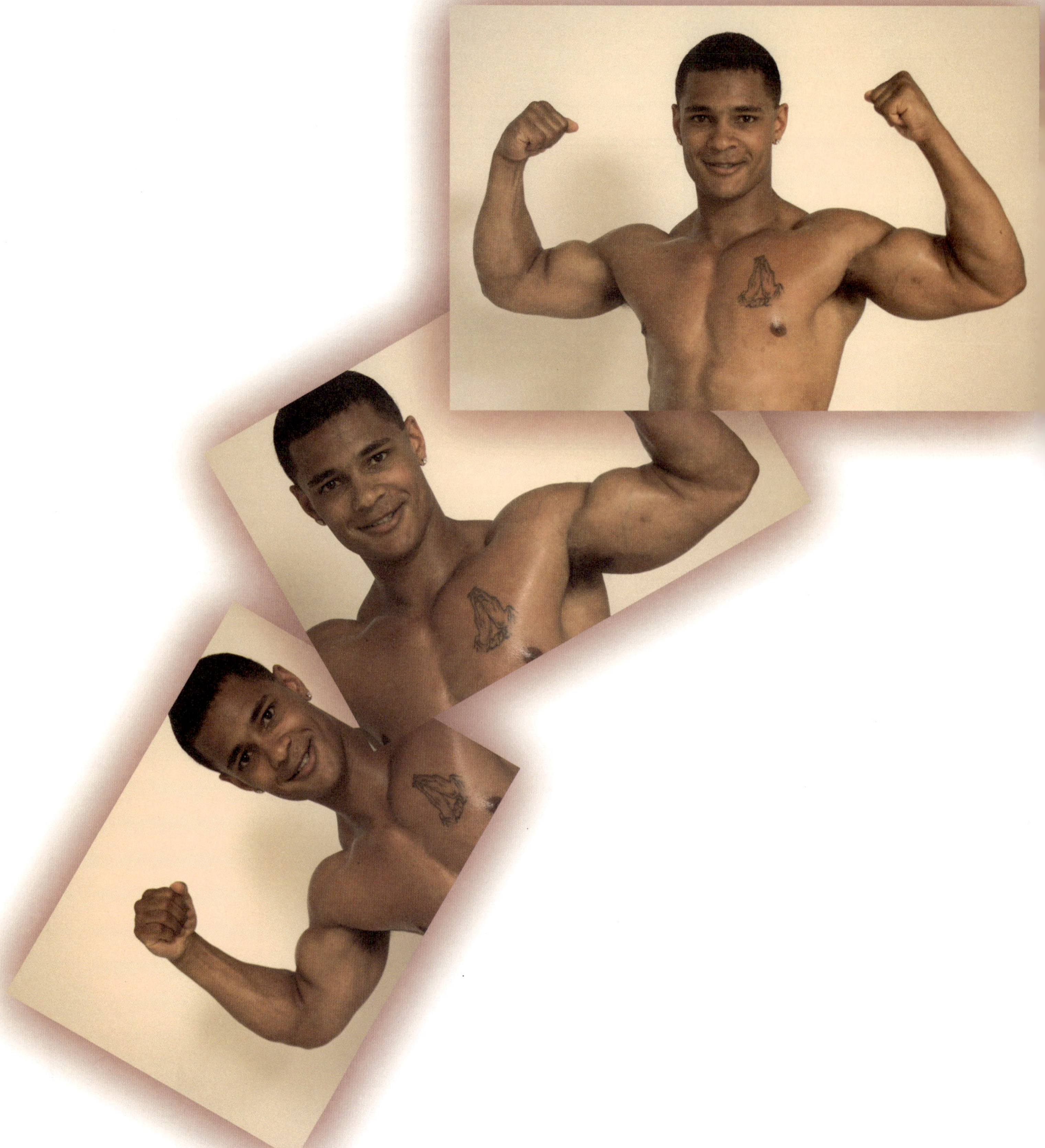

Week 10

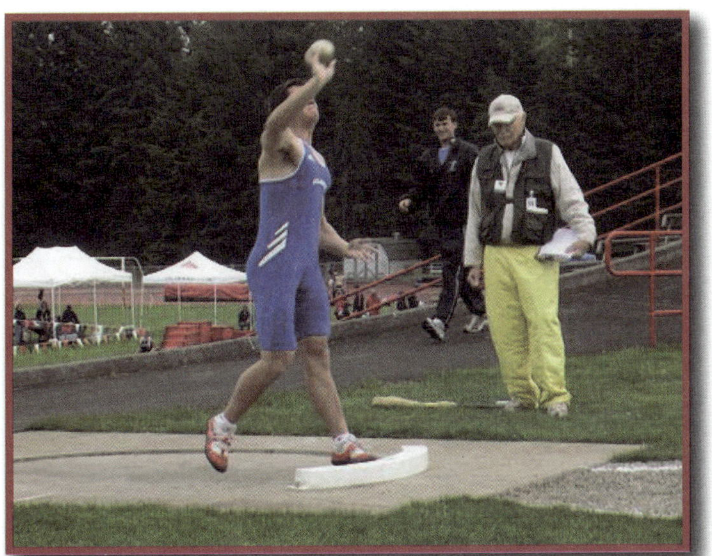

I have been a competitive powerlifter for over two years. I was strong, but I was also fat and had very little energy when it came to everyday life. Kevin taught me the importance of nutrition, cardio, and overall body and mental health. Through everything he has taught me, I not only have a different outlook on fitness and life, but I also have that six-pack I have always dreamed of!

Bob McCabe

Goal:

Maintain healthy eating habits at social gatherings, special events, and during the holidays.

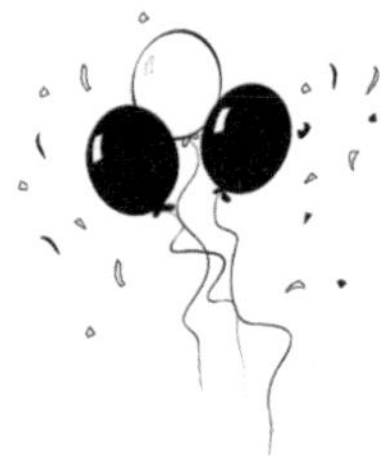

Why?

Social occasions present a big challenge for people who are working to develop healthy eating habits. Weddings, parties, and holidays put us in situations where we face temptations that are not present in our everyday lives. Additionally, it is human nature to eat more when you are with others than when you are alone. Cravings that had disappeared can pop back up. Positive decision-making and staying the course with goals can weaken. Making healthy choices in these situations can be difficult, especially in the early stages of adopting a healthy lifestyle.

How?

The simplest way to approach social situations is with a mind-set for maintaining your weight, not trying to lose weight. This will help you make moderate choices of what you eat and drink in social occasions and will ensure that you continue to make progress towards your goals without feeling deprived. Having a good idea of the PFC and calorie content of typical foods served during these social times is very helpful. It's amazing how calories can add up at social events.

Average Food Consumption at a Wedding Reception	**P**	**F**	**C**	**Calories**
Wedding cake	6	15	65	419
Champagne	.5	0	2.5	160
Cheese Stuffed rolls	27	**35**	**50**	**623**
Chicken and ham	20	15	0	215
Pastry	10	35	65	615
Salad with dressing	0	22	10	238

Average Food Consumption at Thanksgiving	**P**	**F**	**C**	**Calories**
Turkey	30	20	10	340
Stuffing	3	9	25	193
Ham	30	20	10	340
Mashed potatoes	4	9	35	237
Gravy	3	.5	6	38
Roll	4	12	22	200
Cranberry sauce	0	0	22	88
Pumpkin pie	1	3	7	58
Pie	2	13	42	285
Vegetable dish with butter	0	23	0	201
Corn with butter	6	25	42	417

Average Food Consumption at Christmas	P	F	C	Calories
Turkey	30	20	10	340
Chocolate cake	5	30	38	410
Christmas cookies	2	8	17	148
Fruit cake	1	4	26	139
Eggnog	10	19	34	343
Wine	0	0	8	250
Candy	1	3	32	150

Average Food Consumption at New Year's	P	F	C	Calories
Wine	0	0	8	250
Alcohol	0	0	0	192
Cake	5	30	38	410
Candy	1	3	32	150
Chocolate chip cookies	3	21	51	405
Peanut butter and fudge brownies	5	10	40	270

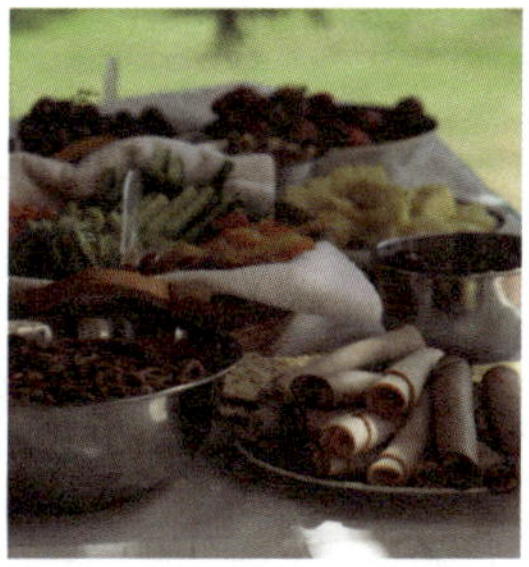

The same guidelines you follow every day still apply in social situations. So, where ever you are, plan to eat balanced meals and snacks. Keep your PFC ratios in mind as you choose what to eat and drink. A typical buffet will have a wide variety of food. Scan what's available and make your PFC choices before you pick up a plate.

At restaurants, it should be fairly easy to make healthy choices.

- Start with a salad. Ask for a low calorie dressing or salsa on the side. This will help control your hunger and you will feel satisfied sooner.

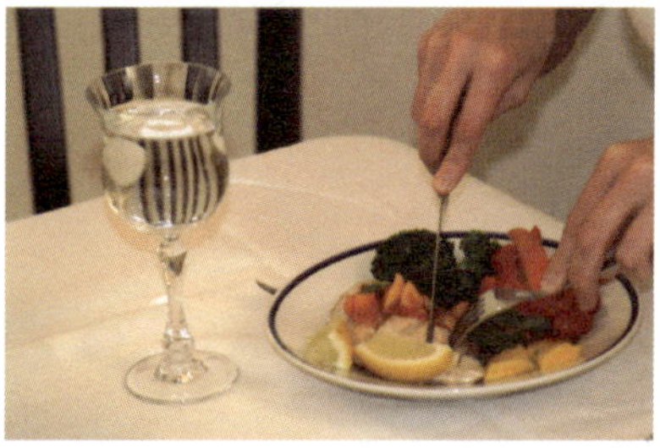

- Stay away from fried foods and cream sauces. Anything crispy, sautéed, or stuffed should be avoided.

- Look for steamed, broiled, baked, grilled, poached or roasted foods.

- You can always request that your meal be prepared with vegetable or olive oil instead of butter and that the visible fat is trimmed from your meat or the skin removed from your poultry before cooking to avoid extra calories.

- Ask for toppings on the side or skip them completely.

These are much healthier options!

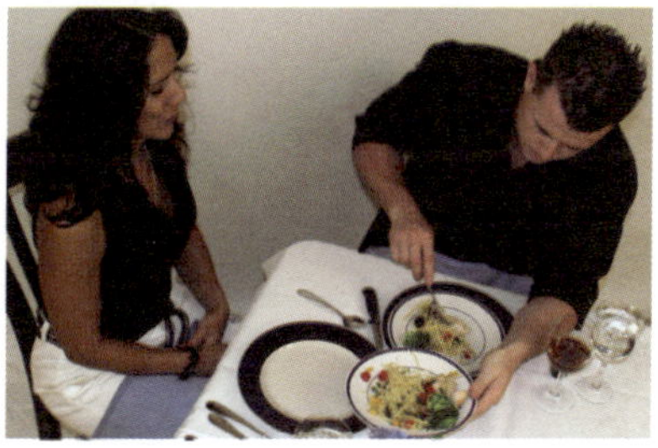

Also, keep in mind that restaurant portions are often two to three times larger than you really need. Share your entree with your dinner partner or ask for a "to go" bag when you order. When your food arrives, cut the serving in half, package it up, and save it for later.

If you order pasta, choose whole wheat and have a tomato-based sauce. Order an appetizer or side dish instead of an entrée. The appetizer menu is more likely to fit your portion sizes. If you are craving dessert, order sorbet or tropical fruit smoothie topped with light cool whip or split a dessert with a friend.

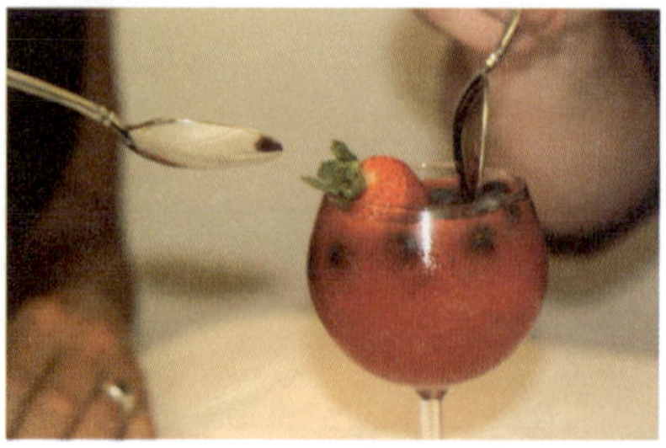

Always remember to drink lots of water. If you order alcohol beverages, drink a glass of water between each alcoholic drink. Remember, although, wine can be part of a healthy diet, all alcoholic beverages are loaded with alcohol calories!

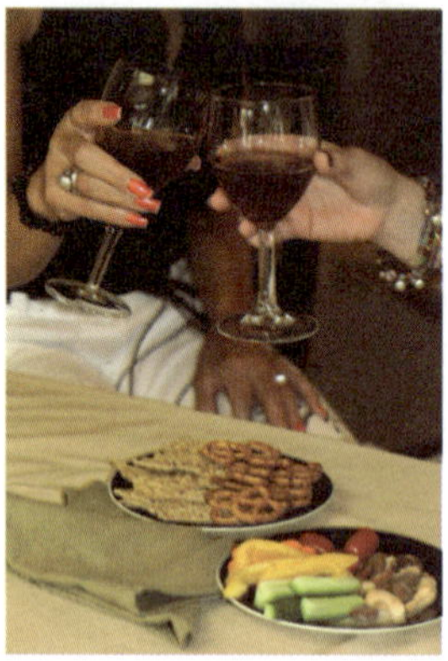

During the holidays, the challenges accelerate because rich food is everywhere! If you are in charge of preparing holiday meals, search the internet for lower calorie/lower fat versions of traditional dishes. Make sure that you prepare plenty of vegetable appetizers and side dishes. If you are a guest, ask to bring a side dish or dessert and make it a healthy one. Focus on the "social" part of the activity rather than the food part of the event. And have fun. If you blow it, get back on track as soon as possible.

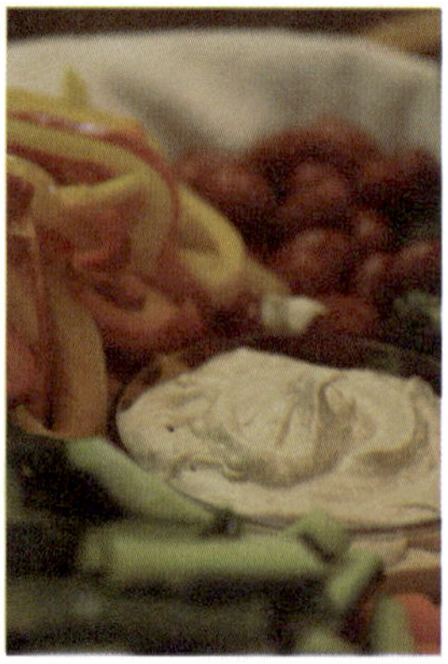

It really is possible to negotiate these challenges and make a successful lifestyle change that includes social eating, but it will take practice and guidance. Here are some social eating tips from several of my clients who faced the same challenges and what they did to find success:

Drink two glasses of water before each meal. I make sure to do this before a party, so that I'm not famished and tempted to overeat rich, high-calorie foods.
-Nina Kolafa

If it's an appetizer-only event, I bring my own platter to add to the offerings. I include edible flowers (nasturtiums are my favorite. The flowers and green seed pods have a light radish flavor.) and slices of fruits, vegetables, and imported hard cheeses. Labeling them makes them more tempting and the platter more intriguing. I also include a variety of whole grain crackers or bread squares. This variety of culinary choices helps the tray to stand out from the usual "carrots, broccoli, and cauliflower" plate that usually remains long after everything else on the table is eaten.
-Sher Jennings

Don't stand by the food. Snack on the veggies, drink lots of water, and visualize how you want to look in those tight jeans.
-Charlotte Williams

I eat before an event and carry a healthy snack with me in my purse in case I get hungry and there are no healthy choices available at the gathering. If there is a buffet or menu I stick with the meat and veggie trays. I've realized that most restaurants are very accommodating with low fat and low carb alternatives if you just ask.
-Cailyn McIntosh

Stay away from the food. If it's a party, keep a drink (water or something) in your hand at all times. It's hard to fill a plate with munchies, and hold a beverage at the same time. At a friend's home, just try a little of everything; politely decline additional portions while complimenting the host or hostess.
-Beth Johnson

I always try to eat a snack at home before dining out or attending a social gathering. An ounce of cheese, an ounce of cooked chicken, hard boiled egg or another protein with equal value. A low fat protein drink is another good way to curb your appetite before attending a function. It also helps prevent alcohol from absorbing so quickly if you choose to have a drink.
-Deborah Goedecke

Social events can be tough because of the amount of food available or the pressure of keeping up with everyone else. I try to limit myself to one glass of wine or a light beer. I also order a glass of water with whatever I order. This keeps me from drinking too fast. With appetizers, I just try to taste something instead of eating. What I mean is, I may try a bit, but I will never load up on appetizers.
-Tim Fetters

Eat and drink in moderation.
-Bob Narciso

I normally try to decrease my calorie intake during the day by eating the same amount of meals with foods that contain fewer calories. Fruit, vegetables, and yogurts are my primary life saver foods. During the "social event," I try to stay away from processed sugar goodies and fill up with vegetables if available.
-Donatella Johanson

I do not actually think about what I eat ALL of the time, but I live life with the motto: Eat in moderation.
-Teri Erickson

One thing that has always helped me in social settings is drinking water. Just having a glass or bottle of water in my hand or in easy reach can mean the difference between success and failure for me. Also, focusing on the fresh vegetables verses the fattier items helps. If I need a little something sweet, fruit has usually satisfied that craving. If I do indulge, I use a smaller plate, so I don't take too much, which helps as well.
-Terri Maxwell

Look for anything that is baked, broiled, or grilled. Typically, these types of meals contain 50% less fat than those that are fried or sautéed. Also, a great way to cut down on calories and saturated fat is to pass on the cheese and mayo. Add extra vegetables and honey mustard!
-Amy Gurske

When I eat out at restaurants, I always eat about half of my meals and take the rest home.
-Heather Cowell

I eat very very slowly. At dessert time, I confess that I am very full, and ask if i can take my portion home. That way I don't offend the hostess, and when I get home, I can do what I want with the dessert.
-Lin Detmers

Remember, if you know that social eating is going to be a huge challenge for you, switch your goals to weight maintenance while at social events and during the holidays. This will eliminate any guilt and set you up for success rather than failure. Afterward, get right back on track. Don't worry if you stumble occasionally. Nobody is perfect. Successful nutrition is a lifestyle change to help you reach YOUR goals.

Questions and Answers

How do I calculate the PFCs when I'm eating out?

Calculating the amount of PFCs was the hard part in Week 7. Now that you have been working with the PFCs for awhile, you should have a good idea of how many PFCs are in certain amounts of foods. Estimate the amount of PFCs in your meal. Eyeballing it should be easy at this point. Nonetheless, here are some additional tips for you:

Protein:
- The size of a deck of cards represents about 4 oz. of any meat, which is about 20 grams of protein.

Fats:
- 2 dice is about 1 oz., which is one serving or slice of cheese.
- One tablespoon of olive oil, butter, avocados, and peanut butter is about 7 grams of fat.

Carbohydrates:
- One slice of thick bread is typically 20 grams of carbohydrates.
- ¾ cup of rice or pasta (about the size of one tennis ball) is about 45 grams of carbohydrates.
- One cup of vegetables (lower sugar) is typically 10 grams of carbohydrates.
- One cup of fruit (lower sugar) is typically 20 grams of carbohydrates.

How do I avoid eating too much when I go out?

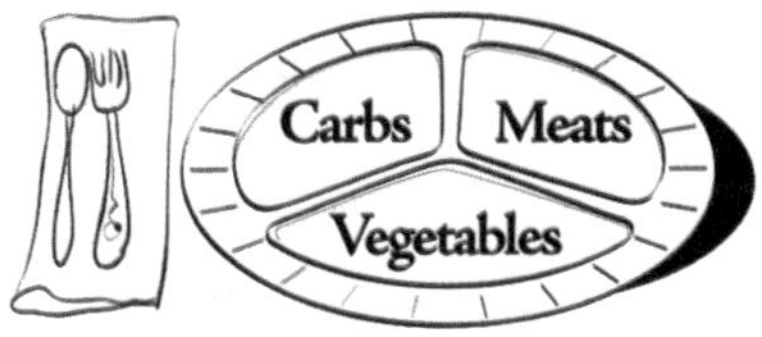

Portion control!
- Select the foods you want to eat in moderation and use a small plate.
- Make your meal last by savoring each bite. Eating slowly will help you feel satisfied sooner.
- Another way to eat more slowly is to take a small bite then set your utensil(s) and plate down, drink some water, wait a minute, then take another bite.
- Converse with your company! Talking keeps your mind off of food.

I'm used to eating every three hours. How do I stay on track at social events?

Timing is the key. Continue to plan to eat every three hours. If you can't eat because you're in a meeting or at an event where you will not have access to food, plan for it in advance. Eat enough to hold you over while you're in the meeting or the event. If you're in a situation where there is food available, but there are not any healthy options, remember that in order to maintain your blood sugar balance, eating something is better than eating nothing. Just be smart and use moderation. Only eat enough to get you by until your next meal or snack.

Food is always the center of attention at my parties. What should I do?

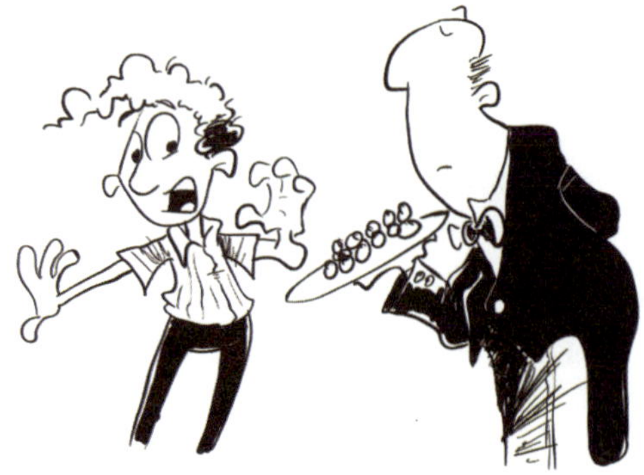

Sight, smells, and tastes are often triggers for eating more than you should. Do yourself a favor and sit as far away from the food as possible. Standing in the kitchen is only going to make matters worse! Keep yourself occupied with the other guests. When it is time to eat, make yourself one small plate of food and stick to drinking water. Start a conversation, bring out the board games, turn on the music and start dancing! Keeping busy should distract you from eating too much.

What can I drink at my social event?

Water should always be your beverage of choice! High-calorie coffee drinks, sodas, juices, and cocktails - including wine - loaded with sugars and empty calories. Iced tea, black decaf coffee, and sparkling water are better choices.

Is it OK to drink alcohol?

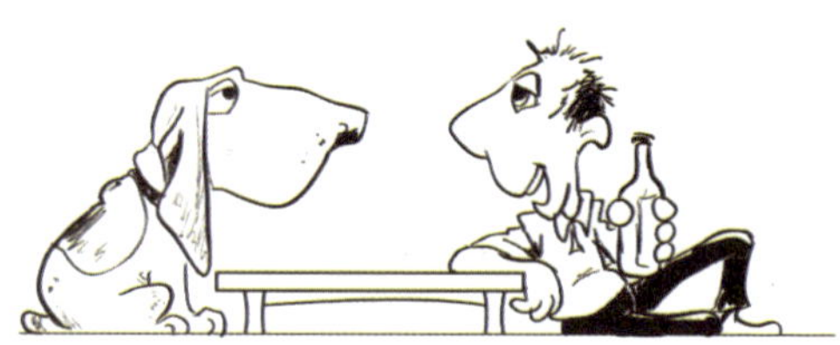

Alcohol can be OK in moderation. Just remember that alcohol is full of high glycemic empty calories. Factor in the alcohol carbohydrates into your PFC ratios to stay balanced and on course. (There are 7 calories per gram of alcohol which works out to approximately 2 grams of carbohydrates.) Red wine has approximately 24 calories and 1 carbohydrate per oz. A typical bottle of beer has approximately 150 calories and 13 carbohydrates. Always eat some food before you drink alcohol. The food will slow the absorption, decrease the glycemic impact, and help to stabilize your blood sugar. Also, to minimize the dehydrating effects of alcohol, you should drink a full glass of water before and after each alcoholic beverage.

What about drinking coffee?

Coffee, in moderation, is fine. Avoid loading it up with cream and sugar. Be aware that coffee contains caffeine, and caffeine is a stimulant. A stimulant is like running on fumes instead of actual fuel. Your blood sugar may take a steep dive after the fumes run out. Look out below!

I crave sweets! Can I drink diet sodas?

Any time you're eating or drinking something sweet, your taste buds and internal chemicals will stimulate cravings for more sweets. Even artificial sweeteners can trigger the cravings for more sweets. Several artificial sweeteners are linked to headaches, dizziness, nervous system disruption, and depression. Sodas contain phosphoric acid, which is known to block calcium absorption. Calcium depletion is associated with osteoporosis (bone loss). It is best to avoid or limit sweets, whether from artificial sweeteners or real, caloric sugars.

Can I have a "free day"?

Free days are dangerous to your mind-set. Your mind and body function best when you have a predictable routine and nutrition pattern. This means you should eat a balanced meal or snack every three hours. The problem with a "free day" is that it is unpredictable and inconsistent. Most individuals view a "free day" as the chance to eat things they wouldn't normally eat: Pizza and beer, burgers and fries, or chocolate sundaes, justifying this counter-productive behavior as a reward for staying disciplined and eating consistently throughout the week. This so-called "free day" will throw your body way out of balance. You will most likely feel foggy, tired, and lethargic. It will take seven-10 days to rebalance your internal hormones and chemicals to function properly and that's if you are able to get right back on track with your healthy eating habits. Unfortunately, most people have a hard time getting back on track after a "free day." Some individuals say they'll indulge in a moderate amount of bad foods on their "free day." They stay very strict with their eating habits during the week, look forward to that "free day", and then go overboard. They feel guilty and become very strict during the week again and then grant themselves another "free day" again. It becomes a vicious cycle. Their progress is sabotaged. My advice is to avoid "free days." It is OK to treat yourself to an indulgence in moderation every once in a while. So, if you're craving something "bad," eat a little of it. Remember, you're not on a diet. Eating healthy is a lifestyle habit.

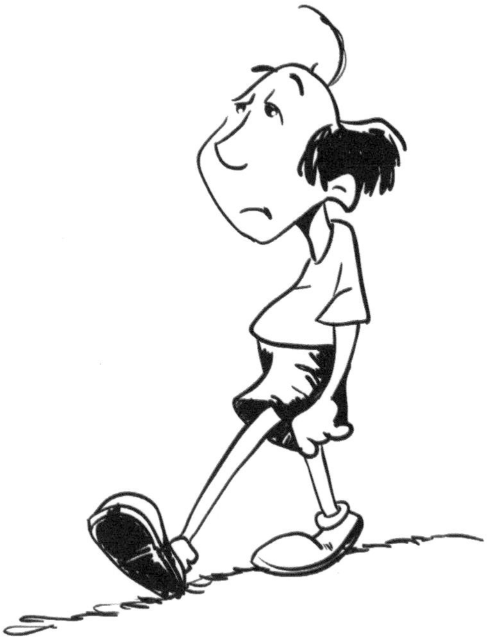

Time to review your nutrition log.

1. Plan and prepare for your social events.

2. Keep your "better choice" food selections simple.

3. Continue to record everything you eat and drink in your nutrition log daily.

For Example:

Time	Event	Better Choice
7:00 AM	Brunch	**Eggs, WW toast, fruit**
10:00 AM	Company meeting	**WW crackers, low-fat cream cheese**
12:30 PM	Luncheon	**Deli wraps, fruits/veggies**
3:00 PM	Kid's sport's event	**Apple, string cheese**
6:00 PM	Family night	**WW Boboli home-made pizzas**
8:00 PM	Movie night	**Veggie plate, low-fat dress-ing**

WW = 100% whole wheat

Nutrition Log

Date:___________	Sun Mon Tues Wed Thurs Fri Sat	
	Food	**PFC**
Meal 1	*Food & Amount*	*P F C*
Time:_____		
Meal 2		
Time:_____		
Meal 3		
Time:_____		
Meal 4		
Time:_____		
Meal 5		
Time:_____		
Meal 6		
Time:_____		

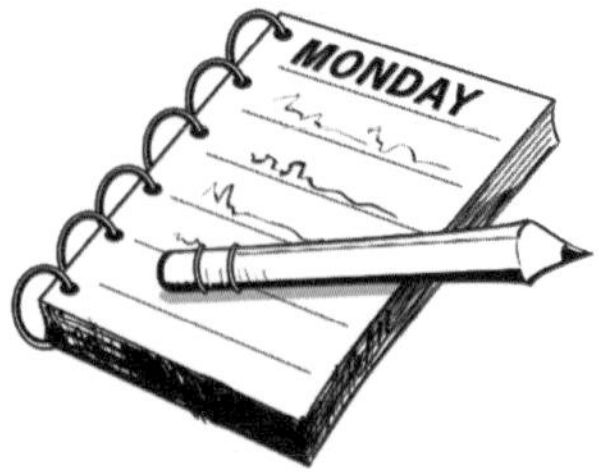

Checklist

Achieved:

- ✓ Consume meal or snack every 3 hours
- ✓ Water every 3 hours
- ✓ Sleep optimal hours
- ✓ Intake multivitamin
- ✓ Weights and cardio
- ✓ Consume PFCs every meal or snack
- ✓ Foods low on the GI
- ✓ PFC ratio balance
- ✓ Planned meals
- ✓ Add nutritional variety
- ✓ **Moderation when social eating**

Avoided:

- ✓ Sugars
- ✓ White flour
- ✓ Processed foods

Key Points

Week 1
- Eat a small meal or snack once every three hours – five to six meals per day.
- Drink at least 1 cup (8 ounces) of water per meal and at least one cup before, during, and after your workouts.
- Keep a nutrition log.
- Sleep is vital!
- Take a daily multivitamin.

Week 2
- Avoid bad sugars.

Week 3
- Avoid white flour and white rice.

Week 4
- Avoid processed foods.

Week 5
- Balance your meals and snacks with a combination of proteins, fats, and carbohydrates.

Week 6
- Eat foods that are low on the Glycemic Index.

Week 7
- Balance your meals and snacks with a specific ratio of proteins, fats, and carbohydrates.

Week 8
- Plan and prepare your foods for meals and snacks ahead of time.
- Keep your prepared food selection simple.
- Continue to record everything you're eating and drinking in your nutrition log daily.

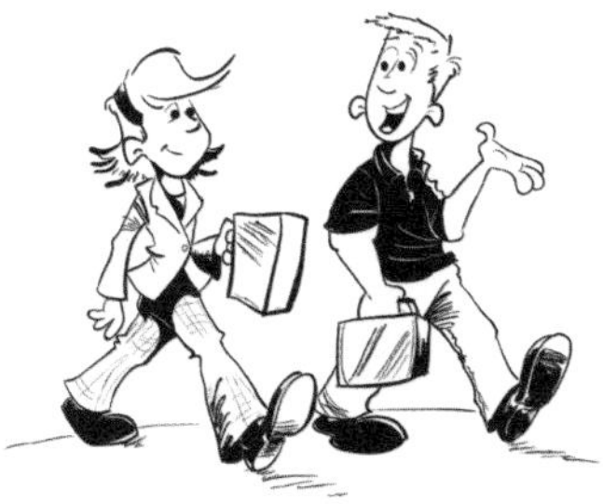

Week 9
- Add a variety of foods to your meal plans.

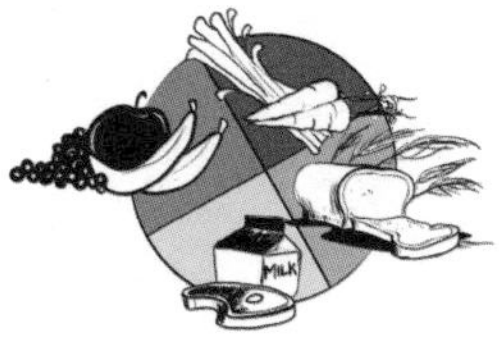

Week 10
- **Eat right and healthy at your social gatherings and events.**
  Most of all, have fun!

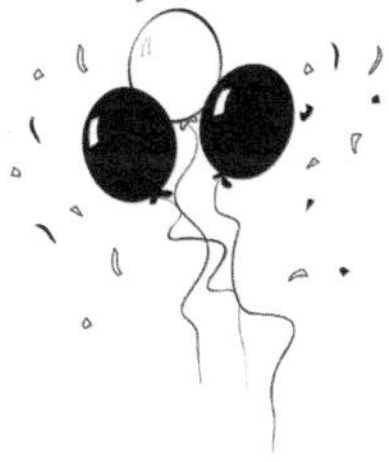

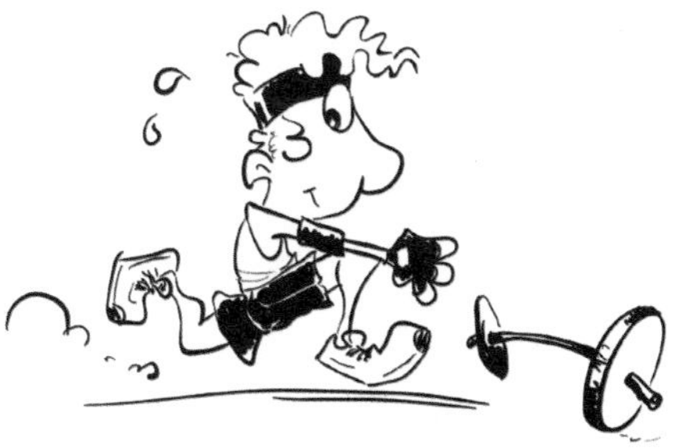

Legs

Goal:

Complete four sets of 20 reps on the **leg press**.

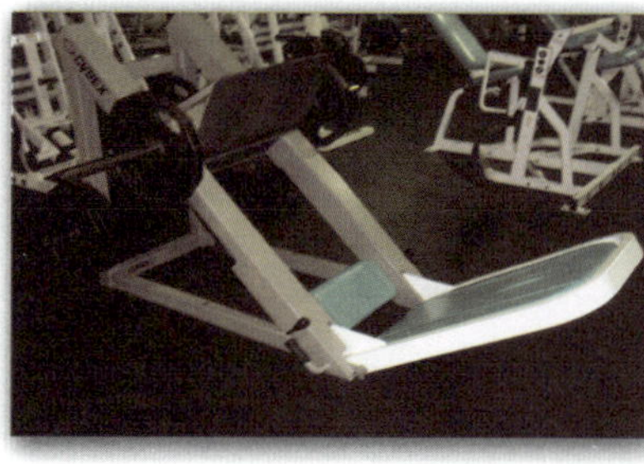

Primary
Glutes
Quads
Hamstrings

Stabilizers
Lower back
Core
Calves

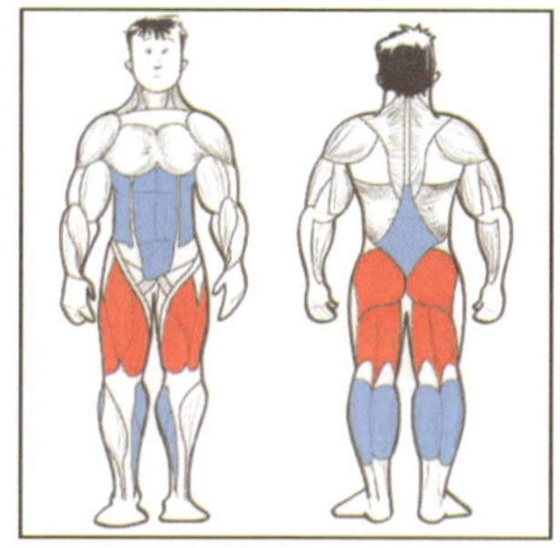

Why?

The leg press is a machine exercise targeting the major muscle groups of your legs. The power behind the leg press comes from your quads, glutes, and hamstrings. The muscle stabilizers include your lower back, calves and core. Machines are specifically designed to relieve tension in your joints while maintaining stability and balance. Unlike squats and lunges, the leg press places less tension in your shoulders, lower back, knees, and ankles.

How?

Step 1 - Sit down. Center yourself on the seat.

Step 2 - Squeeze your abs. Press your back flat against the seat.

Step 3 - Place your feet slightly wider than a shoulder-width stance.

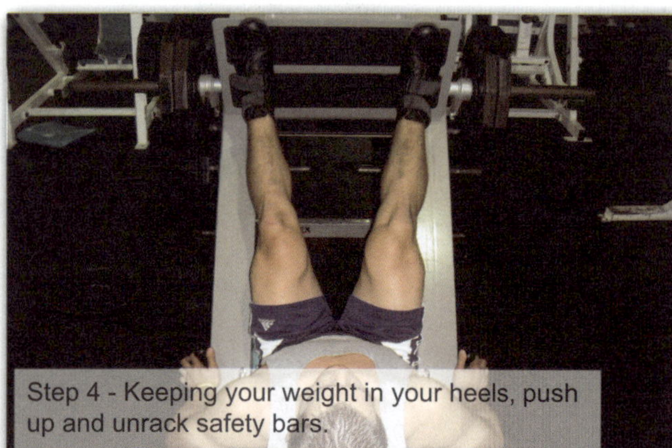

Step 4 - Keeping your weight in your heels, push up and unrack safety bars.

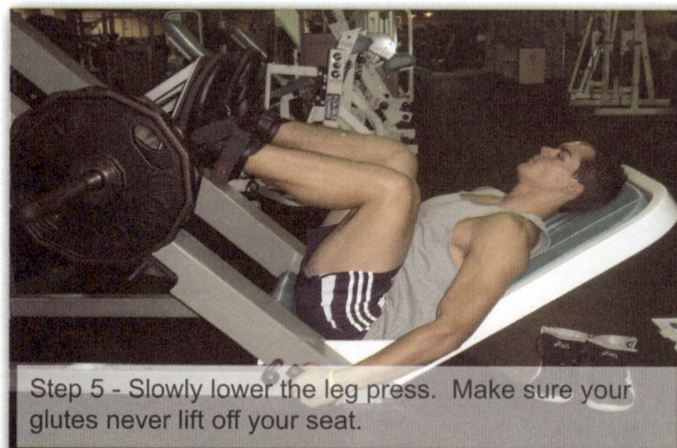

Step 5 - Slowly lower the leg press. Make sure your glutes never lift off your seat.

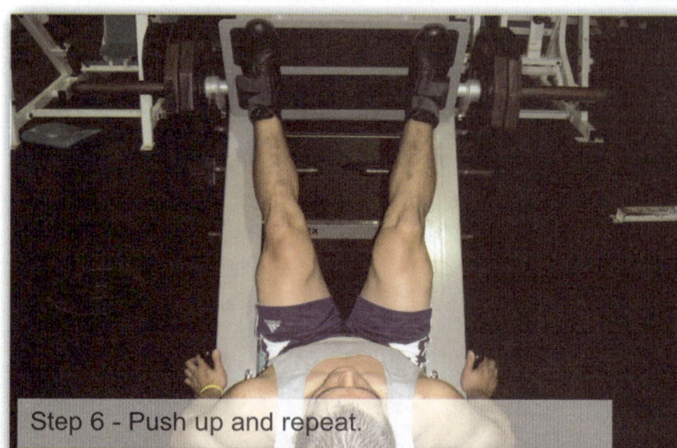

Step 6 - Push up and repeat.

Your goal is to complete four sets of 20 (4 x 20).

Range of Motion Techniques

To Maximize Muscle Tension and Minimize Overcompensation

Dos

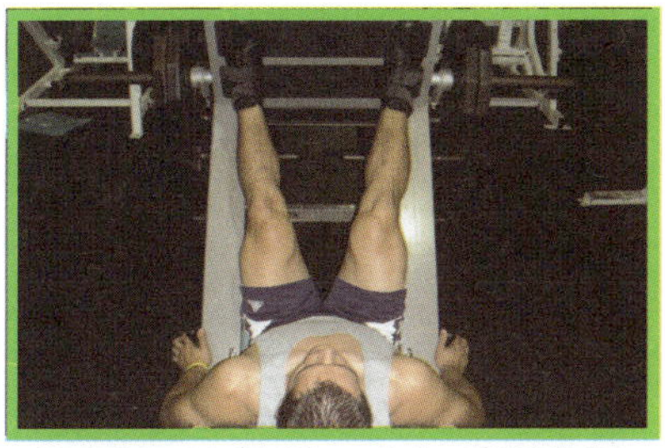

Begin with Shoulder-Width Stance and Knees Bent

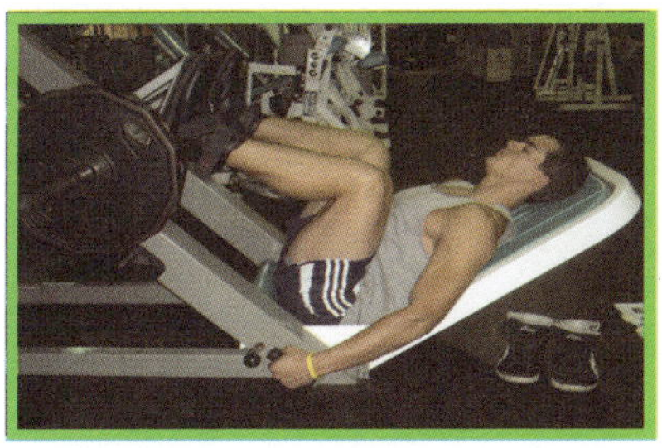

Lower Legs to 90-Degree Angle

Don'ts

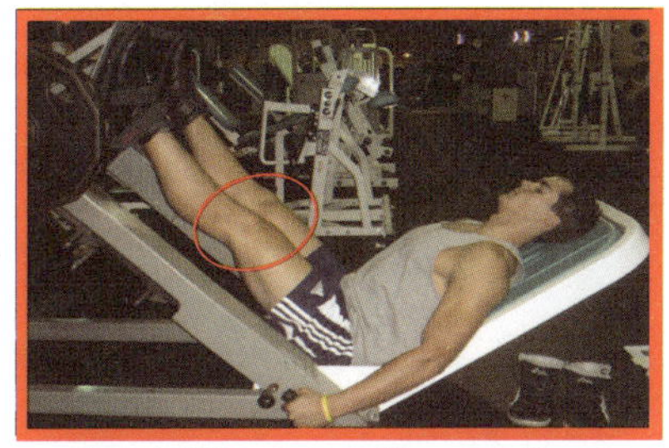

Avoid Locking Knees Out

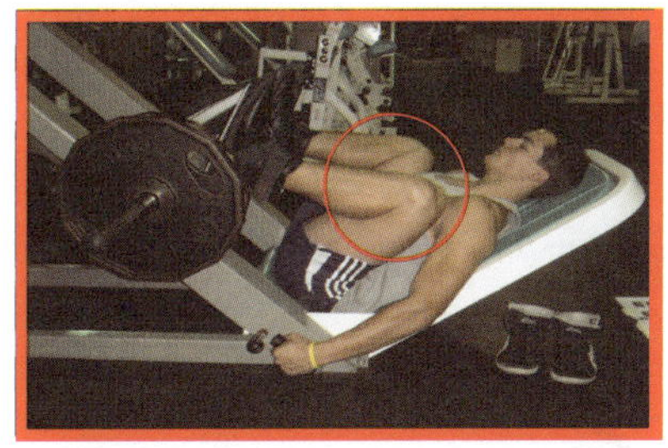

Avoid Coming Down Too Far and Allowing Glutes to Lift off from Seat

Visualize

"Cable and Balloon Effect"

As you lower the leg press down and push it back up, visualize a cable attached to the leg press. The cable is pulling it straight up, guiding you through the leg press motion. This visualization will assist in a smooth, controlled motion. Next, visualize a cable attached to both of your knees, pulling them straight up. This ensures knee stabilization and proper alignment. Last of all, visualize balloons underneath both your feet. Place the least amount of pressure against the leg press. This helps to utilize your leg muscles while decreasing tension in your knees and toes.

Your goal is to resist the leg press as you lower it and when you push it back up without popping the balloons. At the same time, visualize yourself allowing the cables to pull your leg press up to maintain a smooth, controlled motion.

This visualization technique forces your legs to maintain tension and control, while decreasing overcompensation and tension in your hips, knees, and toes.

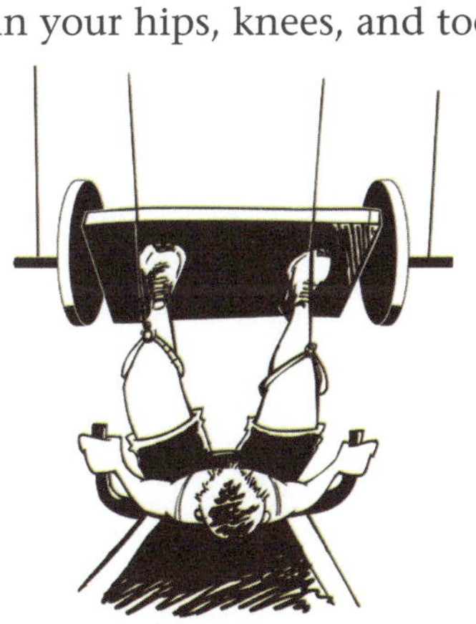

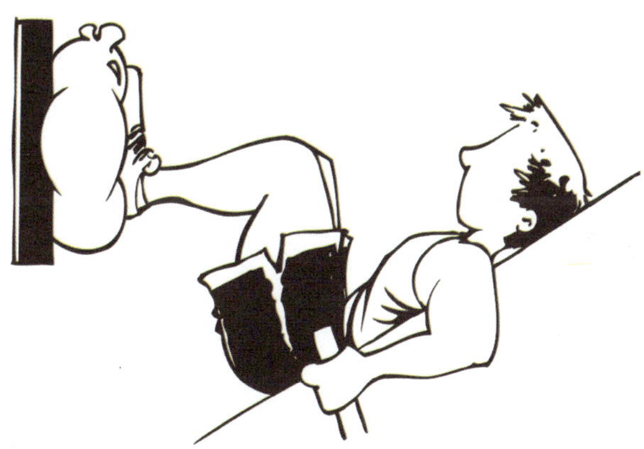

Questions and Answers

Why do I need my weight and pressure on my heels?

By placing your weight in your heels, you will relieve the pressure in your knees, which forces your legs to do the work. One technique to ensure your weight is on your heels, is to lift your toes slightly inside your shoe. Your heels should be flat against the floor. Be sure your knees stay above or behind your toes.

What should I feel after performing leg press?

You should feel a burning sensation by the end of each set. You should also feel a slight pump and/or a "wobble" effect in your legs. This means you're training at optimal intensity.

What if I feel pain in my knees?

Pain in the knees is associated with incorrect form.

1

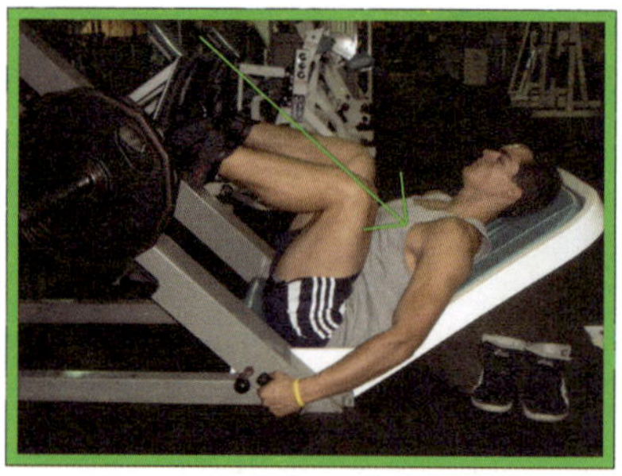

When lowering the leg press, avoid allowing your knees to go beyond your toes

2

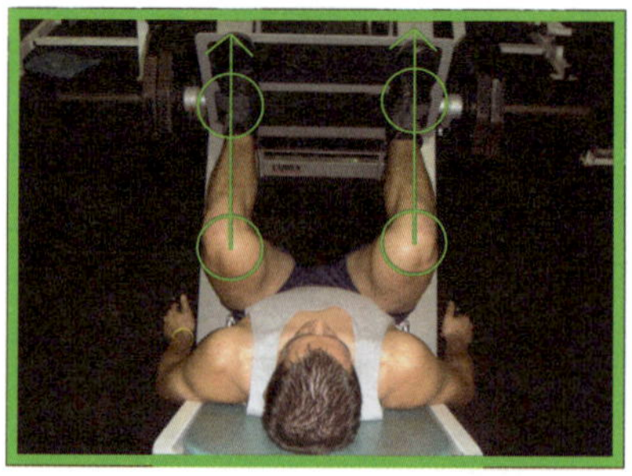

Keep knees in proper alignment. Don't let your knees move in or extend out

Kevin does a great job! He not only shows you how to work the machines, how to target certain muscles, but he educates you on them. He makes you understand the how and why. Just by a simple slide of an elbow, angle of a bar, or intensity of a rep, he shows you how to really get the most out of your workout, at the same time, always making sure you are in touch with your body and mind. When going over nutrition, he reminds you that it is not a diet, but a lifestyle change. He has inspired and touched my life forever.

- Julie Merryman

Calves

Goal:

Complete four sets of 20 reps on the **machine calf raises**.

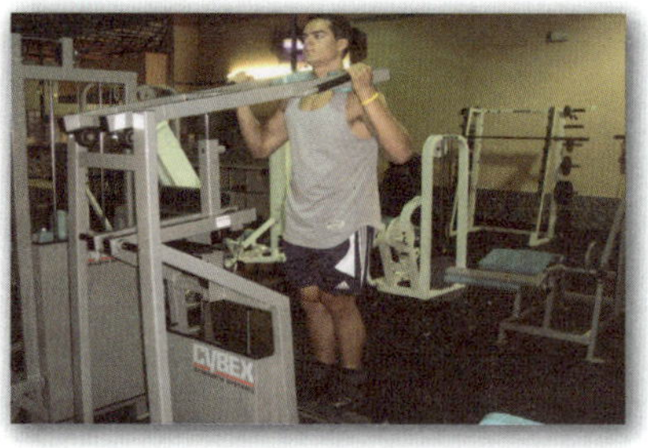

Primary
Calves

Stabilizers
Quads
Hamstrings
Core

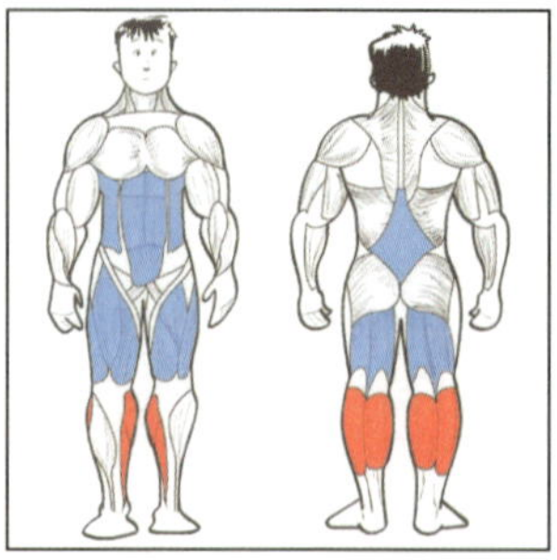

Why?

The machine calf raises are another way to increase the intensity and strength in your calves. This machine adds training variety and guides your motion enabling you to add weight for increased intensity. Machine calf raises use fewer stabilizers than free weight calf raises.

How?

Step 1 - Stand on the edge of the calf raise machine. Place your weight on the balls of your feet.

Step 2 - Squeeze your abs to push your lower back into a neutral position.

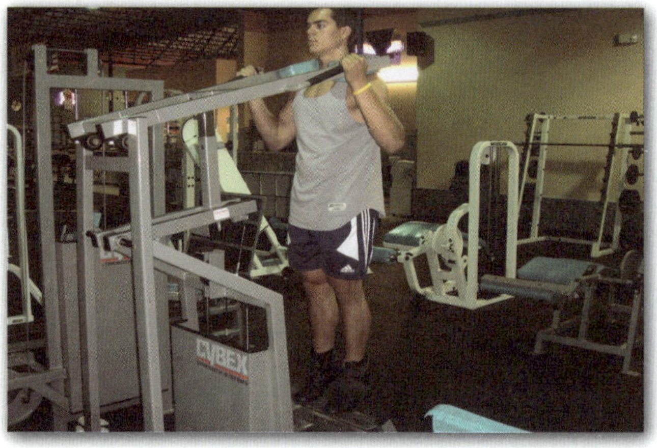

Step 3 - Pull your hips slightly back and lean slightly forward.

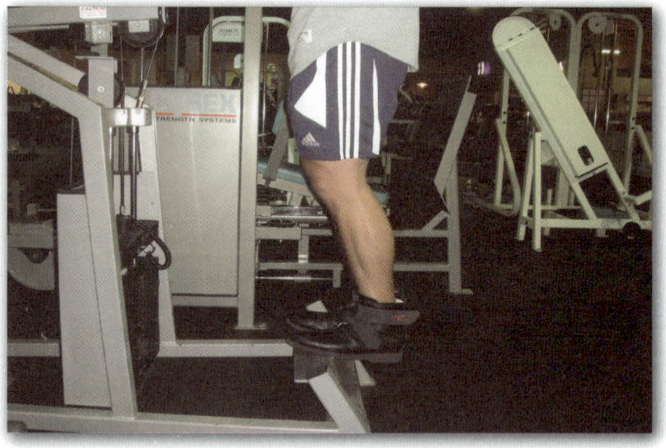

Step 4 - Lower your heels to the point of feeling a slight stretch in your calves.

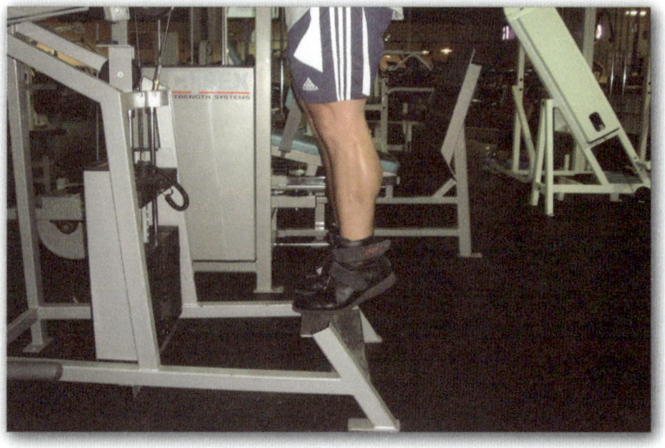

Step 5 - Lift and squeeze up to the peak contraction of your calves and repeat.

Your goal is to complete four sets of 20 (4 x 20).

Range of Motion Techniques

To Maximize Muscle Tension and Minimize Overcompensation

Dos

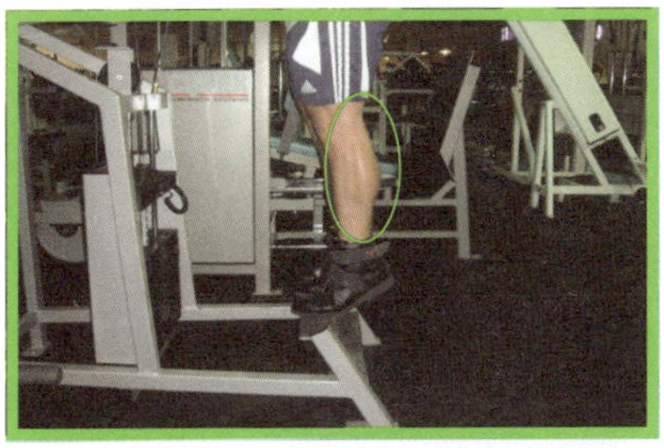

Begin With Squeezing Calves at Top

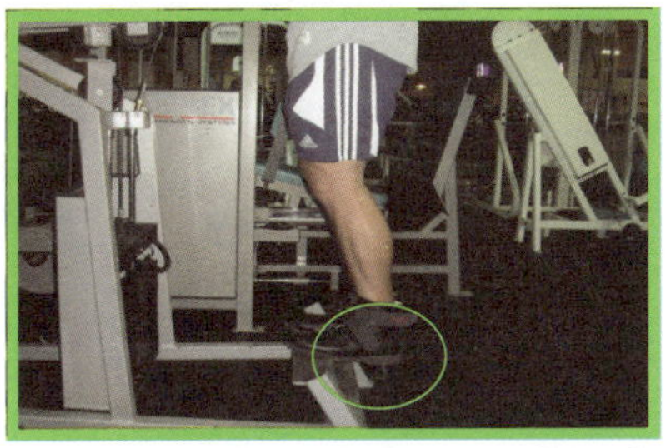

Lower Heels to Resist and Feel Calves Stretching

Don'ts

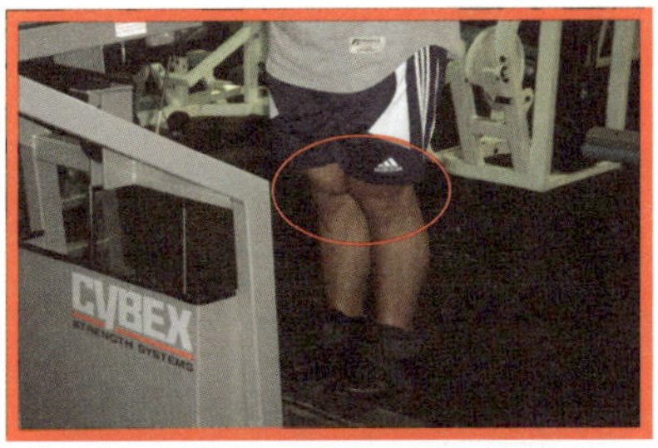

Avoid Locking Out Knees and Arching Lower Back

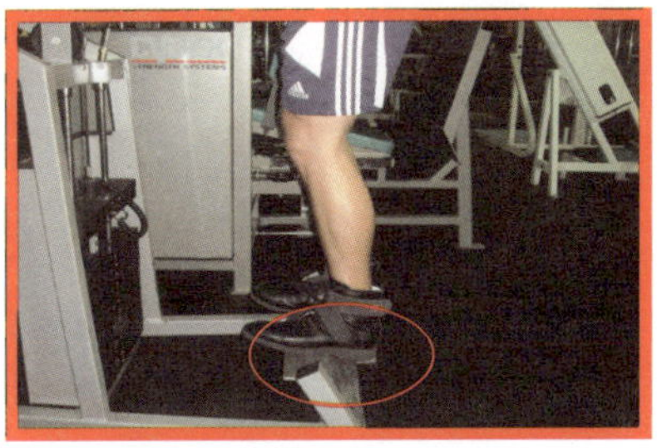

Avoid Too Much Stability by Standing on the Arch of Feet

Visualize

"Balloon Effect"

As you lower your heels down and push yourself up, visualize yourself standing on a balloon that cannot be popped. This will maximize the pressure and tension in your calves while minimizing overcompensation from other muscle groups.

Your goal is to lower your heels to feel a stretch in your calves and push up to contract your calves without popping the balloon.

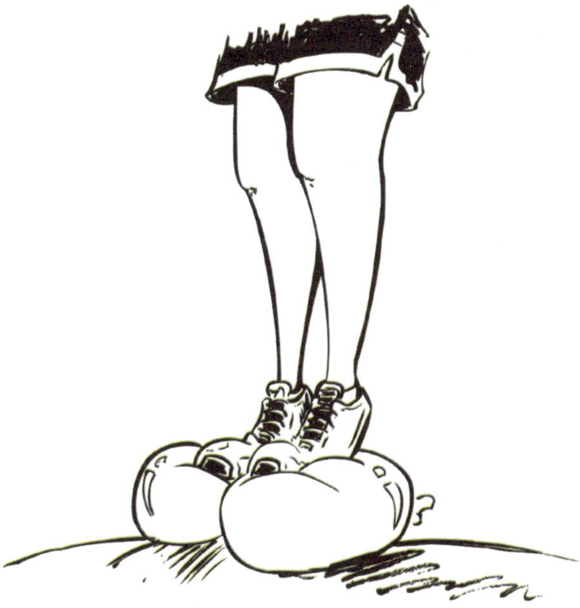

Week 10

Questions and Answers

How do I position my feet for machine calf raises?

Place the balls of your feet on the edge of the stand with your heels hanging slightly off the edge. This forces the calves to do the work and keeps your toes from overcompensating.

Why do I need to maintain a neutral lower back position when I am training my calves?

The neutral lower back position is proper posture, which relieves the pressure in your lower back, helps to prevent overcompensation, and forces your calves to do most of the work. For that reason, pull your hips back, lean slightly forward, and squeeze your abs to push your lower back into a neutral position.

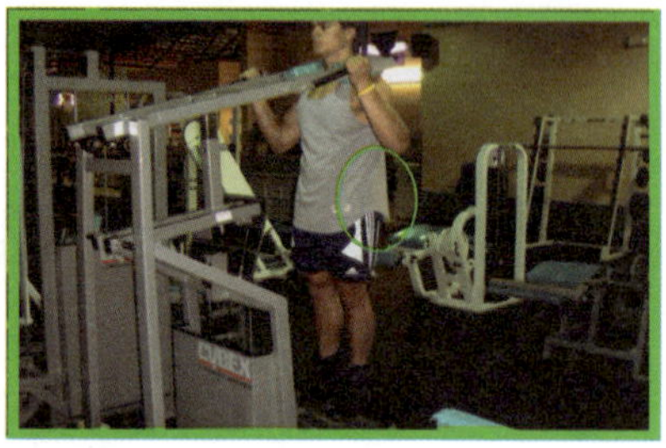

The Secrets to Success!

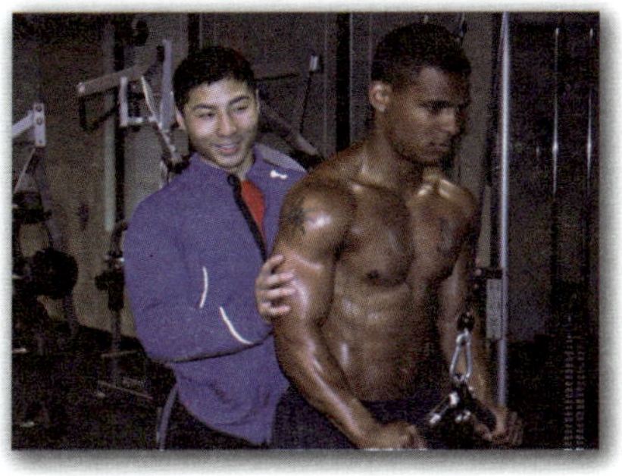

From Your Personal Trainer, Kevin Orr

At parties, gatherings, weddings, and simply hanging out with friends, I'm known to always be the healthy one. Sometimes that encourages others to be conscious of what they eat for the first hour and sometimes it makes others feel a little uncomfortable. No matter what your goals are and where you live, social eating is a fact of life. But, it doesn't necessarily mean you have to eat and drink a lot to enjoy social activities. You now know how to stay in control and still have fun. Furthermore, you never know, by modeling healthy choices in social situations, you could be the catalyst for someone else to decide to make a change to a healthier lifestyle. Thus, a social life is the secret success!

Example Weight & Cardio Routine

Continue to choose a workout routine based on your level of fitness and your schedule before progressing on a weekly basis. Write it down in your schedule, page 249. If none of the example routines work for you, configure a routine that fits your needs, and write it down. Planning ahead will help you set yourself up for success.

Weight Routine 1

Sunday	Monday	Tuesday	Wednesday	Thursday	Friday	Saturday
	Legs 4x20		Chest/Back/ Shoulders 4x15		Legs: 4x20 Arms: 4x15 Abs: 4x20	

Weight Routine 2

Sunday	Monday	Tuesday	Wednesday	Thursday	Friday	Saturday
		Legs 4x20	Chest/Back/ Shoulders 4x15	Arms: 4x15 Abs: 4x20		Legs 4x20

Weight Routine 3

Sunday	Monday	Tuesday	Wednesday	Thursday	Friday	Saturday
	Legs 4x20		Chest/Back/ Shoulders 4x15		Arms: 4x15 Abs: 4x20	Legs 4x20

Continue to choose routine 1, 2, or 3 to begin your weekly cardio routine, or rearrange your cardio training to best fit you.

Cardio Routine 1

Sunday	Monday	Tuesday	Wednesday	Thursday	Friday	Saturday
	Cycle: 15 Stepper: 15		Cycle: 15 Stepper: 15		Cycle: 15 Stepper: 15	

Cardio Routine 2

Sunday	Monday	Tuesday	Wednesday	Thursday	Friday	Saturday
		Cycle: 15 Stepper: 15	Cycle: 15 Stepper: 15	Cycle: 15 Stepper: 15		Cycle: 15 Stepper: 15

Cardio Routine 3

Sunday	Monday	Tuesday	Wednesday	Thursday	Friday	Saturday
	Cycle: 15 Stepper: 15	Cycle: 15 Stepper: 15	Cycle: 15 Stepper: 15	Cycle: 15 Stepper: 15	Cycle: 15 Stepper: 15	

Example Schedule

On your schedule, page 249, continue to write down which cardio machines along with the duration you plan to complete this week.

	Sunday	Monday	Tuesday	Wednesday	Thursday	Friday	Saturday	
Week 9 Weight: Body fat: Cardio: Duration:		209 27% *Arms: 4x15* *Abs: 4x20* *Stepper: 15* *Tread:R 15*	*Legs: 4x20* *Stepper: 15* *Tread:R 15*	~~*Chest/Back*~~ ~~*Shoulders: 4x15*~~ ~~*Stepper: 15*~~ ~~*Tread:R 15*~~	~~*Arms: 4x15*~~ ~~*Abs: 4x20*~~ ~~*Stepper: 15*~~ ~~*Tread:R 15*~~	*Stepper:* ~~*15*~~ ~~*Tread:R*~~ *15*		Why *Vacation* Solution *Make up week?*
Week 10 Weight: Body fat: Weights: Sets: Cardio: Duration:		*208* *Legs: 4x20* *Cycle: 15* *Stepper: 15*	*Chest/Back* *Shoulders: 4x15* *Cycle:: 15* *Stepper: 15*	*Arms: 4x15* *Abs: 4x20* *Cycle: 15* *Stepper: 15*	*Legs: 4x20* *Cycle: 15* *Stepper: 15*	*Cycle: 15* *Stepper: 15*		

Before moving on...

Did you follow through with your plan? If not, cross out what you did not complete on your schedule and write in what you did complete. Continue accomplishing your goals on a weekly basis.

Final Thoughts

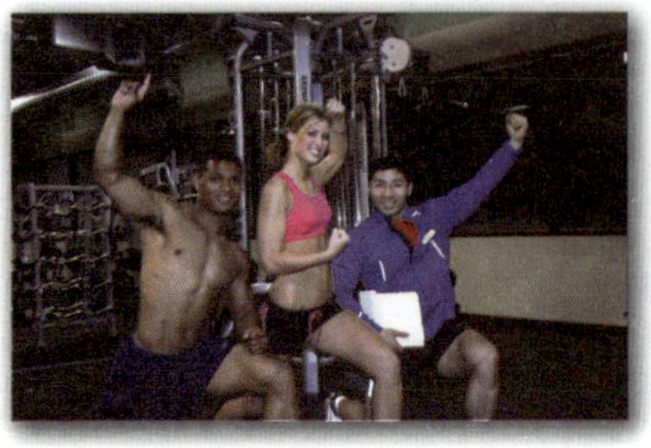

Congratulations! You have completed 10 Weeks to a New You. You feel better. You look better. You have energy and a positive outlook on life. You are confident in your ability to set and meet goals. You did it! But this isn't the ending. It's the starting point for new goals to accomplish. Set your mind to it and all your goals are within your reach. You are dedicated and have passion. You are an inspiration!

Share your before and after success at *www.makeyouhappen.com*. You can be featured as a model and example of positive lifestyle changes!

Before

PASTE PHOTO HERE

Date of Picture: ____________________
Body Weight: ____________________
Body Fat Percentage: ____________________

Lifestyle:

- Hours of Sleep per Night: ____________________
- Frequency of Meals a Day: ____________________
- Energy Levels: ____________________
- Weight Training Frequency: ____________________
  - Duration: ____________________
  - Intensity: ____________________
- Cardio Training Frequency: ____________________
  - Duration: ____________________
  - Intensity: ____________________

After

PASTE PHOTO HERE

Date of Picture: ____________________
Body Weight: ____________________
Body Fat Percentage: ____________________

Lifestyle:

- Hours of Sleep per Night: ____________________
- Frequency of Meals a Day: ____________________
- Energy Levels: ____________________
- Weight Training Frequency: ____________________
  - Duration: ____________________
  - Intensity: ____________________
- Cardio Training Frequency: ____________________
  - Duration: ____________________
  - Intensity: ____________________

Nutrition Log

Date:____________	Sun Mon Tues Wed Thurs Fri Sat			
	Food	**PFC**		
Meal 1	*Food & Amount*	*P*	*F*	*C*
Time:_____				
Meal 2				
Time:_____				
Meal 3				
Time:_____				
Meal 4				
Time:_____				
Meal 5				
Time:_____				
Meal 6				
Time:_____				

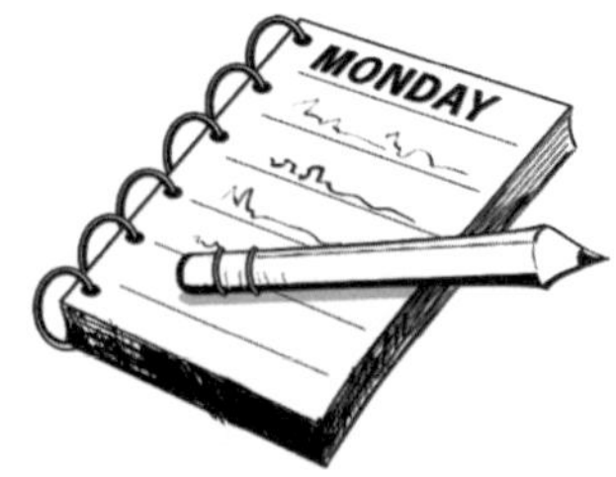

Checklist

Achieved:

- ✓ Consume meal or snack every 3 hours
- ✓ Water every 3 hours
- ✓ Sleep optimal hours
- ✓ Intake multivitamin
- ✓ Weights and cardio
- ✓ Consume PFCs every meal or snack
- ✓ Low glycemic food
- ✓ PFC ratio balance
- ✓ Planned meals
- ✓ Add nutrition variety
- ✓ Moderation when social eating

Avoided:

- ✓ Sugars
- ✓ White flour
- ✓ Processed foods

Workout Schedule

1. Write down the weight and cardio machines you plan to complete this week.

	Sunday	Monday	Tuesday	Wednesday	Thursday	Friday	Saturday
Body Weight: Body fat: Weights: Sets: Cardio: Duration:							
Body Weight: Body fat: Weights: Sets: Cardio: Duration:							
Body Weight: Body fat: Weights: Sets: Cardio: Duration:							
Body Weight: Body fat: Weights: Sets: Cardio: Duration:							
Body Weight: Body fat: Weights: Sets: Cardio: Duration:							

2. Were you able to follow through with your plan? If not, cross out what you did not complete and write in what you did complete before continuing your weekly workout routine.

Grocery List

PROCUCE SECTION

Vegetables

- □ asparagus spears
- □ avocado
- □ bell pepper, green
- □ bell pepper, red
- □ bell pepper, yellow
- □ broccoli florets
- □ broccoli slaw
- □ cabbage, napa
- □ carrots
- □ carrots, baby
- □ celery
- □ coleslaw mix (packaged)
- □ corn
- □ cucumber
- □ garlic
- □ ginger
- □ green beans
- □ jalapeños
- □ lettuce, Bibb
- □ lettuce, iceberg
- □ lettuce, looseleaf
- □ lettuce, romaine
- □ lettuce, romaine salad blend (packaged)
- □ lettuce, baby romaine salad (packaged)
- □ lettuce, salad greens, mixed (packaged)
- □ mushrooms, portabella
- □ mushrooms, shiitake
- □ mushrooms, sliced
- □ mushrooms, whole
- □ onions, red
- □ onions, white
- □ onions, green
- □ parsnips
- □ potatoes, new
- □ potatoes, red
- □ potatoes, russet
- □ potatoes, white
- □ radishes
- □ shallots
- □ snow peas
- □ spinach leaves, baby (packaged)
- □ squash, yellow
- □ tomatoes
- □ tomatoes, grape
- □ tomatoes, Roma
- □ yams or sweet potatoes
- □ zucchini

Fruit

- □ apples, red
- □ bananas
- □ blueberries
- □ cantaloupe
- □ grapefruit
- □ grapes, green seedless
- □ grapes, red seedless
- □ grapes, black seedless
- □ lemon
- □ lime
- □ mango
- □ oranges
- □ papaya
- □ peaches
- □ pears
- □ raspberries
- □ strawberries
- □ watermelon

Fresh Herbs

- □ basil
- □ chives
- □ cilantro
- □ dill
- □ mint
- □ oregano
- □ parsley, curly
- □ parsley, Italian
- □ rosemary
- □ thyme

DELI COUNTER

- □ ham, lean
- □ pastrami, sliced
- □ roast beef, lean, sliced
- □ turkey breast, roasted, sliced
- □ turkey breast, roasted

BAKERY AREA

- □ bread, Italian
- □ bread, rye
- □ bread, whole wheat
- □ bread, whole grain
- □ buns, whole wheat
- □ buns, whole grain
- □ English muffin, whole wheat
- □ pita
- □ pita, whole wheat
- □ roll, whole grain
- □ tortillas, spinach (10")
- □ tortillas, corn
- □ tortillas, flour (6")
- □ tortillas, flour (8")
- □ tortillas, whole wheat (8")

CANNED FOODS

- ☐ applesauce, unsweetened
- ☐ artichoke hearts in water
- ☐ beans, black
- ☐ beans, cannellini
- ☐ beans, chili
- ☐ beans, chili in sauce
- ☐ beans, kidney
- ☐ beans, pinto
- ☐ beans, refried, fat free
- ☐ beef consommé
- ☐ broth, beef, low fat, reduced sodium
- ☐ broth, chicken, fat free, reduced sodium
- ☐ broth, vegetable, reduced sodium
- ☐ capers
- ☐ cherry peppers
- ☐ chicken, white meat
- ☐ chow mein noodles
- ☐ corn, whole kernel
- ☐ cranberry sauce, whole berry
- ☐ cream of mushroom soup, condensed, low fat, reduced sodium
- ☐ evaporated milk, fat free
- ☐ green chilies, diced
- ☐ green chilies, whole
- ☐ green enchilada sauce
- ☐ hominy, white
- ☐ mandarin oranges
- ☐ maraschino cherries
- ☐ marinara pasta sauce, low fat
- ☐ olives, ripe, chopped
- ☐ olives, ripe, sliced
- ☐ pasta sauce, low fat
- ☐ pineapple, tidbits
- ☐ pineapple, chunks
- ☐ pineapple, crushed
- ☐ pizza sauce, low fat
- ☐ pumpkin puree
- ☐ sauerkraut
- ☐ tomato juice
- ☐ tomato paste
- ☐ tomato sauce
- ☐ tomato sauce, no salt added
- ☐ tomatoes, crushed
- ☐ tomatoes, diced
- ☐ tomatoes, pureed
- ☐ tuna, albacore, water packed
- ☐ water chestnuts, sliced

PACKAGED FOODS

Grains

- ☐ bulgur wheat
- ☐ couscous, plain
- ☐ oats, old fashioned, whole grain
- ☐ pearl barley
- ☐ rice, brown
- ☐ rice, jasmine

Pasta

- ☐ bow tie
- ☐ Ditalini
- ☐ egg noodles, wide
- ☐ fettuccini
- ☐ fettuccini, spinach
- ☐ penne, whole wheat
- ☐ rigatoni, whole wheat
- ☐ rotini
- ☐ rotini, tri-color
- ☐ rotini, whole wheat
- ☐ spaghetti

General

- ☐ chai tea concentrate
- ☐ chocolate wafer cookies
- ☐ Cream of Wheat
- ☐ graham crackers
- ☐ instant pudding mix, banana, fat free, sugar free
- ☐ instant pudding mix, butterscotch, fat free, sugar free
- ☐ instant pudding mix, chocolate, fat free, sugar free
- ☐ instant pudding mix, pistachio, fat free, sugar free
- ☐ instant pudding mix, vanilla,
- ☐ fat free, sugar free
- ☐ Kellogg's Complete Oat Bran Flakes
- ☐ Knorr Hunter Mushroom Gravy Mix
- ☐ Knorr Roasted Chicken Gravy Mix
- ☐ Knorr Vegetable Soup Mix
- ☐ malted milk
- ☐ peanut butter, natural
- ☐ protein powder (whey or soy),
- ☐ chocolate
- ☐ protein powder (whey or soy), vanilla
- ☐ raisins
- ☐ Ry Krisp, seasoned
- ☐ stuffing mix, herb flavored
- ☐ teriyaki marinade
- ☐ tortilla chips, baked
- ☐ whey protein, naturally flavored

BAKING AISLE

- ☐ almonds, sliced
- ☐ baking powder
- ☐ baking soda
- ☐ breadcrumbs, Italian seasoned
- ☐ breadcrumbs, plain
- ☐ brown sugar substitute
- ☐ canola oil
- ☐ cherry pie filling, sugar free
- ☐ cocoa powder, unsweetened
- ☐ cooking spray
- ☐ cooking spray, butter
- ☐ flavored
- ☐ cornstarch
- ☐ extract, almond
- ☐ extract, coconut
- ☐ extract, peppermint
- ☐ extract, vanilla
- ☐ flour, all purpose
- ☐ flour, oat
- ☐ flour, soy
- ☐ flour, whole wheat
- ☐ nuts, chopped
- ☐ olive oil, extra virgin
- ☐ pecans, chopped
- ☐ pistachios, chopped
- ☐ pine nuts
- ☐ Ready Crust, reduced fat graham cracker crust
- ☐ sesame oil, toasted
- ☐ sesame oil, light
- ☐ sugar substitute
- ☐ walnut pieces
- ☐ wheat germ

SPICES AND SEASONINGS AISLE

- ☐ allspice
- ☐ basil, dried
- ☐ bay leaves
- ☐ black pepper
- ☐ blackened redfish seasoning
- ☐ Butter Buds
- ☐ Cajun seasoning
- ☐ chili powder
- ☐ cinnamon, ground
- ☐ coriander, dried
- ☐ cumin, ground
- ☐ curry
- ☐ five-spice powder
- ☐ fresh red chili powder
- ☐ ginger, ground
- ☐ Greek seasoning
- ☐ Hungarian paprika
- ☐ Italian seasoning
- ☐ lemon-pepper seasoning
- ☐ Johnny's (no MSG)
- ☐ McCormick Montreal Chicken seasoning
- ☐ McCormick Montreal Steak seasoning
- ☐ McCormick Rotisserie Chicken seasoning
- ☐ Mrs. Dash Extra Spicy
- ☐ Mrs. Dash Original Blend
- ☐ Mrs. Dash Table Blend
- ☐ Mrs. Dash Tomato-Basil-Garlic
- ☐ nutmeg, ground
- ☐ oregano, dried
- ☐ paprika
- ☐ poultry seasoning
- ☐ pumpkin pie spice
- ☐ red pepper flakes
- ☐ red pepper, ground (cayenne)
- ☐ salt
- ☐ sesame seeds
- ☐ Spike seasoning
- ☐ taco seasoning
- ☐ thyme, dried
- ☐ turmeric
- ☐ wasabi, powdered
- ☐ white pepper, ground

CONDIMENTS

- ☐ barbecue sauce
- ☐ chili garlic sauce
- ☐ chili sauce
- ☐ chocolate syrup
- ☐ hoisin sauce
- ☐ horseradish
- ☐ hot pepper sauce
- ☐ ketchup
- ☐ lemon juice
- ☐ maple syrup, sugar free
- ☐ mayonnaise, fat free
- ☐ mayonnaise, reduced fat
- ☐ Miracle Whip Free
- ☐ mustard, Dijon
- ☐ mustard, spicy brown
- ☐ mustard, yellow
- ☐ relish, dill
- ☐ relish, sweet pickle
- ☐ salad dressing, Caesar, low fat
- ☐ salad dressing, honey-Dijon, lite
- ☐ salad dressing, Italian, fat free
- ☐ salad dressing, Italian, low fat
- ☐ salad dressing, Newman's Own Light Balsamic Vinaigrette
- ☐ salad dressing, ranch, fat free
- ☐ salsa
- ☐ soy sauce, lite
- ☐ teriyaki marinade
- ☐ vinegar, balsamic
- ☐ vinegar, cider
- ☐ vinegar, rice
- ☐ vinegar, white
- ☐ Worcestershire sauce

BEVERAGES

- ☐ apple juice, unsweetened
- ☐ bottled water
- ☐ coffee, instant
- ☐ diet soda
- ☐ sherry, dry
- ☐ vermouth, dry
- ☐ wine, red
- ☐ wine, white

HOUSEHOLD

- ☐ aluminum foil, heavy duty
- ☐ foil muffin liners
- ☐ food storage containers
- ☐ plastic wrap
- ☐ Ziploc bags, gallon size
- ☐ Ziploc bags, sandwich size

DAIRY CASE

General

- ☐ buttermilk, low fat
- ☐ egg substitute
- ☐ eggs
- ☐ milk, skim
- ☐ Reddi-wip, fat free
- ☐ sour cream, fat free
- ☐ sour cream, low fat
- ☐ soy milk, vanilla
- ☐ yogurt, blueberry, light, fat free
- ☐ yogurt, orange flavored, light, fat free
- ☐ yogurt, plain, fat free
- ☐ yogurt, raspberry, light, fat free
- ☐ yogurt, vanilla, light, fat free

Cheese

- ☐ blue, crumbled
- ☐ cheddar, reduced fat, shredded
- ☐ cheddar, reduced fat, block
- ☐ cheddar, reduced fat, sliced
- ☐ colby-jack, reduced fat, shredded
- ☐ feta, basil and tomato flavored
- ☐ reduced fat, crumbled
- ☐ feta, reduced fat, crumbled
- ☐ Monterey Jack, reduced fat, block
- ☐ mozzarella, reduced fat, shredded
- ☐ Parmesan, fresh
- ☐ Parmesan, reduced fat, grated
- ☐ provolone, reduced fat, sliced
- ☐ ricotta, low fat
- ☐ string cheese
- ☐ Swiss, reduced fat, sliced
- ☐ cottage cheese, fat free
- ☐ cottage cheese, low fat
- ☐ cream cheese, reduced fat

MEAT AND SEAFOOD COUNTER

Poultry

- ☐ chicken breast (cooked)
- ☐ chicken breast, boneless, skinless
- ☐ chicken breast, tenders
- ☐ turkey bacon, lean
- ☐ turkey breast, slices
- ☐ turkey, ground, lean

Fish/Seafood

- ☐ crab meat (cooked)
- ☐ halibut, fillets
- ☐ halibut, steaks
- ☐ lobster meat (cooked)
- ☐ orange roughy fillets
- ☐ salmon fillets
- ☐ shrimp (cooked)
- ☐ shrimp (raw)
- ☐ swordfish fillet
- ☐ tuna steak, yellowfin

Fish/Seafood

- ☐ beef, boneless bottom round roast
- ☐ beef, filet mignon
- ☐ beef, flank steak
- ☐ beef, lean, ground
- ☐ beef, top loin steak
- ☐ beef, top round steak
- ☐ beef, top sirloin
- ☐ buffalo, lean, ground
- ☐ Canadian bacon
- ☐ pork tenderloin

FREEZER CASE

- ☐ blackberries
- ☐ blueberries
- ☐ broccoli florets
- ☐ cherries
- ☐ Cool Whip Free
- ☐ Cool Whip Lite
- ☐ green beans
- ☐ green beans, cut Italian
- ☐ limeade concentrate
- ☐ mixed vegetables
- ☐ orange juice concentrate
- ☐ peas
- ☐ potatoes, diced
- ☐ potatoes O'Brien
- ☐ raspberries
- ☐ soybeans in pod
- ☐ strawberries
- ☐ vegetable breakfast patties

YOUR WEEKLY GROCERY LIST

Glycemic Index*

PROTEINS

Meats	GI
Lean Beef	0
Lean Ham	0
Lean Pork	0
Round Steak	0
Top Sirloin	0

Poultry	GI
Chicken Breast	0
Ground Turkey	0
Turkey Breast	0
Turkey Sausage	0

Fish	GI
Catfish	0
Cod	0
Clams	0
Crab	0
Haddock	0
Halibut	0
Lobster	0
Tilapia	0
Trout	0
Salmon	0
Scallops	0
Shell Fish	0
Shrimp	0
White Fish	0

Dairy	GI
Cottage Cheese	Low
Eggs	0
Egg Substitutes	0
Egg Whites	0
Milk	Low
String Cheese	0
Yogurt	Low

FATS

Seeds	GI
Avocados	Low
Flax Seeds	Low
Olives	Low
Sunflower Seeds	Low

Oils	GI
Canola Oil	0
Flax Oil	0
Olive Oil	0
Sunflower Oil	0

Nuts	GI
Almonds	Low
Peanuts	Low
Walnuts	Low

Nut Butters	GI
Almond	Low
Cashew	Low
100% Natural PB	Low

*Some food's GI is based on www.nutritiondata.com

CARBOHYDRATES

100% Whole Grain, etc.	GI
Brown Rice	Low
Cream of Wheat	Med
Oatmeal	Low
Popcorn	Low-Med
Wild Rice	Low
Whole Wheat Bagel	Med
Whole Wheat Bread	Low
Whole Wheat Buns	Low
Whole Wheat Crackers	Med
Whole Wheat English Muffins	Med
Whole Wheat Pasta	Low
Whole Wheat Pita	Low
Whole Wheat Rolls	Low
Whole Wheat Tortilla	Low

Fruits	GI
Apples	Low
Apricots, raw	Low
Apricots, dry	Low
Apricots, canned in syrup	Med
Bananas	Low-Med
Cantaloupe	Med
Cherries	Low
Grapefruit	Low
Grapes	Low
Oranges	Low
Papaya	Med
Peaches	Low
Peaches, canned in syrup	Med
Pears	Low
Pineapple	Low
Raspberries	
Strawberries	Low
Watermelon	High

Vegetables	GI
Asparagus	Low
Bell Pepper	Low
Broccoli	Low
Cauliflower	Low
Carrots	Low
Carrots, boiled	High
Celery	Low
Corn	Med
Cucumber	Low
Eggplant	Low
Green Beans	Low
Legumes	Low
Lettuce	Low
Peas	Low
Potato	Low
Potato, boiled	Med
Pumpkin	High
Spinach	Low
Squash	Low
Sweet Potatoes	Low
Sweet Potatoes	High
Tomatoes	Low
Yams	Low
Zucchini	Low

*Some food's GI is based on www.nutritiondata.com

Glossary

accountable (accountability). Responsibility to someone or for some activity.

aerobic (exercise). Based on or using the principles of aerobics; enhancing respiratory and circulatory efficiency; "aerobic dance"; "running is very aerobic.

allergies. A reaction of the body to something that was inhaled, ingested, injected or contacted through skin. Often times symptoms include itchy eyes, runny nose, wheezing, swelling, skin rash or diarrhea.

alpha-carotene. Vitamin A that is found in vegetation such as carrots, pumpkin and red and yellow peppers and oranges, tangerines, peaches, nectarines and papayas. Vitamin A causes many of the red, orange and yellow hues of plant leaves, fruits and flowers.

amino acids. Amino acids are the basic structural building blocks of proteins.

antioxidants. A molecule that is able to slow down or even prevent the appearance of other molecules destruction.

anxiety. Is commonly associated with a fear, anger, sadness or even a happiness that can cause the body to react negatively. Symptoms can include raised blood pressure and heart rate, increased sweating, increased blood flow to major muscle groups, immune and digestive systems could become inhibited. Externally you may notice pale skin, sweating, trembling and pupil dilation as well as nausea and chills.

arthritis. Arthritis is actually an umbrella term used for a group of more than 100 medical conditions that collectively affect nearly 46 million adults and 300,000 children in America alone. Arthritis affects the musculoskeletal system and specifically the joints–where two or more bones meet. Arthritis-related joint problems include pain, stiffness, inflammation and damage to joint cartilage (the tough, smooth tissue that covers the ends of the bones, enabling them to glide against one another) and surrounding structures.

atherosclerosis. A hardening of the arteries that is caused mostly by cholesterol sticking to the inner walls causing them to become inflamed; narrowing the ability to pass blood through efficiently and effectively.

beta-carotene (carotenoid n flavonoid). β-Carotene is the more common form and can be found in yellow, orange, and green leafy fruits and vegetables. These can be carrots, spinach, lettuce, tomatoes, sweet potatoes, broccoli, cantaloupe, oranges, and winter squash. As a rule of thumb, the greater the intensity of the colour of the fruit or vegetable, the more β-carotene it contains.

bicep. This is the large muscle mass on top of your upper arm between the elbow and shoulder.

bloating. Bloating is any abnormal general swelling, or increase in diameter of the abdominal area. As a symptom, the patient feels a full and tight abdomen, which may cause abdominal pain sometimes accompanied by borborygmus. Bloating may have several causes, the most common being accumulation of liquids and intestinal gas.

blood pressure. The amount of compression in the blood vessels from each heart beat. Measured in systolic and diastolic pressure. The American Heart Association says that pressure around 120/80 is ideal when in a relaxed state.

blood sugar. The amount of glucose or sugar that is flowing through your bloodstream. Glucose is a primary source of energy for you body's cells and rise after eating and are usually lower before the first meal of the day.

borborygmus. The rumbling sound you hear that comes from your stomach, typicaly when you are hungry or have intestinal gas.

brain swelling. Brain swelling is the displacement of brain tissue, cerebrospinal fluid, and blood vessels outside the compartments in the head that they normally occupy.

brown rice. Rice from which the bran layers and germs have not been removed by polishing or grinding.

calorie. A calorie is a unit of measurement for energy.

carbohydrates. Any of a group of organic compounds that includes sugars, starches, celluloses, and gums and serves as a major energy source in the diet of humans. These compounds are produced by photosynthetic plants and contain only carbon, hydrogen, and oxygen, usually in the ratio 1:2:1.

carcinogens. Is a substance or chemical that promotes cancer within the body.

cardio. Cardio is the medical term used to reference the heart.

cardio training. Cardio training or cardiovascular training can be defined simply as your body's ability to get oxygen and blood to the muscles by increasing ones heart rate.

Cardiorespiratory capacity. Cardiorespiratory capacity is the highest amount of oxygen consumed during maximal exercise in activities that use the large muscle groups in the legs or arms and legs combined. Other terms that are used in place of cardiorespiraty capacity are: Aerobic capacity, aerobic power, functional capacity, functional aerobic capacity, maximal functional capacity, cardiorespiratory fitness, cardiovascular fitness, maximal oxygen intake, and maximal oxygen uptake.

cardiovascular (conditioning). Cardiovascular conditioning is regular physical training in aerobic activities over an extended period of time.

carotenoid. See beta-carotene or alpha-carotene.

cholesterol. Cholesterol is a soft, waxy substance found among the lipids (fats) in the bloodstream and in all your body's cells.

chronic disease. Is a disease that lasts a long time or that keeps recurring. Often times a debilitating or life-threatening disease.

circadian rhythm. A circadian rhythm is a roughly-24-hour cycle in the physiological processes of living beings, including plants, animals, fungi and cyanobacteria.

colon cancer. A bad tumor or growth inside the large intestine that is capable of spreading to other parts of the body.

coma. Is a state of being unconscious or non-responsive to external stimuli. A person in a coma cannot be awakened, fails to respond normally to pain or light, does not have sleep-wake cycles, and does not make voluntary actions.

complex carbohydrate. Consists of two or more single sugars (monosaccharides) like glucose or fructose.

conditioning. Conditioning is the process of modifying a person's behavior, mentally physically or emotionally.

contaminants. Any chemical that is impure or not suitable to ingest, inhale or put on ones body so as to cause harm.

contraction. The change in a muscle by which it becomes thickened and shortened.

coronary heart disease. A condition where hardening of the arteries make it difficult to supply oxygen and blood to the heart.

cortisol. Also known as hydrocortisone; it's a chemical that is produced by the adrenal cortex that helps regulate carbohydrate metabolism and maintains blood pressure.

dehydrated. where ones body loses too much water or does not have enough water to get enough blood to ones organs.

depressed. Sad and gloomy; dejected; downcast.

detoxifies. To remove the effects of poison from.

diabetes/diabetic. A polygenic disease characterized by abnormally high glucose levels in the blood; any of several metabolic disorders marked by excessive urination and persistent thirst.

durations. The length of time something continues or exists.

eating disorder. A condition where eating habits are not normal (i.e. bulimia or anorexia).

EFX: The elliptical fitness crosstrainer, EFX, is a non-impact, all-in-one cardio machine that incorporates the motions of running, cycling, and stair climbing. It simulates your natural movement while targeting the muscles of your lower body, which is the key to effective aerobic exercise and cardiovascular conditioning.

energy. The sustenance of life itself is critically dependent on energy transformations; living organisms survive because of exchange of energy within and without. In a living organism chemical bonds are constantly broken and made to make the exchange and transformation of energy possible. These chemical bonds are most often bonds in carbohydrates, including sugars.

enzymes. Any of numerous proteins produced in living cells that accelerate or catalyze the metabolic processes of an organism.

exercise. Bodily or mental exertion, esp. for the sake of training or improvement of health.

exercise duration. The amount of time you spend exercising for the sake of training or improving ones health.

exercise frequency. The number of times that you spend exercising.

exercise intensity. The amount of energy, strength or concentration one puts into exercising, as of activity, thought or feeling.

fatique/muscle fatigue. A feeling from ones body when you exercise a muscle(s) to the point that they feel weak or can do no more.

fiber. It is a type of carbohydrate that passes through the human digestive system without being broken down into nutrients that is mainly found in the outer layers of plants.

flavonoid. See beta-carotene.

flax seed. Comes from the Flax Flower that are pale blue with five petals. The seeds are shaped like an apple pip that are 4-7mm long.

fructose. A very sweet sugar occurring in many fruits and honey and used as a preservative for foodstuffs and as an intravenous nutrient.

glucose. A monosaccharide sugar that has several forms; an important source of physiological energy.

glutes. The muscles of the buttocks.

Glycemic Index. A system that ranks foods by the speeds at which their carbohydrates are converted into glucose in the body; a measure of the effects of foods on blood-sugar levels.

glycogen. A polysaccharide stored in the liver and muscle cells that is easily converted to glucose to meet metabolic energy requirements. Most of the carbohydrate energy stored in body cells is in the form of glycogen.

goal. The result or achievement toward which effort is directed; aim; end.

headaches. A pain located in the head, as over the eyes, at the temples, or at the base of the skull.

hip flexor. Group of muscles attached from the hip to the top of ones leg that make the thighs move toward the abdomen.

homeostasis. The ability of the body to maintain a balance within its own self even when encountering outside changes (i.e. the ability of the body to maintain a temperature of around 98.6 degrees).

hormonal balance. The act of evening out the various secreted chemicals in ones body, through diet and nutrition, that affect functions of various organs and tissues.

hormone. The secretion of a chemical(s) by the endocrine glands put directly into the bloodstream. In turn the chemical(s) travels to distant organs to regulate a specific organs function.

humidity. The amount of water vapor in the air.

hydration. The act of providing an adequate amount of liquid to ones body (i.e. drinking water or other liquid).

hydrogenation. A process in which hydrogen is added or combined to carbon.

hyperglycemia. Higher than normal amount of glucose or blood sugar in the bloodstream.

hypertension. A common condition where blood pressure remains abnormally high (a reading of 140/90 or greater).

hypoglycemia. Lower than normal amount of glucose or blood sugar in the bloodstream.

hyponatremia. A condition of drinking an overly excessive amount of water and of not having enough sodium available in the bloodstream.

immune system. The system of organs, tissues and cells that attack harmful bacteria and viruses to aid in keeping the human body free from illness or harm.

impact. 1) The striking of one thing against another; forceful contact; collision 2) to have an effect on; influence or alter ones mind-set.

infections. An invasion of the body by microorganisms, including bacteria, viruses, or fungi causing change in ones cells.

inflammation. Redness, swelling, pain, tenderness, heat, and disturbed function of an area of the body.* It is a defense mechanism that helps protect from infection and injury. Its purpose is to localize and remove damaged tissue so that the body can begin to heal.

infrequently. Not constant, habitual, or regular.

insulin. Is used to help regulate the amount of glucose (sugar) in the blood by having the body absorb and convert glucose into glycogen and fat for the bodies use of stored carbohydrates.

joint degeneration. Is a condition where cartilage around a joint begins to deteriorate and unless corrected the cartilage can erode or disappear altogether causing the bone to rub against the opposite bone causing pain and stiffness.

lactose intolerance. The inability to digest or consume dairy products.

Latissimus Dorsi (lats). The muscle that is attached to the back and side of the ribs under the armpit regions and allows for lifting pulling and rotating the shoulder/arm.

legumes. Beans or peas.

lethargic. Of, pertaining to, or affected with lethargy; drowsy; sluggish.

lubricates. Act of making something slippery or smooth.

lutein. A yellow carotenoid pigment found in body fats, egg yolk, and green plants.

lycopene. A red carotenoid found chiefly in blood, the reproductive organs, tomatoes, and palm oils. It is an antioxidant and is the parent substance from which all natural carotenoids are derived.

lymphomas. A growth or tumor that spreads through or onto lymph nodes.

macronutrients. Elements, such as carbon, hydrogen, oxygen, or nitrogen, that are required in large amounts for normal growth and development. Refers to proteins, fats, and carbohydrates.

mental fatigue. Desire to just want to rest, tendency to withdraw and sleep rather than seek activity.

metabolism. The chemical processes by which cells produce the substances and energy needed to sustain life.

microorganism. An organism that can be seen only with the aid of a microscope and that typically consists of only a single cell.

minerals. Any of the inorganic elements, as calcium, iron, magnesium, potassium, or sodium, that are essential to the functioning of the human body and are obtained from foods.

minimize. To reduce to the smallest possible amount or degree.

motivation. The psychological feature that arouses an organism to action toward a desired goal.

multivitamin. A compound of several vitamins.

muscle mass. The amount of muscle (tissue) you have between joints, ligaments and tendons.*

muscle stabilizer. Muscles that hold a joint in place so that a particular exercise may be performed while maintaining balance or level exercise.

mutagens. A physical or environmental change that causes cells to mutate or change their originally intended design.

nausea. A feeling of sickness in the stomach characterized by an urge to vomit.

nutrient-dense. (of food) Relatively rich in nutrients for the number of calories contained.

nutrients. A substance that provides nourishment for growth or metabolism.

nutrition. Study of the relationship between the diet and health of what we consume to use for growth and replacing tissues.

nutritional value. The amount of nourishment an individual food and amount has on ones body; How good is it for you?

obesity. Excessively overweight due to having too much fat stored within the body and cells.

optimal metabolism. The chemical processes by which cells produce the substances and energy needed to sustain life in the best way possible.

overcompensate. Make excessive corrections for fear of making an error.

PFC. Protein, Fat, Carbohydrate.

physical conditioning. The process of modifying a person's behavior physically.

physical fatigue. You want to be active and have ambitious plans but cannot implement them.

phytonutrients (phytochemicals). A nonnutritive bioactive plant substance, such as a flavonoid or carotenoid, considered to have a beneficial effect on human health.*

primary muscles. Muscles of the neck, traps (trapezius), lats (Latissimus Dorsi), biceps, triceps, chest, shoulders, stomach/abdominal muscles, lower back, thighs/butt, calves.

probiotic. Dietary supplements containing potentially beneficial bacteria or yeast, with lactic acid bacteria (LAB) as the most common microbes used.

pump effect. The result of one's ability to exercise to fatigue causing a greater blood flow and swelling to the muscle groups trained.

quads. The quadriceps femoris (quadriceps, quadriceps extensor, quads or guads) includes the four prevailing muscles on the front of the thigh. It is the great extensor muscle of the knee, forming a large fleshy mass which covers the front and sides of the femur.

range of motion. The area through which a joint may normally be freely and painlessly moved, the range of flexion and extension of a joint.

regulate (water temp). To control.

REM sleep. Rapid Eye Movement: A stage in the normal sleep cycle during which dreams occur and the body undergoes marked changes including rapid eye movement, loss of reflexes, and increased pulse rate and brain activity.

replenishment. The act of ingesting nutrients that have been used up. The act of making one full or complete again by giving back to the body what it needs.

respiratory arrest. Is the cessation of the normal tidal flow of the lungs due to paralysis of the diaphragm, collapse of the lung or any number of respiratory failures.

rhomboids. Any of several muscles of the upper back that help move the shoulder blade.

rotator cuff. A set of muscles and tendons that secures the arm to the shoulder joint and permits rotation of the arm.

satiates. To satisfy (an appetite or desire) fully.

sensory receptor. An organ having nerve endings (in the skin or viscera or eye or ear or nose or mouth) that respond to stimulation.

session. A period of time during which a group of persons meets to pursue a particular activity.

sleep deprivation. The condition of being robbed of sleep, in real life or in experiment, as opposed to being able to sleep.

stabilizer/muscle stabilizer. Stabilizer muscles are those that hold a joint in place so that the exercise may be performed.

stimulant. Something that temporarily quickens some vital process or the functional activity of some organ or part.

stride. A single coordinated movement of the four legs of a horse or other animal, completed when the legs return to their initial relative position.

stroke. A blockage or hemorrhage of a blood vessel leading to the brain, causing inadequate oxygen supply and, depending on the extent and location of the abnormality, such symptoms as weakness, paralysis of parts of the body, speech difficulties, and, if severe, loss of consciousness or death.

technique. Skillfulness in the command of fundamentals deriving from practice and familiarity; "practice greatly improves proficiency."

tension/muscle tension. The act or process of stretching a muscle tight by either pushing or pulling.

testosterone. A steroid hormone that is the most potent naturally occurring androgen and that regulates the development of the male reproductive system and male secondary sex characteristics. Testosterone is produced mainly in the testes and is also used as a drug in the treatment of certain medical disorders.

tofu. A soft, bland, white cheese-like food, high in protein content, made from curdled soybean milk: used originally in Oriental cooking but now in a wide variety of soups and other dishes.

trapezius. The muscle that goes from the inside of your spine from your cranium down to your tailbone inside of the shoulder blade on both sides of ones body.

tricep. The large muscle on the back of your arm in between your elbow and shoulder.

visualize/visualization. A process by which you create a mental picture and/or imagine accomplishing a certain task or goal.

vitamin A. A fat-soluble vitamin important for normal vision, tissue growth, and healthy skin. It is found in fish-liver oils, milk, green leafy vegetables, and red, orange, and yellow vegetables and fruits. A deficiency of Vitamin A in humans causes poor vision at night and damage to the skin and mucous membranes.

vitamin B. Contains eight water-soluble vitamins (B1, B2, B3, B5, B6, B7, B8, B9, B12) that play an important role in cell metabolism. Vitamin B helps manufacture blood for the body, help neural functions and promotes growth from within.

vitamin C. A water-soluble vitamin important for healthy skin, teeth, bones, and blood vessels.

It is found especially in citrus fruits, tomatoes, potatoes, and green leafy vegetables.

vitamin D. Vitamin D is essential for normal bone growth and is often found in milk, fish and eggs. Interesting Fact: Vitamin D can be produced on the skin when exposed to sunlight.

vomiting. To eject part or all of the contents of the stomach through the mouth, usually in a series of involuntary spasmic movements.

weight training. The amount or quantity of heaviness or mass one uses when exercising.

whole-grain. Natural or unprocessed grain containing the germ and bran.

whole-wheat. Prepared with the complete wheat kernel.

yoga. Any of the methods or disciplines prescribed, especially a series of postures and breathing exercises practiced to achieve control of the body and mind.

zeaxanthin. A yellow crystalline carotenoid alcohol C40H56O2 that is isomeric with lutein and occurs widely with it and that is the chief pigment of yellow Indian corn.

*Most definitions were found on www.dictionary.com

Index

My Notes

My Notes

My Notes

My Notes